Phagocytosis - Main Key of Immune System

Edited by Seyyed Shamsadin Athari and Entezar Mehrabi Nasab

Published in London, United Kingdom

Phagocytosis - Main Key of Immune System
http://dx.doi.org/10.5772/intechopen.104359
Edited by Seyyed Shamsadin Athari and Entezar Mehrabi Nasab

Contributors
Victory Ibigo Poloamina, Amy L. Ryan, Ben A. Calvert, Alok Mishra, Laban Turyamuhika, Musinguzi Benson, Agaba Bosco, Asiimwe Moses, Okek Erick, Filex Odhiambo Otieno, Gianluca Cipriani, Magdalini Mischopoulou, Gabriela Echeverria-Valencia, Antonia Isabel Castillo Rodal, Claudia I. Rivas-Ortíz, María Cristina Vanrell, Patricia Silvia Romano, Ken Shirato, Keisuke Kasuga, Shogo Sato, Haruyuki Ishii, Jeanet Serafin-Lopez, Ursino Pacheco García, María Eugenia Castro Mussot, Ernesto Pacheco Ramírez, Kazuki Santa

First published in London, United Kingdom, 2023 by IntechOpen
IntechOpen is the global imprint of INTECHOPEN LIMITED, registered in England and Wales, registration number: 11086078, 5 Princes Gate Court, London, SW7 2QJ, United Kingdom
Printed in Croatia

British Library Cataloguing-in-Publication Data
A catalogue record for this book is available from the British Library

Additional hard and PDF copies can be obtained from orders@intechopen.com

Phagocytosis - Main Key of Immune System
Edited by Seyyed Shamsadin Athari and Entezar Mehrabi Nasab
p. cm.

This title is part of the Physiology Book Series, Volume 19
Topic: Cell Physiology
Series Editor: Tomasz Brzozowski
Topic Editor: Angel Catala

Print ISBN 978-1-83768-739-8
Online ISBN 978-1-83768-740-4
eBook (PDF) ISBN 978-1-83768-741-1
ISSN 2631-8261

For EU product safety concerns:
IN TECH d.o.o., Prolaz Marije Krucifikse Kozulić 3, 51000 Rijeka, Croatia,
info@intechopen.com or visit our website at intechopen.com.

IntechOpen Book Series

Physiology

Volume 19

Aims and Scope of the Series

Modern physiology requires a comprehensive understanding of the integration of tissues and organs throughout the mammalian body, including the cooperation between structure and function at the cellular and molecular levels governed by gene and protein expression. While a daunting task, learning is facilitated by identifying common and effective signaling pathways mediated by a variety of factors employed by nature to preserve and sustain homeostatic life. As a leading example, the cellular interaction between intracellular concentration of Ca+2 increases, and changes in plasma membrane potential is integral for coordinating blood flow, governing the exocytosis of neurotransmitters, and modulating gene expression and cell effector secretory functions. Furthermore, in this manner, understanding the systemic interaction between the cardiovascular and nervous systems has become more important than ever as human populations' life prolongation, aging and mechanisms of cellular oxidative signaling are utilised for sustaining life. Altogether, physiological research enables our identification of distinct and precise points of transition from health to the development of multimorbidity throughout the inevitable aging disorders (e.g., diabetes, hypertension, chronic kidney disease, heart failure, peptic ulcer, inflammatory bowel disease, age-related macular degeneration, cancer). With consideration of all organ systems (e.g., brain, heart, lung, gut, skeletal and smooth muscle, liver, pancreas, kidney, eye) and the interactions thereof, this Physiology Series will address the goals of resolving (1) Aging physiology and chronic disease progression (2) Examination of key cellular pathways as they relate to calcium, oxidative stress, and electrical signaling, and (3) how changes in plasma membrane produced by lipid peroxidation products can affect aging physiology, covering new research in the area of cell, human, plant and animal physiology.

Meet the Series Editor

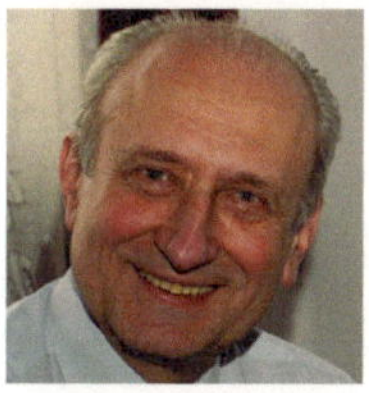

Prof. Dr. Thomas Brzozowski works as a professor of Human Physiology and is currently a Chairman at the Department of Physiology and is V-Dean of the Medical Faculty at Jagiellonian University Medical College, Cracow, Poland. His primary area of interest is physiology and pathophysiology of the gastrointestinal (GI) tract, with a major focus on the mechanism of GI mucosal defense, protection, and ulcer healing. He was a postdoctoral NIH fellow at the University of California and the Gastroenterology VA Medical Center, Irvine, Long Beach, CA, USA, and at the Gastroenterology Clinics Erlangen-Nuremberg and Munster in Germany. He has published 290 original articles in some of the most prestigious scientific journals and seven book chapters on the pathophysiology of the GI tract, gastroprotection, ulcer healing, drug therapy of peptic ulcers, hormonal regulation of the gut, and inflammatory bowel disease.

Meet the Volume Editors

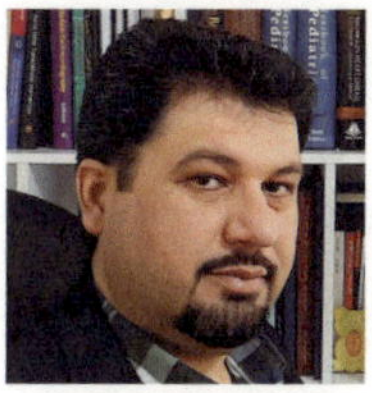

Dr. Seyyed Shamsadin Athari is an Assistant Professor of Immunology in the Department of Immunology, School of Medicine, Zanjan University of Medical Sciences, Iran. He has more than 170 journal papers and 35 books to his credit. He is also an editorial board member of more than eighty international journals. He has several medical inventions to his credit and has recorded gene sequences in gene banks. Dr. Athari has been invited as a speaker to more than fifty international congresses and symposia. He is the recipient of several awards from scientific societies.

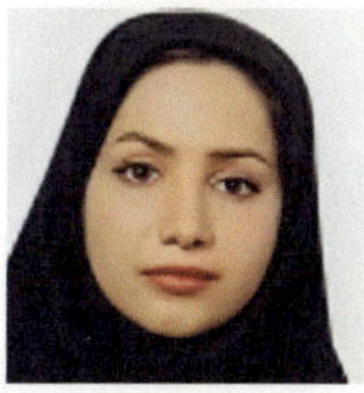

Dr. Entezar Mehrabi Nasab is a cardiologist who completed her residency at the Tehran Heart Center, Tehran University of Medical Sciences, Iran. She has published more than twenty-five scientific articles in international journals. She has been invited as a speaker to more than twenty-five international congresses. Dr. Nasab has received several awards from different scientific societies.

Contents

Preface

Infections are immune-mediated illnesses that can range from mild to serious. In recent years, new pathogens have appeared, such as the COVID-19 virus, which caused a worldwide pandemic. Due to the appearance of new and serious pathogens, the human immune response is continually being tested.

Phagocytosis is one of the main mechanisms in innate immune defense and the first process to respond to pathogens. It is also one of the initiating branches of an adaptive immune response. In the immune system, the cells that are capable of phagocytosis are called "professional phagocytes." These include neutrophils, macrophages, monocytes, dendritic cells, and eosinophils. In these cells, the phagosome is the organelle formed by phagocytosis of material. It then moves toward the centrosome of the phagocyte and is fused with lysosomes, forming a phagolysosome and leading to degradation. Progressively, the phagolysosome is acidified, activating degradative enzymes and killing all pathogens.

This book discusses the main aspects of phagocytosis and related cells in the human immune response. It also examines the molecular mechanisms involved in infections and related pathogens, providing a comprehensive review of infectious diseases and their pathophysiology, diagnosis, management, and treatment.

As educators, we are frequently faced with probing questions from students who are confused by the paradoxical functions of the immune system. We think this book can help students to understand the molecular pathways of phagocytosis. Thus, it is a useful resource not only for undergraduate and graduate students but also for immunology specialists and clinicians.

Dr. Seyyed Shamsadin Athari
Department of Immunology,
School of Medicine,
Zanjan University of Medical Sciences,
Zanjan, Iran

Dr. Entezar Mehrabi Nasab
Department of Cardiology,
School of Medicine,
Tehran Heart Center,
Tehran University of Medical Sciences,
Tehran, Iran

Department of Cardiology,
School of Medicine,
Valiasr Hospital,
Zanjan University of Medical Sciences,
Zanjan, Iran

Section 1

Phagocytosis Process

Chapter 1

Functioning and Control of Phagocytosis

Laban Turyamuhika, Agaba Bosco, Asiimwe Moses, Musinguzi Benson and Okek Erick

Abstract

Phagocytosis is a very complex and versatile process that contributes to immunity through a series of events that is it's sometimes referred to the Come and Eat me process. Due to the recognition ingestion and digestion then destruction. It's also central to tissue homeostasis and remodeling by clearing dead cells. This ability of phagocytes to perform such diverse functions rests in large part on their vast repertoire of receptors. In this book chapter we looked at the processes used by phagocyte to perform there phagocytosis function. This is made possible by the binding of opsonins on the microbes like the C3b of the complement. This works as a chemo attractant to the phagocytes to come and initiate the process of eating. On recognition this microbe or dead cell interacts with the phagocyte with the help of a very big repertoire of receptors the microbe is engulfed with in the phagosome. As microbes interact with the phagocyte receptors a cascade of signaling events downstream that then activate phagocytosis. This membrane and cytoskeleton remodulation lead to the formation of pseudopods that cover the entire microbe forming a phagocytic cup which closes a few minutes to take up the microbe completely. The signal cascade is most known for the Fc receptor activities. Crosslinking of the Fc receptor on the surface of phagocyte activate phagocytosis and any other effector functions such as activation of the oxidative burst, degranulation, antibody dependent cell mediated cytotoxicity and activation of genes for cytokine/chemokine production that are beneficial in microbe destruction and initiation of inflammation. This starts once the interaction of phagocytes receptors and their ligands on the target microbes takes place appropriately. The phagocyte receptors will then aggregate to activate a series of pathways that regulate actin cytoskeleton which helps in the formation of a new vesicle which comes out of the membrane to enclose the microbe. In here a number of processes and stages take place all aimed at killing and denaturing the particle. They include early phagosome, intermediate phagosome, phagolysosome formation and the late phagosome all these participate in eliminating the phagocytized microbe. However with all the above phagocytic efficiency, some pathogens evade phagocytosis using different means and presence of certain capacities that facilitate evasion examples of organisms that evade phagocytosis include *Mycobacterium tuberculosis, Listeria monocytogens Escherichia coli* etc. all these use different means in evasion. Therefore the concept and science of Phagocytes used to be studied more to explore more pharmaceutical products based on the evasion mechanisms.

Keywords: phagocytes, recognition, internalization, degranulation, signaling evasion

1. Introduction

It's a century since a great discovery by Elie Metchnikoff which championed the role of phagocytosis in cellular immunity. Although some other group had observed the uptake of particles from simple to complex organisms he understood and stated better its significance in the host response to injury and infection. This made our understanding of inflammation and homeostasis much better, with more improved tools for cellular and molecular biology the study of the role of phagocytosis and its contribution to physiological and pathological processes, including receptor function in innate and acquired immunity.

2. Professional phagocytes

Neutrophils and macrophages both have a key role in innate immunity because they recognize ingest and destroy pathogens without the assistance of the adaptive immune response. Usually macrophages are the first to encounter microbes in the tissues but are soon replaced but a large number of neutrophils to sites of infection [1].

Our bodies are made of strong epithelial layers of defense however some pathogens have evolved strategies to penetrate these defense and therefore epithelia can be disrupted by wound, insect bites or abrasions that may lead to entry of pathogens.

Phagocytosis is fundamental for host defense against invading pathogens and contribute to the immune and inflammatory response. Phagocytosis is done majorly in specialized cells in multicellular organisms and is facilitated by a number of cells called phagocytes preferably professional phagocytes and these include neutrophils, macrophages, monocytes, dendritic cells. In this process a cell uses its plasma membrane to engulf a large particle giving rise to an internal compartment called the phagocytosis. Microbes are recognized by phagocytes that have a number of receptors on their surfaces which directly recognize conserved molecules on the microbe surfaces called PAMPs. This particulate matter must be opsonized (coated) with IgG, complement fragments C3b or iC3b, fibrinoctin or other proteins before being recognized and engulfed by PMNs. This process is essential for tissue balance and involve several steps that include particle recognition, particle ingestion early phagosome formation, late phagosome formation and phagolysosome formation [2].

3. Receptors involved in phagocytosis

Variety of ligands can be recognized by most phagocytic cells, with their efficient recognition requiring a great number of receptor types with distinct selectivity. Multiple receptor types are co expressed and this helps display a diverse array of adherent opsonins, some phagocytic receptors engaged in the process of phagocytosis may not be phagocytic receptors. The most commonly engaged receptors are listed in the **Table 1** [13]. Macrophages recognize and identify the phagocytic targets using this array of receptors that are normally displayed on the plasma membrane of microbes.

This happens through a coordinated signaling cascade that is initiated once a phagocytic receptor binds its ligand [14].

The recognition and identification were the first known functions of phagocytosis.

Receptor	Ligands	references
Pattern-recognition receptors		
Dectin-1	Polysaccharides of some yeast cells	[3]
Mannose receptor	Mannan	[4]
CD14	Lipopolysaccharide-binding protein	[5, 6]
Scavenger receptor A	Lipopolysaccharide, lipoteichoic acid	[6]
CD36	*Plasmodium falciparum*-infected erythrocytes	[7]
MARCO	Bacteria	[8]
Opsonic receptors		
FcγRI (CD64)	IgG1 = IgG3 > IgG4	[9]
FcγRIIa (CD32a)	IgG3 ≥ IgG1 = IgG2	[9]
FcγRIIIa (CD16a)	IgG	[9]
FcαRI (CD89)	IgA1, IgA2	[10]
FcεRI	IgE	[11]
CR1 (CD35)	Mannan-binding lectin, C1q, C4b, C3b	[12]

Table 1.
Shows human phagocytic receptors found on phagocytes.

4. Receptor synergy during phagocytosis

The engagement of apoptotic cells for example is achieved by action of CD36 that binds oxidized PS, and integrins that bind PS-bridging proteins, including MFG-E8. Signaling by integrins to the main actin cytoskeleton at sites of apoptotic corpse engagement involves Rac activation and completion of internalization which requires myosin [13]. The avidity of an interaction is normally thought of as the proportion pf the number of copies of a single receptor type engaged at a time. Therefor in the context of phagocytosis myriad different receptors exist and physiological targets expose a variety of ligands. This phenomenon raises the chances of combined avidity,

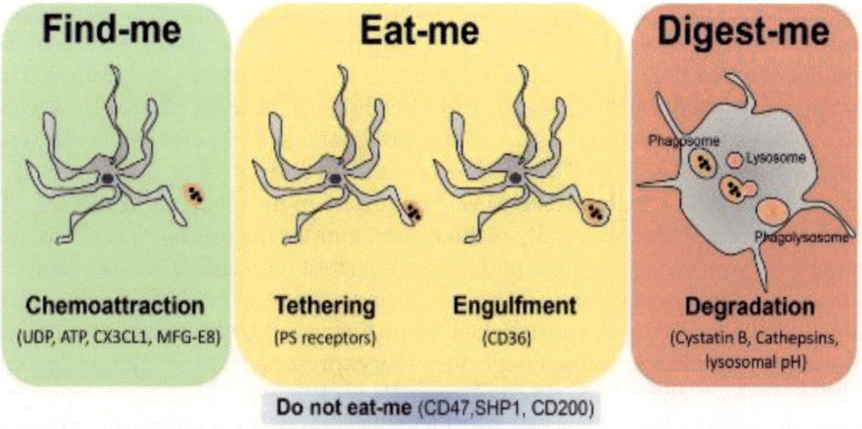

Figure 1.
The figure show the main steps of phagocytosis in dead cells and microbes.

conferred by simultaneous engagement of multiple unrelated receptor types. Thus a microbe exposed in serum is likely to be recognized immediately by pattern recognition receptors like Dectin (**Figure 1**) [15].

4.1 The Phagocytosis Process

These are the main steps that facilitate phagocytosis of microbes and dead cells.

To what extent does the phagocyte decode the microbial genetics to be able to mount an appropriate response? There is a clue on the fact that there are cations like magnesium and calcium. These cations must be present in in the extracellular fluid in sufficient quantities for macrophages to ingest a variety of microbes with ease, however C3 opsonized particles are more easily ingested with a much lower divalent amounts of cations than unopsonised ones. Therefore C3 seem to have increase ingestion by potentiating the effect of cations [16].

5. The schematic shows the process of phagocytosis

IMAGE FROM Molecular and Cellular Immunology by Saunders 4th edition. page35. Pathogens could be ingested by different membrane receptors on the phagocytes. Some receptors bind microbes directly while others will only bind opsonized pathogens. But remember that the Mac-1 integrins binds microbes opsonized with complement protein e.g. C3. The pathogens are internalized in the phagosome which then fuse with lysosomes to form phagolysosomes. Where the microbes are killed by ROS and nitrogen intermediate enzymes. (NO, nitric oxide, ROS, reactive oxygen species).

5.1 Step one: recognition of the microbe

Neutrophils and other macrophages are always exposed to cells that they ignore but instead will specifically take on different microbes and particles. The specificity is due to the presence of different of receptors on these cells that recognize microbes [17]. Despite the various differences all phagocytic targets have a common characteristic that is they present the phagocyte multivalent arrays of ligands, a critical feature for the activation of most phagocytic receptors that are invariably activated by clustering laterally in the plane of the membrane therefore unlike GPCRs or growth factor receptors that undergo trans membrane remodulation upon binding with their ligands, phagocytic receptors are stimulated when their fluid cation quantities are elevated as they get immobilized by closely apposed stationary ligands [17]. Pathogen ligands for most phagocytic receptor include various protein receptor and complex lipids such as lipopolysaccharides, teichoic acids and mycobacterial lipids [18]. The none opsonic receptors that are expressed by professional phagocytes include lectin like recognition molecules such as CD169, CD33 and the related receptors specifically for sialylated membrane residues [19]. You recall that some receptors may bind these pathogen associated molecules) PAMPs (and still fail to initiate phagocytosis majorly due to poor preparation or priming. TLRs and some G-protein coupled receptors prime the cell for phagocytosis by inducing inverted activation of phagocytic integrins [20]. Phagocytes also express some other types of receptors like the Dectin-1 which for fungal betaglucan [21] with well-defined signaling capacity, other related lectin include MICL, Dectin 2,Mincle and DNGR-1 with other group of scavenger receptors like SR-A, MARCO and CD36 that have different domain structures which work by overlapping of recognition apoptotic [22].

5.2 Step two: particle internalization

When a particle binds with a phagocyte receptor, various signaling pathway events are triggered to activate phagocytosis. Most changes in membrane conformation and the actin cytoskeleton take place which leads to the formation of pseudopods that the engulf the microbe [23]. The Fcy receptors get activated in the plane of the phagocyte membrane when they aggregate after binding to their IgG ligands which then cover the particle to be ingested [24].

5.3 Step three: phagocyte formation

Signaling events are triggered to start phagocytosis immediately when the phagocyte receptors engage the microorganism. This is followed by membrane remodeling and the cytoskeleton leading to the formation of pseudopods that engulf the microbes. This causes lipids to associate and dissociate from the membrane of phagosome in orderly way [25]. A depression of the membrane (a phagocytic up) is made at the point of contact of the phagosome with the microbe, then the membrane protrusions fuse at the distal end to finally seal off the new phagosome [26, 27]. When the Fcy Receptors aggregate after binding to their IgG ligands that cover the particle to be ingested. Clustering of activating receptors FcyRs results in phosphorylation of the immunoreceptor tyrosine based activation motifs (ITAMs) present in the cytoplasmic domain of the receptors in the case of FcyRIIa and FcyRIIc or in an FcR common Y-chain [24, 28].

A number of receptors are attached on the phagocyte that cooperate to facilitate phagocytosis and ingestion. The interactions of receptors are improved with possible targets by (i) creating active protrusions that allow the cell to explore larger area increasing the chances for receptors to engage their ligands. (ii) selectively removing of the larger glycoproteins allowing the receptors to diffuse more freely on the membrane [29]. The phosphatase CD45 can extend more than 40 nm from the cell membrane [30] and it's a real obstacle for most phagocytic receptors, therefore removing these large molecules could drastically improve receptor binfding.CD45 was first identified during the Dectin 1 mediated phagocytosis in a phagocytic synapse [31] for its resemblance with the T lymphocyte immune synapse. When the T cell receptor TCR molecules on the T lymphocyte interact with the MHC molecules on an antigen presenting cell APC, a central cluster of engaged TCRs are surrounded by a ring of integrin LFA-1 molecules and CD45 is excluded from the center [32].

6. Phagosome maturation

The newly formed phagosome changes its membrane composition very fast to become a microbicial vacuole called the phagolysosome. The process used to transfer endocytosed material from endosomes to lysosome is complex and has been described hypothetically to explain the process of phagolysosome formation [33]. Phagosome maturation can be divided into three stages namely early phagosome late phagosome and phagosome.

7. Early phagosome

The newly formed phagosome rapidly gets the characteristics of the early endosome by fusing with sorting and recycling endosomes [34]. The interior becomes acidic but not very destructive, the small GTPase Rab5 regulates the membrane fusion events between endosome and early endosome. This ATPase on the membrane is useful for the transition from the early to a late phagosome, Rab5 then works through the recruitment of EEA1 (early endosome antigen 1), that promotes the fusion of the new phagosome with early endosomes [35, 36]. Rab5 also recruits the classic PI-3 K human vacuolar protein-sorting 34, which then generates phosphatidylinostol3-phosphate [37]. The acidity of the early phagosome is activated by the recruitment of and action of V-ATPase accumulating on its membrane and also by accumulating on its membrane and also by transient fusions with more acidic vesicles. The V-ATPase Trans locates protons (H) lumen of the phagosome using cytosolic ATP as an energy source.

8. The late phagosome

Rab5 is lost as the phagosome matures and Rab7 appears on the membrane which mediates the fusion of the phagosome with late endosomes [38]. Similarly proteins that will be recycled are separated through sorting of vesicles whereas the proteins intended for degradation are eliminated in intraluminal vesicles and dare directed into the lumen of the phagosome [39], which will make it a little acidic due to the

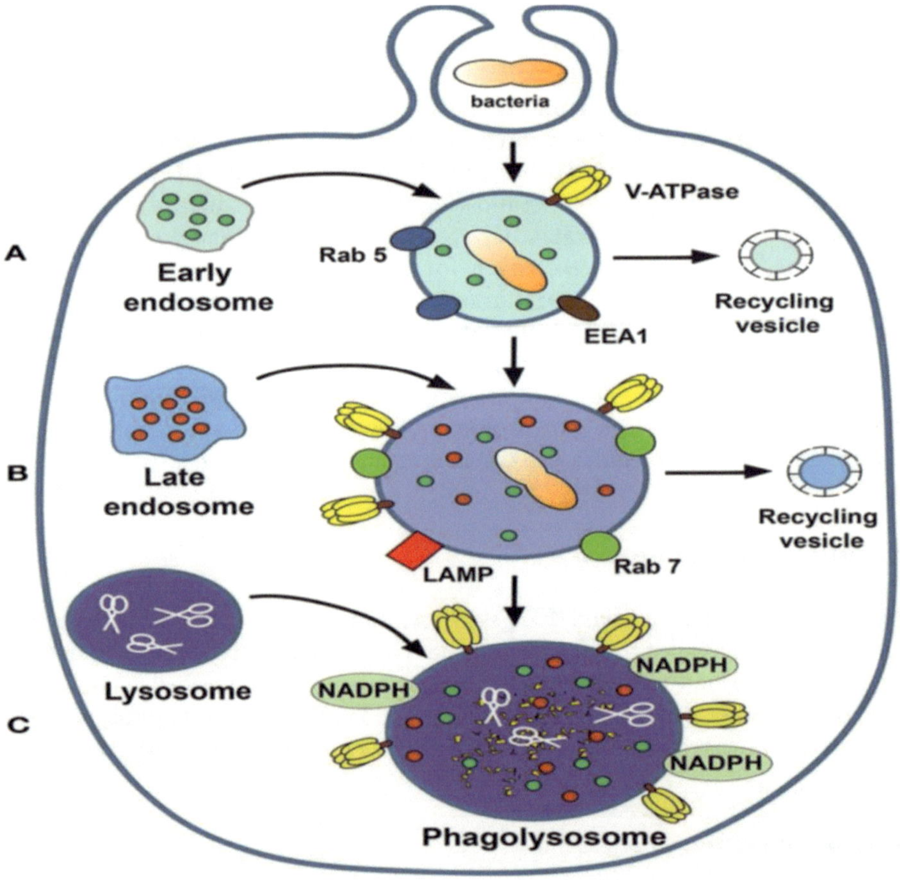

Figure 2.
The phagolysosome.

action of V-ATPase molecules on the membrane [40]. The lysosomal associated membrane proteins (LAMPS) and luminal proteases cathepsins and hydrolases) are incorporated from fusion with late endosomes or from the Golgi apparatus [41]. This well-illustrated in the **Figure 2**.

To mature to phagolysosomes these late phagosome fuse with lysosomes, which are the definitive microbicial organelles [42, 43]. Phagolysosomes have many sophisticated mechanisms that eliminate and degrade microorganism. They usually contain degradative enzymes like proteases, lysozymes, lipases and cathepsins, they are also acidic (ph. 5–5.5), due to the presence of V-ATPase molecules on their membrane [44]. This phagolysosome also presents with NADPH oxidase responsible for producing reactive oxygen species that are bactericidal like the superoxide (02-) [45] superoxide dismutase to H2O2 that can react Cl- ions to form hypochlorous acid, a very potential microbicial substance. This final reaction is catalyze by enzyme myeloperoxidase [46]. The best anti microbicial agent of neutrophils is hydrogen peroxide despite it being bactericidal, in its own way it can be anti-fungal and antiviral using myeloperoxidase in presence of hyalide ions [47].

9. Strategies pathogens use to evade phagocytosis

The importance of phagocytosis cannot be under scored in the prevention and clearance of infection and its because of this that mic robes have devised different means to dodge recognition and eventually phagocytosis **Table 2.**

Mostly the microbes interfere with opsonins binding of polysaccharide-based capsules which shield the deposition of opsonins, while other bacteria express some surface proteins that inhibit binding for example Group A streptococci escape complement mediated phagocytosis using M proteins that are lacking in higher organisms [48]. These PAMPs are usually detected by receptors on the phagocyte particularly Toll like receptors. fc and complement receptors are the best studied receptors and there signaling is quite known more phagocytic receptors studies are ongoing.

Effectors	Importance	Species involved
Protein A	Binds Fc region, preventing normal interaction with FcyR	*Cryptococcus aureus*
Capsule	Prevents complement deposition	*Cryptococcus neoformans,streptococcus pneumonia,Eschericia coli KI,Klebsiela pneumonia,Neiseria meningitides,S,aureus Haemopholus influenza Treponema pallidium*
M proteins	Prevents binding to CRs	*Streptococcus pyogens*
YadA	Prevents deposition of C3b	*Yersinia entercolitica*
Organisms that inhibit signaling		
YopE	GAP for RhoA,Rac and CDC42	*Yersinia sp.*
ExoT	Cysteine protease of Rho,Rac and Cdc42	*Yersinia sp.*
YOPH	Tyrosin phosphatase for Cas,Fyb,SKAP,-HOM,paxillin and FAK	*YERSINIA SP.*

Effectors	Importance	Species involved
Espj	Inhibits FcyR and CR3 mediated phagocytosis	*Eschericia coli*
EspB	Inhibits myosin actin interactions	*Eschericia coli*
EspH	Inactivates Rho GEFs	*Eschericia coli.*
T4SS	Delays phagocytosis	*Helicobacter pyroli*
Nef	Inhibits membrane delivery to the phagosome	*HIV*

Abbreviations: CR, complement receptor, GAP, GTPase-activating proteins, GEF, guanine nucleotide exchange factor, HIV, human immunodeficiency virus, T4SS, type 4 secretion system.

Table 2.
Shows different virulent factors microbes use to dodge uptake by phagocytosis.

10. Efficiency of phagocytosis

Many phagocytes have a relatively low phagocytosis capacity at rest and when inflammation gets in, phagocytes get exposed to a variety of activating stimuli which increase the efficiency of the cell to phagocytose. The activating stimuli include, bacterial products, cytokines and inflammatory mediators, the signals induced by these substances lead to increased activation of molecules involved I phagocytosis e.g. leukotrieneB4 increases Syk activation and consequently antibody dependent phagocytosis [49]. Also the action of P13K and ERK, which are essential enzymes for bacterial peptide, glanulocyte colony stimulating factor, leukotrienes and cytokines such as interleukin [50]. Phagocytosis can be regulated by cell differentiation, e.g. monocytes have lower phagocytic capability than neutrophils and macrophages, however they can enhance their phagocytic capacity after cell differentiation [51]. The capacity of monocytes to phagocytose diverse targets alter with the state of differentiation. Therefore during monocyte to macrophage differentiation the e most important signaling enzymes are reorganized in order to achieve increased phagocytosis [51, 52].

Author details

Laban Turyamuhika[1*], Agaba Bosco[2], Asiimwe Moses[3], Musinguzi Benson[4] and Okek Erick[5]

1 Makerere University, Uganda

2 Malaria Control Programme, Ministry of Health, Uganda

3 Mountains of the Moon University, Fort Portal, Uganda

4 Muni University, Arua, Uganda

5 Uganda Virus Research Institute, Entebbe, Uganda

*Address all correspondence to: labanturyamuhika74@gmail.com

References

[1] Murphy K, Weaver C. Janeway's Immunobiology. USA: Garland Science, Havard Medical School; 2016

[2] Seeberg JC, Loibl M, Moser F, Schwegler M, Büttner-Herold M, Daniel C, et al. Non-professional phagocytosis: A general feature of normal tissue cells. Scientific Reports. 2019;**9**(1):1-8

[3] Herre J, Marshall AS, Caron E, Edwards AD, Williams DL, Schweighoffer E, et al. Dectin-1 uses novel mechanisms for yeast phagocytosis in macrophages. Blood. 2004;**104**(13):4038-4045

[4] Ezekowitz R, Sastry K, Bailly P, Warner A. Molecular characterization of the human macrophage mannose receptor: Demonstration of multiple carbohydrate recognition-like domains and phagocytosis of yeasts in Cos-1 cells. The Journal of Experimental Medicine. 1990;**172**(6):1785-1794

[5] Schiff DE, Kline L, Soldau K, Lee J, Pugin J, Tobias PS, et al. Phagocytosis of gram-negative bacteria by a unique CD14-dependent mechanism. Journal of Leukocyte Biology. 1997;**62**(6):786-794

[6] Peiser L, Makepeace K, Plüddemann A, Savino S, Wright JC, Pizza M, et al. Identification of Neisseria meningitidis nonlipopolysaccharide ligands for class a macrophage scavenger receptor by using a novel assay. Infection and Immunity. 2006;**74**(9):5191-5199

[7] Patel SN, Serghides L, Smith TG, Febbraio M, Silverstein RL, Kurtz TW, et al. CD36 mediates the phagocytosis of plasmodium falciparum–infected erythrocytes by rodent macrophages. The Journal of Infectious Diseases. 2004;**189**(2):204-213

[8] van der Laan LJ, Döpp EA, Haworth R, Pikkarainen T, Kangas M, Elomaa O, et al. Regulation and functional involvement of macrophage scavenger receptor MARCO in clearance of bacteria in vivo. The Journal of Immunology. 1999;**162**(2):939-947

[9] Anderson CL, Shen L, Eicher DM, Wewers MD, Gill JK. Phagocytosis mediated by three distinct fc gamma receptor classes on human leukocytes. The Journal of Experimental Medicine. 1990;**171**(4):1333-1345

[10] Bakema J, Van Egmond M. The human immunoglobulin a fc receptor FcαRI: A multifaceted regulator of mucosal immunity. Mucosal Immunology. 2011;**4**(6):612-624

[11] Daëron M, Malbec O, Bonnerot C, Latour S, Segal DM, Fridman WH. Tyrosine-containing activation motif-dependent phagocytosis in mast cells. Journal of Immunology (Baltimore, Md: 1950). 1994;**152**(2):783-792

[12] Ghiran I, Barbashov SF, Klickstein LB, Tas SW, Jensenius JC, Nicholson-Weller A. Complement receptor 1/CD35 is a receptor for mannan-binding lectin. The Journal of Experimental Medicine. 2000;**192**(12):1797-1808

[13] Freeman SA, Grinstein S. Phagocytosis: Receptors, signal integration, and the cytoskeleton. Immunological Reviews. 2014;**262**(1):193-215

[14] Joffe AM, Bakalar MH, Fletcher DA. Macrophage phagocytosis assay with reconstituted target particles. Nature Protocols. 2020;**15**(7):2230-2246

[15] Miyanishi M, Tada K, Koike M, Uchiyama Y, Kitamura T, Nagata S. Identification of Tim4 as a phosphatidylserine receptor. Nature. 2007;**450**(7168):435-439

[16] Stossel TP. Phagocytosis. New England Journal of Medicine. 1974;**290**(14):774-780

[17] Abbas AK, Lichtman AH, Pober JS. Cellular and Molecular Immunology. san Francisco California: Saunders; 1991

[18] Wilson GJ, Marakalala MJ, Hoving JC, Van Laarhoven A, Drummond RA, Kerscher B, et al. The C-type lectin receptor CLECSF8/CLEC4D is a key component of anti-mycobacterial immunity. Cell Host & Microbe. 2015;**17**(2):252-259

[19] Levine AP, Segal AW. What is wrong with granulocytes in inflammatory bowel diseases? Digestive Diseases. 2013;**31**(3-4):321-327

[20] Rosales C, Uribe-Querol E. Phagocytosis: A fundamental process in immunity. BioMed Research International. 2017;**2017**:23-32

[21] Drummond RA, Dambuza IM, Vautier S, Taylor JA, Reid DM, Bain CC, et al. CD4+ T-cell survival in the GI tract requires dectin-1 during fungal infection. Mucosal Immunology. 2016;**9**(2):492-502

[22] Gordon S. Phagocytosis: An immunobiologic process. Immunity. 2016;**44**(3):463-475

[23] Rosales C. Molecular Mechanisms of Phagocytosis. calos Rosales Mexico city: Springer; 2005

[24] Dale B. Enhanced Fcγ receptor signaling in Cbl-/-macrophages reveals surprising insights into the mechanism of phagocytosis. Columbia University; 2008

[25] Uribe-Querol E, Rosales C. Control of phagocytosis by microbial pathogens. Frontiers in immunology. 2017;**8**:1368

[26] Araki N, Hatae T, Furukawa A, Swanson JA. Phosphoinositide-3-kinase-independent contractile activities associated with Fcγ-receptor-mediated phagocytosis and macropinocytosis in macrophages. Journal of cell science. 2003;**116**(2):247-257

[27] Dart AE, Tollis S, Bright MD, Frankel G, Endres RG. The motor protein myosin 1G functions in FcγR-mediated phagocytosis. Journal of cell science. 2012;**125**(24):6020-6029

[28] Rosales C, Uribe-Querol E. Antibody-fc receptor interactions in antimicrobial functions. Current Immunology Reviews. 2013;**9**(1):44-55

[29] Freeman SA, Goyette J, Furuya W, Woods EC, Bertozzi CR, Bergmeier W, et al. Integrins form an expanding diffusional barrier that coordinates phagocytosis. Cell. 2016;**164**(1-2):128-140

[30] Chang VT, Fernandes RA, Ganzinger KA, Lee SF, Siebold C, McColl J, et al. Initiation of T cell signaling by CD45 segregation at'close contacts'. Nature Immunology. 2016;**17**(5):574-582

[31] Goodridge HS, Reyes CN, Becker CA, Katsumoto TR, Ma J, Wolf AJ, et al. Activation of the innate immune receptor Dectin-1 upon formation of a 'phagocytic synapse'. Nature. 2011;**472**(7344):471-475

[32] Dustin ML. Signaling at neuro/immune synapses. The Journal of Clinical Investigation. 2012;**122**(4):1149-1155

[33] Luzio JP, Pryor PR, Bright NA. Lysosomes: Fusion and function. Nature reviews Molecular Cell Biology. 2007;**8**(8):622-632

[34] Levin R, Grinstein S, Canton J. The life cycle of phagosomes: Formation, maturation, and resolution. Immunological Reviews. 2016;**273**(1):156-179

[35] Gutierrez M. Functional role (s) of phagosomal Rab GTPases. Small GTPases. 2013;**4**:148-158

[36] Kitano M, Nakaya M, Nakamura T, Nagata S, Matsuda M. Imaging of Rab5 activity identifies essential regulators for phagosome maturation. Nature. 2008;**453**(7192):241-245

[37] Vieira OV, Botelho RJ, Rameh L, Brachmann SM, Matsuo T, Davidson HW, et al. Distinct roles of class I and class III phosphatidylinositol 3-kinases in phagosome formation and maturation. The Journal of Cell Biology. 2001;**155**(1):19-26

[38] Rink J, Ghigo E, Kalaidzidis Y, Zerial M. Rab conversion as a mechanism of progression from early to late endosomes. Cell. 2005;**122**(5):735-749

[39] Hanson PI, Roth R, Lin Y, Heuser JE. Plasma membrane deformation by circular arrays of ESCRT-III protein filaments. The Journal of Cell Biology. 2008;**180**(2):389-402

[40] Kinchen JM, Ravichandran KS. Phagosome maturation: Going through the acid test. Nature Reviews Molecular Cell Biology. 2008;**9**(10):781-795

[41] Canton J. Phagosome maturation in polarized macrophages. Journal of Leukocyte Biology. 2014;**96**(5):729-738

[42] Pryor PR, Luzio JP. Delivery of endocytosed membrane proteins to the lysosome. Biochimica et Biophysica Acta (BBA)-molecular. Cell Research. 2009;**1793**(4):615-624

[43] Bright NA, Gratian MJ, Luzio JP. Endocytic delivery to lysosomes mediated by concurrent fusion and kissing events in living cells. Current Biology. 2005;**15**(4):360-365

[44] Marshansky V, Futai M. The V-type H+-ATPase in vesicular trafficking: Targeting, regulation and function. Current Opinion in Cell Biology. 2008;**20**(4):415-426

[45] Minakami R, Sumimoto H. Phagocytosis-coupled activation of the superoxide-producing phagocyte oxidase, a member of the NADPH oxidase (nox) family. International Journal of Hematology. 2006;**84**(3):193-198

[46] Nauseef WM. Myeloperoxidase in human neutrophil host defence. Cellular Microbiology. 2014;**16**(8):1146-1155

[47] Klebanoff S, Rosen H. The role of myeloperoxidase in the microbicidal activity of polymorphonuclear leukocytes. Oxygen Free Radicals and Tissue Damage. 1978:263-284

[48] Flannagan RS, Jaumouillé V, Grinstein S. The cell biology of phagocytosis. Annual Review of Pathology: Mechanisms of Disease. 2012;**7**:61-98

[49] Wang J-P, Chang L-C, Lin Y-L, Hsu M-F, Chang C-Y, Huang L-J, et al. Investigation of the cellular mechanism of inhibition of formyl-methionyl-leucyl-phenylalanine-induced superoxide anion generation in rat neutrophils by 2-benzyloxybenzaldehyde. Biochemical Pharmacology. 2003;**65**(7):1043-1051

[50] Knall C, Worthen GS, Johnson GL. Interleukin 8-stimulated

phosphatidylinositol-3-kinase activity regulates the migration of human neutrophils independent of extracellular signal-regulated kinase and p38 mitogen-activated protein kinases. Proceedings of the National Academy of Sciences. 1997;**94**(7):3052-3057

[51] Newman SL, Tucci MA. Regulation of human monocyte/macrophage function by extracellular matrix. Adherence of monocytes to collagen matrices enhances phagocytosis of opsonized bacteria by activation of complement receptors and enhancement of fc receptor function. The Journal of clinical investigation. 1990;**86**(3):703-714

[52] Kambayashi T, Koretzky GA. Proximal signaling events in FcεRI-mediated mast cell activation. Journal of Allergy and Clinical Immunology. 2007;**119**(3):544-552

Chapter 2

Macrophages: Phagocytosis, Antigen Presentation, and Activation of Immunity

Kazuki Santa

Abstract

Macrophages are phagocytes and one of the white blood cells discovered by Ilya I. Mechnikov in 1892. They engulf and digest foreign substances like pathogens and conduct antigen presentation, mature from haematopoietic stem cells in bone marrow, moving into blood vessels and become monocytes, and differentiate into macrophages in the tissue. Macrophages have intracellular granules called lysosome accumulating digestive enzymes. Their life span is several months and proliferates by cell division. There are three roles: First one is phagocytosis. Macrophages incorporate pathogens and work in natural immunity. In inflammation, macrophages aggregate after neutrophils recruitment and engulf pathogens into cellular phagosomes, fused with lysosomes and degrade. Second role is antigen presentation. Macrophages present fragment of digested foreign substances on cell surface MHC class II molecules and release cytokines. Dendritic cells and B cells are also APCs expressing MHC class II. $CD4^+$ T cells recognize antigens presented on macrophages by using TCR. Only well-matched helper T cells *via* MHC class II-TCR interaction are activated. The third is activation of immunity. Cytokines produced by T cells activate macrophages and differentiate them into inflammatory M1 and wound-healing M2 macrophages.

Keywords: macrophages, phagocytosis, antigen presentation, activation of immunity, tissue regeneration

1. Introduction

1.1 Development of macrophages

Macrophages are originated from variety of cells. In the early development, it depends on the tissues; however, macrophages are derived from yolk sac and replaced by the macrophages derived from liver and bone marrow [1]. Tissue resident macrophages are divided into two types, macrophages derived from circulating monocytes and having other origins including yolk sac, embryonic liver, and embryo near dorsal aorta-derived macrophages. In the adulthood, they are independently kept from their original monocytes. Tissue-specific macrophages differentiate from circulating monocytes by the ability of migration at the time of inflammation. Dendritic cells differentiate from monocytes as well as macrophages. Macrophages have variety of morphologies and phenotypes because they distribute in many organs and tissues. Instead of neutrophils that live only few days, the life span of the macrophages is several months. The diameter of the human macrophage is about 21 μm.

1.2 Differentiation and subtypes

Macrophages differentiate from premature M0 to M1 or M2 phenotypes depending on various factors from the signal transduction molecules, growth factors, transcription factors, and epigenetic or post-transduction changes to cytokines, cell adherence molecules, and metabolites [2]. Furthermore, macrophages change their activation state in response to microbes and microbial products like LPS. Recently, it is said that the classifications of macrophages are not easy because of the plasticity of the macrophages.

M1 macrophages are the so-called classically activated macrophages, pro-inflammatory macrophages, and killer macrophages. M1 macrophages produce high levels of IL-12 after the stimulation of LPS and IFN-γ. The feature of M1 macrophages is possessing specific pathways which converts arginine into "killer molecules" nitric oxide. M1 macrophage is the phenotype observed in early inflammation phase activated by IFN-γ, TNF, and damage-associated molecular patterns (DAMPS). They show high antigen presenting ability, producing high amounts of NO and reactive oxygen spices (ROS), showing increased expression of IL-12 and IL-23, and decreased IL-10 expression. In addition, M1 macrophages express high levels of MHC class II molecules, CD68, CD80, and Th1 cell-inducing chemokine CXCL9 and CXCL12 [3].

M2 macrophages are called alternatively activated macrophages and wound healing macrophages divided into M2a, M2b, M2c, and M2d phenotypes. They are a typical phenotype of tissue-resident macrophages and participate in constructive process including wound healing and tissue repair. These macrophages are stimulated by several factors including parasitic and fungal infection, immune complexes, apoptotic cells, macrophage colony stimulation factors (M-CSF), IL-13, TGF-β, and Th2 cytokine IL-4, and cytokines produced by Th2 cells like IL-25 and IL-33. Signal transduction pathways including STAT6, IRF4, PPARδ, and PPARδ are required for the differentiation of M2 macrophages. Generally, M2 macrophages produce low IL-1, IL-6, and TNF-α, whereas producing low IL-12. A typical feature of M2 macrophages is converting arginine to ornithine "repair molecules." Ornithine is important for wound healing and required for vascular and endothelial regeneration. M2 macrophages are also important for clearance of pathogens, anti-inflammation, metabolism, wound healing, tissue regeneration, immune regulation, and progression of tumours. On the other hand, M2 macrophages induce tissue fibrosis in the lung and liver, and progressively stimulate tumour growth as tumour-related macrophages. M2 phenotypes are characterised by the expression of CD206, CD163, FIZZ1, and Ym1/2. There are four types of M2 macrophages a, b, c, and d. These are different by their cell surface markers, secreting cytokines, and biological function. However, the common feature of these M2 macrophages is the production of IL-10 [4].

M2a macrophages are activated by IL-4 or IL-13. IL-4 induces the expression of the mannose receptor (CD206). Upregulation of IL-10, TGF-β, CCL17, CCL18, and CCL22 induces cell proliferation, cell repair, and endocytosis of M2a macrophages.

Immune complex, toll-like receptor (TLR) and their ligands, and IL-1β activate M2b macrophages. When activated, these subtypes of macrophages produce both proinflammatory and anti-inflammatory cytokines TNF-α, IL-1β, IL-6, and IL-10. M2b macrophages work on immune response and regulation of inflammation. High IL-10-producing and low IL-12-producing M2b macrophages are the so-called regulatory macrophages (Mreg). Mregs are recently focused on their ability to induce regulatory T cells (Treg) [5].

M2c macrophages are activated by glucocorticoid, IL-10, TGF-β, and inactivated macrophages. The feature of M2c macrophages is high expression of anti-inflammatory IL-10, TGF-β, CCL16, CCL18, and tyrosine-protein kinase MER (MerTK), which enhance phagocytosis activity.

TLR antagonist, IL-6, and adenosine activate M2d macrophages. Adenosine induces the expression of IL-10 and vascular endothelial growth factor (VEGF) and enhances angiogenesis and tumour progression.

M2 macrophages are important for the stability of blood vessels because they produce VEGF-A and TFG-β. In acute lesion, macrophages change their phenotype from M1 to M2; however, these changes will be lost in chronic lesion. This dysregulation results in insufficient M2 macrophages and induces the deficiency of growth factor. The lack of growth factors and anti-inflammatory cytokines from M2 macrophages and excess production of proinflammatory cytokines from M1 macrophage prevent sufficient repair of wound healing. Normally, depletion of neutrophils by apoptosis after eating debris and pathogens induces the switch of macrophages from M1 to M2, but inflammation is unnecessary at that time. Then, M1 macrophages cannot eat apoptosis-inducing neutrophils, and this phenomenon increases the numbers of macrophages and inflammation because of the dysregulation [6].

2. Classification of macrophages by the tissue

2.1 Adipose tissue macrophages: Adipose tissue

Macrophages exist in body fat and increase in case of obesity.

2.2 Monocytes: bone marrow, blood

The largest white blood cells in the blood. They develop into macrophages and dendritic cells.

2.3 Kupffer cells: liver

Kupffer cells exist in the liver and also known as stellate macrophages. Kupffer cells were named after Karl Wilhelm von Kupffer. They work as the first defence against gut bacteria and endotoxin in the liver.

2.4 Alveolar macrophages: pulmonary alveoli

Macrophages exist in alveoli and bronchus. Alveolar macrophages have high activity to get rid of dusts and microbes in the lung.

2.5 Microglia: central nerve system

A family of glial cells with different origin from other family of cells. Most of glial cells developed from ectoderm; however, alveolar macrophages are developed from mesoderm and haematopoietic stem cells. Microglia have phagocytic activity in the nerve and participate in the repair of neural tissue after the tissue damage.

2.6 Hofbauer cells: placenta

Eosinophilic histocytes found in the placenta, often seen in early pregnancy, named after J. Isfred Isidore Hofbauer. Hofbauer cells are considered as a type of macrophage.

2.7 Intraglomerular mesangial cells: kidney

Intraglomerular mesangial cells exist in basement membrane surrounded by glomerular capillaries. They are considered as a type of fibroblast.

2.8 Osteoclasts: bone

Osteoclasts are the specialist of absorbing or destroying bone in the process of bone regeneration. They are usually polygonal giant cells with 5–20 nuclei, but sometimes mononuclear osteoclast can be found. Bone marrow-derived monocyte progenitors differentiate into osteoclasts. The marker of osteoclasts is tartrate-resistant acid phosphatase. On the other hand, the marker of osteoblast is alkaline phosphatase.

2.9 Langerhans cells: skin

Langerhans cells are named after Paul Langerhans. Usually, they are regarded as dendritic cells other than macrophages.

2.10 Epithelioid cells: granulomas

Activated macrophages similar to epithelial cells. They have a thin eosinophilic cytoplasm with small granules and nucleus less dense than lymphocytes. They are found in granulomatous inflammation and participate in arthritis.

2.11 Red pulp macrophages (sinusoidal lining cells): red pulp in spleen

Macrophages found in red pulp in spleen are necessary for the blood homeostasis by depleting damaged or aged red blood cells with the phagocytosis.

2.12 Intestinal macrophages: intestine

Macrophages specifically evolved in intestinal environment. Intestinal macrophages do not induce inflammation to coexist with intestinal microbiome. They do not excrete proinflammatory cytokines such as IL-1, IL-6, and TNF-α. TGF-β produced by surrounding environment changes these macrophages from proinflammatory phenotype to non-inflammatory phenotype. Intestinal macrophages conduct phagocytosis, but they do not produce cytokines after phagocytosis nor express receptors for LPS, IgA, and IgG.

2.13 Others

Sinus histiocytes: lymph nodes
Tissue macrophages leading to giant cells: connective tissue
Peritoneal macrophages: peritoneal cavity
LysoMac: Peyer's patch

3. Function of macrophages

3.1 Phagocytosis

Macrophages are one of the three professional phagocytes with other phagocytes including granulocytes (eosinophils, neutrophils, and basophils) and dendritic cells (DC). Phagocytosis is the process that microorganisms entering the host and recognised by phagocytes and incorporated and destroyed. This process starts after the interaction with pathogen-specific receptors (usually pathogen-specific sugar or lipid structures) on phagocytes and the surface molecular on pathogens. Typical phagocyte receptors are dectin-1 and mannose receptor (CD206), and both are the family of members of c-type lectin. Dectin-1 expressed on macrophages and neutrophils connects with glucose polymers on the cell walls of fungus. On the other hand, CD206 expressed on macrophages and DCs connects with variety of ligands on fungus, bacteria, and virus. Generally, macrophages exist in all of tissues and monitor potential pathogens with amoebic motility. Most of macrophages are strategically placed where microbes invade or debris accumulate [7].

After starting interaction with pathogens, phagocytic plasma membrane in macrophages engulfs pathogens into phagosomes, large membrane-enclosed endocytic vesicles (endosomes). Phagosomes enclose pathogens, merged with lysosomes containing antimicrobial peptides and enzymes, and form phagolysosomes. Toxic peroxides like superoxide radicals in phagolysosomes kill and digest pathogens after acidification and enzymic processes. Macrophages ultimately digest over 100 bacteria through digestive compounds in their lifetime. However, some bacteria have resistant properties to these digestive methods. Mycobacterium tuberculosis survives within the macrophages through inhibiting the fusion to phagosomes. To reproduce themselves, Salmonella enterica serovar Typhi induces phagocytosis to incorporate into macrophages, inhibits lysosomal digestion, and triggers apoptosis of macrophages. Furthermore, leishmaniasis causes Leishmania parasitises in macrophages.

3.2 Activation of natural immunity

Macrophages participate in natural immunity by engulfing and digesting pathogens. They protect hosts from the infections and damages through phagocytosis [8]. Macrophages are the first defence against pathogens working with neutrophils and are specific phagocytes with long life. After the invasion of pathogens, neutrophils are firstly recruited to the site of infection, die after phagocytosis of pathogens, and generate neutrophil traps (NETs). Then, macrophages are recruited and digest NETs after approximately 48 hours later. Recruited macrophages digest pathogens and dead cells through phagocytosis. Finally, they initiate immune responses through releasing factors like TNF-α to recruit other immune cells such as lymphocytes.

3.3 Adaptive immunity and antigen presentation

Macrophages are the most important antigen-presenting cells (APC) as well as dendritic cells (DC), which have important roles in the initiation of immune responses. Furthermore, they produce strong modification factors and chemical substances, such as enzymes, complement proteins, and IL-1. At the same time, macrophages activate to seek microorganisms and tumour cells through their lymphokine receptors.

Antigen-digested macrophages present pathogen antigens to helper T cells, most of which are protein molecules expressed on the surface of pathogens. Antigen presentation is conducted by MHC class II molecules (MHCII) on the surface of macrophages presenting antigens incorporated. Antibody production attaching to the pathogenic antigens starts from plasma B cells after the antigen presentation by APCs and making macrophages easy to adhere to cell membrane of pathogens the so-called opsonisation.

In lymph nodes, antigen presentation *via* macrophages through MHCII stimulates Th1 cells to start proliferation. B cells recognise same unprocessed antigen by the cell surface antibodies and then incorporate and process them through endocytosis. MHCII molecules on the surface of B cells present processed antigens. T cells that recognise antigen-MHCII complex with co-stimulatory factor CD40-CD40L help B cells to produce antibodies. Then, macrophages incorporate opsonised pathogens by antibodies and eliminate them from the body. However, regarding phagocytosis, recently dendritic cells are more focused than macrophages.

Macrophages provide another defence pathway against fungus and parasites. After the recognition of specific antigen on the cell surface, activated T cells differentiate into effector cells and produce lymphokines. Produced lymphokines stimulate macrophages to more offensive form.

4. Role of macrophages in tissue regeneration and homeostasis

4.1 Wound healing

Macrophages have significant roles in wound healing. By 2 days after the injury, they replace neutrophils and become the dominant cells in the place where injured. Monocytes are attracted to the wound site by the growth factors released from platelets and other cells and then enter the site from bloodstream through the blood vessel wall. The number of monocytes in the injured sites peaks at 1.5 days. At the site of injury, monocytes mature into macrophages. In addition, spleen contains half the numbers of macrophages as a spare, and they are sent to the wound sites when injured [9].

The main role of macrophages is conducting phagocytosis to the microbes and injured tissues. In addition, protease released from macrophages induces tissue necrosis. After 3 to 4 days of injury, macrophages secrete variety of factors including cytokines, which proliferate and attract cells involved in wound healing. Under the stimulation of low oxygen environment, macrophages induce and generate accelerating factors of angiogenesis. These factors stimulate cells to promote the growth of epithelial cells, create granulation tissues, and form new extracellular matrix. Then, macrophages direct the next stage of wound healing *via* the secretion of these factors.

4.2 Muscle regeneration

There are two waves in muscle regeneration by macrophages. The first wave is the increased population of phagocytes after the damage of muscular fibre with development of rhabdomyolysis and muscle membrane inflammation by the use of muscle. This population peaks after 24 hours of recruitment to the muscle damage and rapidly decreases after 48 hours. The second wave is non-phagocytic macrophages distributes near the close region of regenerative fibres. These cells peak at 2 to 4 days, and the numbers of the cells remain increased for few days whilst muscle tissue is reconstituted. The first groups of cells do not have any benefits for muscle repair, but second croups are beneficial. They release soluble factors related to the muscle growth, differentiation, repair, and regeneration [10].

4.3 Foot regeneration

In salamanders, macrophages participate in not only consume debris but also a typical regeneration of limbs. Depletion of macrophages in salamanders resulted in the failure of limb regeneration [11].

4.4 Macrophages related with the maintenance of homeostasis

All of tissues have residential macrophages interacting with stromal and functional tissue. These macrophages are unmovable, protecting tissues from inflammatory injuries and provide essential factors to support tissue physiological functions [12].

4.5 Maintenance of pigments

Melanophages, a tissue-resident macrophages, absorb pigments from organ specific or exogenous out-cellular environment. In contrast to melanocytes, melanophages only accumulate melanin incorporated from lysosome-like phagosomes. This phenomenon occurs by which melanophages conduct phagocytosis of tissues from dead skin macrophages. This occurs because melanophages conduct phagocytosis of tissue from dead skin macrophages.

4.6 Nerve-associated macrophages

Nerve-associated macrophages are macrophages related to neurone. They have elongated morphology and stretch up to 200 μm.

5. Macrophages in disorders

5.1 Pathogen hosting macrophages

Generally, macrophages destroy pathogens by phagocytosis. However, some pathogens live in macrophages by interrupting this phagocytosis processes. This phenomenon hides pathogens from immune system and provides them environment to reproduce themselves. Tuberculosis-inducing mycobacterium and Leishmania species are well known [13].

5.2 Heart diseases and cardiovascular diseases

Macrophages are main cause in the onset of progressive plaque lesions in atherosclerosis. Residential M2 macrophages incorporate oxidised LDL in the cells and become form cells which clogging blood vessels. In addition, both M1 and M2 macrophages participate in the progression of atherosclerosis. M1 macrophages enhance atherosclerosis through inflammation induction. M2 macrophages eliminate cholesterol, but incorporated oxidised cholesterol induces apoptotic form cells from macrophages [14].

On the other hand, macrophages are recruited to the place where tissue regeneration is required after acute myocardial infraction, removing apoptotic cells and debris.

5.3 Tissue fibrosis

M2 macrophages induce tissue fibrosis by the production of TGF-β in the damaged lung and liver.

5.4 HIV

Macrophages participate in HIV infection. In addition to CD4+ T cells, macrophages become the storage of reproductive virus. Gp120 protein on HIV couples with chemokine receptor CCR5 to invade into cells.

5.5 Cancer

Some macrophage subtypes participate in the progression of cancer. Cancer-related macrophages participate in tumour cell growth and invasion, progression of angiogenesis, and suppression of anti-tumour immune cells.

5.6 Obesity

Proinflammatory macrophages in fat tissues participate in obesity-related complications such as insulin resistance and type-2 diabetes.

5.7 Inflammatory bowel disease (IBD)

Macrophages participate in inflammatory bowel diseases (IBD) including Crohn's disease (CD) and ulcerative colitis (UC). In healthy intestine, macrophages suppress the inflammation; however, in the patients with IBD, the numbers and diversity of macrophages change and cause adverse effects on the onset of disorders.

Author details

Kazuki Santa
Tokyo College of Biotechnology, Tokyo, Japan

*Address all correspondence to: kazuki_santa@hotmail.com

References

[1] Schulz C et al. A lineage of myeloid cells independent of Myb and hematopoietic stem cells. Science. 2012;**336**(6077):86-90

[2] T'Jonck W et al. Niche signals and transcription factors involved in tissue-resident macrophage development. Cellular Immunology. 2018;**330**:43-53

[3] Biswas SK et al. Macrophage plasticity and interaction with lymphocyte subsets: Cancer as a paradigm. Nature Immunology. 2010;**11**(10):889-896

[4] Yao Y et al. Macrophage polarization in physiological and pathological pregnancy. Frontiers in Immunology. 2019;**10**:792

[5] Riquelme P et al. TIGIT+ iTregs elicited by human regulatory macrophages control T cell immunity. Nature Communications. 2018;**9**(1):2858

[6] Hesketh M et al. Macrophage phenotypes regulate scar formation and chronic wound healing. International Journal of Molecular Sciences. 2017;**18**(7):1545

[7] Murphy K et al. Janeway's Immunobiology. 9th ed. New York: Garland Science; 2017

[8] Germic N et al. Regulation of the innate immune system by autophagy: Monocytes, macrophages, dendritic cells and antigen presentation. Cell Death & Differentiation. 2019;**26**(4):715-727

[9] Swirski FK et al. Identification of splenic reservoir monocytes and their deployment to inflammatory sites. Science. 2009;**325**(5940):612-616

[10] Bréchot N et al. Modulation of macrophage activation state protects tissue from necrosis during critical limb ischemia in thrombospondin-1-deficient mice. PLoS One. 2008;**3**(12):e3950

[11] Godwin JW et al. Macrophages are required for adult salamander limb regeneration. Proceedings of the National Academy of Sciences of the United States of America. 2013;**110**(23):9415-9420

[12] Okabe Y et al. Tissue-specific signals control reversible program of localization and functional polarization of macrophages. Cell. 2014;**157**(4):832-844

[13] Herb M et al. Functions of ROS in macrophages and antimicrobial immunity. Antioxidants (Basel). 2021;**10**(2):313

[14] Santa K et al. Prevention of metabolic syndrome by phytochemicals and vitamin D. International Journal of Molecular Sciences. 2023;**24**(3):2627

Chapter 3

Phagocytosis of *Mycobacterium tuberculosis*: A Narrative of the Uptaking and Survival

Gabriela Echeverría-Valencia

Abstract

Mycobacterium tuberculosis is the causal agent of human tuberculosis. The initial events of the establishment of the infection include the phagocytosis by several innate immune response cells. This chapter will discuss the immune cells involved, the phagocytic pattern recognition receptors (PPRs) that recognize and mediate bacteria phagocytosis (such as C-type lectin receptors, Toll-like receptors, complement receptors, and scavenger receptors), and the outcome of this initial interaction. Additionally, the bacterial strategies to evade the immune response—which includes the inhibition of the phagosome maturation and arresting of phagosome acidification, the mechanisms to survive to the reactive nitrogen species and reactive oxygen species, and finally, the resistance to the apoptosis and autophagy—will be reviewed. Finally, the host-pathogen interaction of *M. tuberculosis* with the phagocytic human cells during the primary events of the tuberculosis infection will also be reviewed.

Keywords: phagocytosis, tuberculosis, macrophages, receptors, phagosome

1. Introduction

Mycobacterium tuberculosis (MTB) is a human pathogen, which belongs to a group of nine species phylogenetically related, called *M. tuberculosis* complex [1]. MTB is the causative agent of tuberculosis: An infectious disease that causes mainly a pulmonary infection although, renal, meningeal, genital tuberculosis, and other anatomical sites have been affected. Is a human pathogen and both (human hosts and MTB) have co-evolved together for an extended period of time of approximately 70,000 years [2].

Before the COVID-19 pandemic, tuberculosis (TB) was the first cause of death from a single infectious agent. It is estimated that 25% of the global population is infected with the bacteria, but only 10% of them will develop the disease during their lifetime. TB continues to be a public health problem due to the increased number of co-infections in HIV patients and the augmented antimicrobial resistance by MTB [3].

The mycobacterial infection in humans originates by the inhalation of aerosols containing the bacteria on *flügge* droplets, which is dispersed by the sneeze or cough of infected individuals. Once in the alveolus, the microorganism interacts with the innate immune response cells; the receptors at the macrophage identify the bacteria through pathogen-associated molecular patterns called PAMPs, and the said PAMPs are composed of lipids, carbohydrates, and protein characteristic of the mycobacteria and other pathogens [4]. During this initial immune response against tuberculosis, various cell types interact with the bacteria, such as dendritic cells, NK cells, neutrophils, and macrophages [5–7].

The phagocyted MTB can survive inside the macrophages through specific strategies. Namely, evasion of the immune response by phagosome, arresting inhibition of phagosome acidification [8], resistance to nitrogen species and reactive oxygen species [9], and also apoptosis and autophagy evasion [10]. The previously mentioned survival mechanisms are live-defining determinants on which mycobacterial efficiency to invade, establish, and survive inside macrophages depends. The phagocytosis constitutes a fundamental event during host-pathogen interaction in TB because this initial interplay determines the outcome of the disease.

As described before, MTB evades the immune response inside the macrophages, it uses the cell as a niche to survive latently, and it even multiplies efficiently within the phagocytic cell during reduced immune containment. The host search for containment and isolation produces cytokines and chemokines, which induce the migration of cells, and thus, granuloma formation. At the beginning of granuloma formation, the immune cells that constitute the granuloma are monocytes, neutrophils, and macrophages; subsequently after, the development of the acquired immune response induces the migration of lymphocytes. At times, the presence of extracellular matrix components and fibroblasts has been found around the mycobacterial granuloma [11, 12].

In the next sections, the initial process of human tuberculosis infection by MTB will be reviewed, focusing on:

1. The interaction with a variety of cells can phagocyte and exert the innate immune response against the bacteria.

2. The earliest events of the immune response: recognition and phagocytosis.

3. MTB's strategies to evade the immune response successfully, and the importance of said strategies for its survival, latency, and persistence.

2. The innate immune response against tuberculosis and the host-pathogen interaction with mycobacteria

The main entrance gate of MTB to the human body is the lung. There, air particles can be cleared by sneezing and coughing. Also, the presence of cilia and mucus contributes to the removal of particles allocated in deeper locations. In addition to that, the epithelia at the lung provide biochemical mechanisms to battle pathogens; among them the hydrolytic enzyme Lysozyme, and peptides (such as cathelicidins and defensins) contribute to the innate immune response through pathogen membrane destruction [13]. Microorganisms that cannot be cleared by these means will be phagocyted by alveolar macrophages (AM). During MTB infection, macrophages become a cellular niche of survival and bacterial multiplication. However, AM are not the only innate immune cells that interplay with MTB, neutrophils, dendritic cells, NK cells (natural killer) also interact with the pathogen.

Mycobacterial recognition by macrophages begins with the cell expression of a variety of phagocytic pattern recognition receptors (PPRs) that identify MTB through PAMPs. Cellular receptors of the C-type lectin receptors (CLRs) recognize microorganisms through carbohydrate patterns; among these receptors are mannose receptor (MR), Mincle, dendritic cell-specific intercellular adhesion molecule-3 grabbing non-integrin (DC-SIGN), and Dectin-1. Also, complement receptors (CR) and immunoglobulin receptors assist in the recognition of opsonized mycobacteria. Likewise, receptors that contribute to mycobacterial interaction are Toll-like receptors (TLRs), Scavenger receptors (SRs), NOD-like receptors (NLRs), and CD14 [14, 15]. These PPRs (which intervened and were stimulated during the interaction with MTB) determine the outcome of the acquired immune response, survival, autophagy, and apoptosis [16].

2.1 Dendritic cells

Dendritic cells originate from bone marrow progenitor cells and migrate as immature cells to different anatomical locations in order to detect pathogens. Part of their function as presenting cells is being an important link between the innate and acquired immune response. After recognition and phagocytosis of antigens (Ag) or pathogens, they increase the expression of MHC I and II [17]. Then, dendritic cells migrate through lymphatic circulation to lymph nodes after antigen processing [18]. At this location, dendritic cells induce T-cell activation through antigen presentation to lymphocytes [19]; however, MTB limits the response of dendritic cells as part of the immune response evasion [20], and moreover, the increased number of MTB found inside the dendritic cells suggests the replication of it (event associated with an increased expression of IL-10) [21]. Additionally, dendritic cells infected with MTB induce the expression of cytokines such as IFN alpha and beta, which contribute to the cell migration of NK cells and T cells, and might promote granuloma formation [22].

2.2 Neutrophils

If neutrophils are present in the lungs before infection, they reduce the bacterial number; however, if they are absent immediately after infection, the bacterial count increases [23, 24]. During MTB infection, neutrophils are recruited to the site of infection due to the cytokine and chemokine expression [25]. Neutrophils exert the innate immune response against MTB through diverse mechanisms, such as bacterial phagocytosis, production of hypochlorous acid, expression of enzymes that destroy bacteria and human cells indiscriminately, and the release of the neutrophil extracellular traps (NETs) [26].

2.3 NK cells

NK cells are lymphocytes that contribute directly to the innate immunity. As part of their capabilities, they produce cytokines to assist the acquired and innate immune response. NK cells destroy infected cells through chemical weapons such as perforin, granzyme, defensin, and NO (nitric oxide). It has been observed that during MTB infection in T cells-deficient mice, NK cells contribute to the resistance against the bacteria. In that regard, in T cell-deficient individuals, the expression of IFN gamma enhances the mycobacterial control [27].

2.4 Macrophages

Macrophages are hematopoietic-derived cells from bone marrow, which are distributed almost throughout the human body. They eliminate foreign particles and microorganisms, remove cell debris, and contribute to homeostasis. When MTB is present in the lungs, alveolar macrophages constitute the central place of survival, growth, and control of it. Furthermore, macrophages comprise the tie with the acquired immune response (which is the responsibility of the outcome of the pathology).

During infection, AM regulate precisely the inflammatory and anti-inflammatory response in order to reduce tissue damage [28].

The mycobacterial recognition through PAMPs, identified by PPRs in the macrophage, induces immune response and phagocytosis. MTB recognition is mediated by TLR, NLRs, and CTLs [29, 30]. On the other hand, phagocytosis is dependent on the interaction of bacteria with macrophage receptors such as MR and DC-SIGN [31]. Additionally, the macrophage activation has been related to the intervention of the NOD2, MR, Mincle, DC-SIGN, Dectin, and TLR 2, 4, and 9 receptors [32].

Mycobacteria phagocytosis is dependent on the movement of cytoskeleton proteins; after the bacteria is located in the phagosome, ATPases are engaged in order to acidify it. Then, the phagosome merges with the lysosome and the content is poured. However, these microbicidal mechanisms (and some others that will be discussed later) are manipulated by MTB in order to survive and replicate inside the macrophage.

3. Innate immune receptors involved in phagocytosis

The interaction of cells of the innate immune response with MTB is based on the contact of PPRs with it and the recognition of PAMPs. The outcome of this encounter will define the response and development of the infection. Among the innate immune PPRs involved in the MTB phagocytosis are: MR, DC-SIGN, Dectin, Mincle TLR, SR, and CR.

3.1 Mannose receptor

MR (CD206) belongs to the C-type lectin receptors that recognize polysaccharides such as mannose, fucose, and N-acetylglucosamine. MR can be found in monocyte-derived macrophages (MDMs), and AM and dendritic cells, but it is absent in monocytes [33, 34].

MR is a transmembrane protein constituted by protein domains that recognize carbohydrates, and a cytoplasmatic region enriched with tyrosine and related to phagocytosis [35]. MR binds lipoarabinomannan (LAM), phosphatidylinositol manosides (PIM), mannoproteins, mannans, and arabinomannans from mycobacteria [36, 37]. Cytokine production in response to MTB recognition through MR, in immature monocyte-derived dendritic cells, induces the expression of an anti-inflammatory profile [38]; furthermore, it inhibits the production of ROS and reduces the expression of IL-12 [39, 40]. In addition, the recognition ofmannosylated LAM by MR prevents phagosome-lysosome fusion and prevents phagosome maturation [36].

3.2 DC-SIGN

Also known as CD209, it is a C-type lectin receptor that can be found in some populations of macrophages and dendritic cells, whereas in AM it is induced after infection with MTB [41, 42]. CD209 is an important link between the innate and acquired immune response, and after the encounter with MTB, it mediates the mycobacterial entry. DC-SIGN identifies glycoproteins, lipomannan (LM), arabinomannan, PIM, and ManLAM from MTB, and discriminates from species with arabinofuranosyl-terminated LAM (AraLAM) such as *Mycobacterium smegmatis* [43]. MTB ManLAM recognized by DC-SIGN induces the expression of the anti-inflammatory cytokine IL-10, where it also counteracts the TLR-4 response [44]. Moreover, the interaction of DC-SIGN with MTB reduces the expression of IL-12, which has caused a decrease in the activity of T cells [45].

3.3 Dectin-1

Dectin is a group of C-type lectin PPR involved in cellular activation, found in neutrophils, dendritic cells, monocytes, and some clusters of T cells [46]. Dectin-1 recognizes beta-glucans and mannosylated lipids and discriminates between mycobacteria species and its strains, such as MTB Ra, *Mycobacteruim bovis* BCG (BCG), *Mycobacterium phlei,* and *Mycobacterium abscessus* [47–50]. MTB triggers the production of IL-17A through the response produced by its interaction with Dectin-1 and TLR4 dependent on IL-1 signaling [51]. Also, it has been found that murine macrophages derived from bone marrow, which contain Dectin-1, showed an increased expression of IL-6, TNF alpha, and G-CSF, when infected with virulent mycobacteria such as BCG, *M. smegmatis, M. phlei*, or *Mycobacterium avium* [49]. Dectin-1 contribution seems to be important during MTB infection in splenic dendritic cells; it is involved with the production of IL-12p40 an important subunit to granuloma development [52].

3.4 Mincle

Macrophage-inducible C-type lectin (Mincle) is a C-type lectin receptor found in leucocytes and macrophages after stimulation [53]. Mincle intervention during MTB infection showed to be fundamental to the recognition of TDM, with an increased production of inflammatory cytokines by macrophages, which contribute to granuloma development [54, 55]. In AM from Mincle deficient mice, the exposure to BCG revealed a reduction in the proinflammatory cytokines, a decreased number of leucocytes in lung tissue, and an increased bacterial count inside and outside the lungs [56]. However, during MTB infection in Mincle-deficient mice, the animals developed a protective immune response T_H1, T_H17, and a granulomatous response [57].

3.5 TLR

TLRs are a family of 10 human PPRs involved in recognition and phagocytosis of intra- and extracellular pathogens. TLRs are composed of a transmembrane domain of leucine-rich repeats that identify the PAMPs; in their structure can also be identified the intramembrane domain that allows the assembly of signaling-related components [58].

TLRs are found in a variety of human cells, such as dendritic cells and AM. These PPRs can be intracellular (such as TLR-3, TLR-7, TLR-8, and TLR-9) or extracellular (such as TLR-1, TLR-2, TLR-4, TLR-5, and TLR-6). TLR-10 can be found in plasmacytoid dendritic cells and B cells. TLR 10 can be found in plasmacytoid dendritic cells and B cells [59]. During MTB infection, TLR triggers the antibacterial response dependent on vitamin D addition [60]. Multiple mycobacterial Ag can be recognized by TLR receptors. The mycobacterial lipoprotein 19 kDa, phosphor-myo-inositol-capped LAM, lipomannans and PIM, are recognized through TLR-2 [61, 62]. The CpG motives of MTB are recognized by TLR-9 [63]. TLR-4 recognizes the MTB heat shock protein 65 (Hsp-65).

The intracellular signaling of MTB recognition by TLR is dependent on the production of the myeloid differentiation factor 88 (MyD88). However, TLR 2, 4, and 9 deficient mice controlled the inflammation during MTB infection and developed a T cell response [64].

3.6 SR

Scavenger receptors are a group of transmembrane glycoproteins found on the surface of dendritic cells, some endothelial cells, macrophages, and monocytes. SR are classified in SR sub-group A and SR sub-group B. The A group comprehends MARCO (a macrophage receptor), SR-A1, and SR-A2, whereas the B group includes SR-B1 and CD36 [65]. The absence of SR-A in infected mice with MTB H37Rv prolonged the life of this animal above the average lifespan of a wild type [66]. MARCO recognizes TDM and this receptor, accompanied by CD14 and TLR-2, mediates cytokine production [67]. However, MARCO-deficient mice had no difference in acute and chronic infection with MTB in comparison with the wild type [68]. In contrast, a MARCO polymorphism is associated with an augmented susceptibility to the infection with MTB in Gambian population [69]. *Cd36*$^{-/-}$ macrophages had an increased capacity to destroy *Mycobacterium marinum* and MTB, whereas CD36-deficient mice had a reduced susceptibility to the BCG infection [70].

3.7 CR

Complement receptors are a group of extracellular receptors that mediate the phagocytosis of non-opsonized, and opsonized bacteria, covered with fragments of proteins of the complement cascade. There are three types of CRs: CR1, CR3, and CR4 located in macrophages, neutrophils, monocytes, NK cells, and lymphocytes. CRs recognize glycopeptolipids from non-opsonized MTB and PIMs [71, 72]. Also, CR3 from monocytes recognize phagocyte microbeads coated with the 85C antigen from BCG and MTB [73]. MTB can be recognized by CR1, CR3, and CR4; however, 80% of the phagocytosis mediated by complement is dependent on the recognition by CR3 [74].

4. Evasion of the immune response in macrophages

Macrophages developed a variety of strategies to destroy bacteria: production of ROS and nitrogen intermediates, iron restriction, use of heavy metals, production of antimicrobial peptides, phagosome acidification, and fusion of the phagosome with the lysosome.

MTB evades and endures the strategies to eliminate bacteria and survive inside the macrophages; this attribute allows them to multiply and increase the population in order to establish the infection or trigger latency. The basic mycobacterial mechanisms to evade the immune response and survive inside the macrophages will be briefly described below.

4.1 Phagosome maturation arresting and inhibition of the phagosome acidification

The phagosome is described as a membrane structure vacuole containing the microorganism; this structure is formed immediately after the phagocytosis. The phagosome maturation is dependent on the actin-mediated movement and is supported by the reactions and delivery of the late and lysosomal constituents [75].

Throughout the establishment of the pathogenic mycobacterial infection, and soon after the bacterial recognition by PPRs, the arresting of the phagosome maturation constitutes a strategy that MTB employs to evade the immune response; specifically, the phagosomal molecule migration pathway is modified in order to avoid the microbicidal activity. During the phagosome maturation, Rab GTPases proteins are recruited to the phagosome membrane; they regulate the membrane fusion and the sorting of lipids and proteins to the organelles. The presence of these molecules is a marker of the phagosome/endosome maturation status. Also, Rab molecules allow identification of the maturity of the structure, specifically Rab5 (which is present on early endosomes) and Rab7 (present on late endosomes) [76–79].

The recruiting of Rab effectors, the endosomal tethering molecule (EEA1), and the phosphatidylinositol 3 kinase hVPS34 to mycobacteria-infected phagosomes are inhibited by mycobacterial PIM and LAM, leading to an arresting of the phagolysosome development [80–82]. Also, MTB ManLAM inhibits the augmentation of Ca^{2+} in the cytosol, avoiding the phosphatidylinositol 3-phosphate fusion with calmodulin at the phagosomal membrane, driving the inhibition of the recruitment of GTPases to the phagosome [81].

The mycobacterial antigens—early secretory antigen target 6 (ESAT-6), culture filtrate protein 10 (CFP10), the eukaryotic-like serine/threonine protein kinase G (PknG), and the SecA1 and SecA2—arrest the phagosome maturation and contribute to the mycobacterial survival inside the macrophages [83–85]. *M. avium* keeps the phagosomal pH between 6.2 and 6.5, due to the exclusion of the proton ATPase in phagosomal acidification [86]. MTB protein tyrosine phosphatase (PtpA) contributes to the survival of the bacteria inside the phagosome, as a consequence of the inhibition of the complex V-ATPase + H with the phagosomal membrane [8].

MTB permits the V-ATPase catalytic subunit A proteasome degradation because of ubiquitination signaling, while also regulating the reduction of the phagosome pH [87]. Glycolipid TDM recognition by the receptor Mincle induces the blockage of signaling involved in the phagosomal formation [88].

4.2 Resistance to reactive nitrogen species and reactive oxygen species

Reactive nitrogen species (RNS) and ROS are short-lived chemical compounds that mediate and contribute to the innate immune response through microbicidal mechanisms [89]. The ROS generation is dependent on the phagosomal acidification. Among the effects of the oxidative stress due to the ROS activity, can be described the oxidation of lipids, proteins and DNA damage. During the MTB infection, the sigma factor and the stress response factor SigH, produced during ROS and RNS action, contribute to the infection [90–92]. The mycobacterial mycothiol has an antioxidant activity and keeps the cell reduced. The MTB mutation of the gene that encodes for the mycothiol synthase, *mshD,* had an increased susceptibility to H_2O_2 [93, 94]. MTB Cu, Zn superoxide dismutase SodC contributes to the resistance to the oxidative burst produced by the ROS of macrophages; also, the MTB *sodC* mutant was sensitive to the superoxide and was susceptible to IFN-gamma too [95]. Similarly, the alkyl hydroperoxide reductase (AphC) contributes to the resistance to ROS of the innate immune response [96].

MTB exposed to NO had a bacteriostatic effect and induced the expression of genes related to dormancy [9]. The expression of inducible nitric oxide synthase (iNOS) confers alveolar macrophages with the ability to kill MTB, and the latency of MTB in macrophages from healthy subjects was dependent on the production of the NO [97]. MTB controls the production of ROS by the increased expression of host histamine receptor H1 (HRH1), by regulating the GRK2-p38MAPK signaling pathway [98].

4.3 Apoptosis and autophagy evasion

Cell apoptosis is a hosting strategy to destroy the intracellular niche of the bacteria. The evasion of apoptosis is related to the mycobacterial virulence. The avirulent strains like *Mycobacterium kansasii*, *M. tuberculosis* H37Ra, and BCG induced more human alveolar macrophages apoptosis, whereas *Mycobacterium bovis*, *M. tuberculosis* H37Rv, and the MTB clinical isolated, named as BMC 96.1, did not [99]. Virulent MTB stimulates the cell necrosis of macrophages by the mitochondrial inner membrane rupture, favoring the release of the microorganism [100].

The autophagy leads to the destruction of damaged cell parts resulting in the cell survival. In MTB infection, the autophagy development conducts a defense mechanism against it. In macrophages infected with MTB or BCG, the autophagy induces the phagolysosomal formation and mycobacterial death [101]. Finally, the foamy phenotype in macrophages protects the cell and reduces autophagy of MTB-infected macrophages [102].

5. Conclusions

The phagocytosis of MTB is the clue event during the development of tuberculosis. The knowledge of human cells involved and the receptors that recognize the strains and species are vital for the understanding of the disease. In addition to that, the information of the variety of mycobacterial strategies to resist cellular control constitutes a contribution to the same aim. Investigative efforts to comprehend the mechanisms involved in MTB survival are important because they contribute to the development of vaccines, therapeutic strategies, and new, more efficient, drugs.

Author details

Gabriela Echeverría-Valencia[1,2]

1 Universidad Técnica de Ambato, Ambato, Ecuador

2 Pontificia Universidad Católica del Ecuador Sede Ambato, Ambato, Ecuador

*Address all correspondence to: gfecheverria81@gmail.com

References

[1] Kanabalan RD, Lee LJ, Lee TY, Chong PP, Hassan L, Ismail R, et al. Human tuberculosis and *Mycobacterium tuberculosis* complex: A review on genetic diversity, pathogenesis and omics approaches in host biomarkers discovery. Microbiological Research. 2021;**246**:126674. DOI: 10.1016/j.micres.2020.126674

[2] Brites D, Gagneux S. Co-evolution of *Mycobacterium tuberculosis* and *Homo sapiens*. Immunological Reviews. 2015;**264**(1):6-24. DOI: 10.1111/imr.12264

[3] Bagcchi S. WHO's global tuberculosis report 2022. Lancet Microbe. 2023;**4**(1):e20. DOI: 10.1016/S2666-5247(22)00359-7

[4] Killick KE, Ní Cheallaigh C, O'Farrelly C, Hokamp K, MacHugh DE, Harris J. Receptor-mediated recognition of mycobacterial pathogens. Cellular Microbiology. 2013;**15**(9):1484-1495. DOI: 10.1111/cmi.12161

[5] Prendergast KA, Kirman JR. Dendritic cell subsets in mycobacterial infection: Control of bacterial growth and T cell responses. Tuberculosis (Edinburgh, Scotland). 2013;**93**(2):115-122. DOI: 10.1016/j.tube.2012.10.008

[6] Allen M, Bailey C, Cahatol I, Dodge L, Yim J, Kassissa C, et al. Mechanisms of control of *Mycobacterium tuberculosis* by NK cells: Role of glutathione. Frontiers in Immunology. 2015;**6**:508. DOI: 10.3389/fimmu.2015.00508

[7] Niazi MK, Dhulekar N, Schmidt D, Major S, Cooper R, Abeijon C, et al. Lung necrosis and neutrophils reflect common pathways of susceptibility to Mycobacterium tuberculosis in genetically diverse, immune-competent mice. Diseases Models and Mechanics. 2015;**8**(9):1141-1153. DOI: 10.1242/dmm.020867

[8] Wong D, Bach H, Sun J, Hmama Z, Av-Gay Y. *Mycobacterium tuberculosis* protein tyrosine phosphatase (PtpA) excludes host vacuolar-H+-ATPase to inhibit phagosome acidification. Proceedings of the National Academy Science U S A. 2011;**108**(48):19371-19376. DOI: 10.1073/pnas.1109201108

[9] Voskuil MI, Bartek IL, Visconti K, Schoolnik GK. The response of *Mycobacterium tuberculosis* to reactive oxygen and nitrogen species. Frontiers in Microbiology. 2011;**1**:105. DOI: 10.3389/fmicb.2011.00105

[10] Jurcic Smith KL, Lee S. Inhibition of apoptosis by Rv2456c through Nuclear factor-κB extends the survival of *Mycobacterium tuberculosis*. International Journal of Mycobacteriology. 2016;**5**:426-436. DOI: 10.1016/j.ijmyco.2016.06.018

[11] Schorey JS, Schlesinger LS. Innate immune responses to tuberculosis. Microbiology Spectrum. 2016;**4**(6). DOI: 10.1128/microbiolspec.TBTB2-0010-2016

[12] Elkington P, Polak ME, Reichmann MT, Leslie A. Understanding the tuberculosis granuloma: The matrix revolutions. Trends in Molecular Medicine. 2022;**28**(2):143-154. DOI: 10.1016/j.molmed.2021.11.004

[13] Ryu JH, Kim CH, Yoon JH. Innate immune responses of the airway epithelium. Molecules and Cells. 2010;**30**(3):173-183. DOI: 10.1007/s10059-010-0146-4

[14] Ernst JD. Macrophage receptors for *Mycobacterium tuberculosis*. Infection and Immunity. 1998;**66**(4):1277-1281. DOI: 10.1128/IAI.66.4.1277-1281.1998

[15] Guirado E, Schlesinger LS, Kaplan G. Macrophages in tuberculosis: Friend or foe. Seminars in Immunopathology. 2013;**35**(5):563-583. DOI: 10.1007/s00281-013-0388-2

[16] Queval CJ, Brosch R, Simeone R. The macrophage: A disputed fortress in the Battle against *Mycobacterium tuberculosis*. Frontiers in Microbiology. 2017;**8**:2284. DOI: 10.3389/fmicb.2017.02284.

[17] Mellman I, Steinman RM. Dendritic cells: Specialized and regulated antigen processing machines. Cell. 2001;**106**(3):255-258. DOI: 10.1016/s0092-8674(01)00449-4

[18] Vermaelen KY, Carro-Muino I, Lambrecht BN, Pauwels RA. Specific migratory dendritic cells rapidly transport antigen from the airways to the thoracic lymph nodes. The Journal of Experimental Medicine. 2001;**193**(1):51-60. DOI: 10.1084/jem.193.1.51

[19] Marino S, Pawar S, Fuller CL, Reinhart TA, Flynn JL, Kirschner DE. Dendritic cell trafficking and antigen presentation in the human immune response to *Mycobacterium tuberculosis*. Journal of Immunology. 2004;**173**(1):494-506. DOI: 10.4049/jimmunol.173.1.494

[20] Hanekom WA, Mendillo M, Manca C, Haslett PA, Siddiqui MR, Barry C 3rd, et al. *Mycobacterium tuberculosis* inhibits maturation of human monocyte-derived dendritic cells in vitro. The Journal of Infectious Diseases. 2003;**188**(2):257-266. DOI: 10.1086/376451

[21] Förtsch D, Röllinghoff M, Stenger S. IL-10 converts human dendritic cells into macrophage-like cells with increased antibacterial activity against virulent *Mycobacterium tuberculosis*. Journal of Immunology. 2000;**165**(2):978-987. DOI: 10.4049/jimmunol.165.2.978

[22] Lande R, Giacomini E, Grassi T, Remoli ME, Iona E, Miettinen M, et al. IFN-alpha beta released by *Mycobacterium tuberculosis*-infected human dendritic cells induces the expression of CXCL10: Selective recruitment of NK and activated T cells. Journal of Immunology. 2003;**170**(3):1174-1182. DOI: 10.4049/jimmunol.170.3.1174

[23] Pedrosa J, Saunders BM, Appelberg R, Orme IM, Silva MT, Cooper AM. Neutrophils play a protective nonphagocytic role in systemic *Mycobacterium tuberculosis* infection of mice. Infection and Immunity. 2000;**68**(2):577-583. DOI: 10.1128/IAI.68.2.577-583.2000

[24] Blomgran R, Ernst JD. Lung neutrophils facilitate activation of naive antigen-specific CD4+ T cells during *Mycobacterium tuberculosis* infection. Journal of Immunology. 2011;**186**(12):7110-7119. DOI: 10.4049/jimmunol.1100001

[25] Craig A, Mai J, Cai S, Jeyaseelan S. Neutrophil recruitment to the lungs during bacterial pneumonia. Infection Immunity. 2009;**77**(2):568-575. DOI: 10.1128/IAI.00832-08

[26] Parker HA, Forrester L, Kaldor CD, Dickerhof N, Hampton MB. Antimicrobial activity of neutrophils against mycobacteria. Frontiers in Immunology. 2021;**12**:782495. DOI: 10.3389/fimmu.2021.782495

[27] Feng CG, Kaviratne M, Rothfuchs AG, Cheever A, Hieny S, Young HA, et al. NK cell-derived IFN-gamma differentially regulates innate

resistance and neutrophil response in T cell-deficient hosts infected with *Mycobacterium tuberculosis*. Journal of Immunology. 2006;**177**(10):7086-7093. DOI: 10.4049/jimmunol.177.10.7086

[28] Hussell T, Bell TJ. Alveolar macrophages: Plasticity in a tissue-specific context. Nature Reviews. Immunology. 2014;**14**(2):81-93. DOI: 10.1038/nri3600

[29] Jo EK. Mycobacterial interaction with innate receptors: TLRs, C-type lectins, and NLRs. Current Opinion in Infectious Diseases. 2008;**21**(3):279-286. DOI: 10.1097/QCO.0b013e3282f88b5d

[30] Reiling N, Ehlers S, Hölscher C. MyDths and un-TOLLed truths: Sensor, instructive and effector immunity to tuberculosis. Immunology Letters. 2008;**116**(1):15-23. DOI: 10.1016/j.imlet.2007.11.015

[31] Kleinnijenhuis J, Oosting M, Joosten LA, Netea MG, Van Crevel R. Innate immune recognition of *Mycobacterium tuberculosis*. Clinical & Developmental Immunology. 2011;**2011**:405310. DOI: 10.1155/2011/405310

[32] Jo EK, Yang CS, Choi CH, Harding CV. Intracellular signalling cascades regulating innate immune responses to mycobacteria: Branching out from toll-like receptors. Cellular Microbiology. 2007;**9**(5):1087-1098. DOI: 10.1111/j.1462-5822.2007.00914.x

[33] McGreal EP, Miller JL, Gordon S. Ligand recognition by antigen-presenting cell C-type lectin receptors. Current Opinion in Immunology. 2005;**17**(1):18-24. DOI: 10.1016/j.coi.2004.12.001

[34] Stahl PD, Ezekowitz RA. The mannose receptor is a pattern recognition receptor involved in host defense. Current Opinion in Immunology. 1998;**10**(1):50-55. DOI: 10.1016/s0952-7915(98)80031-9

[35] Taylor PR, Gordon S, Martinez-Pomares L. The mannose receptor: Linking homeostasis and immunity through sugar recognition. Trends in Immunology. 2005;**26**(2):104-110. DOI: 10.1016/j.it.2004.12.001

[36] Kang PB, Azad AK, Torrelles JB, Kaufman TM, Beharka A, Tibesar E, et al. The human macrophage mannose receptor directs *Mycobacterium tuberculosis* lipoarabinomannan-mediated phagosome biogenesis. The Journal of Experimental Medicine. 2005;**202**(7):987-999. DOI: 10.1084/jem.20051239

[37] Torrelles JB, Azad AK, Schlesinger LS. Fine discrimination in the recognition of individual species of phosphatidyl-myo-inositol mannosides from *Mycobacterium tuberculosis* by C-type lectin pattern recognition receptors. Journal of Immunology. 2006;**177**(3):1805-1816. DOI: 10.4049/jimmunol.177.3.1805

[38] Chieppa M, Bianchi G, Doni A, Del Prete A, Sironi M, Laskarin G, et al. Cross-linking of the mannose receptor on monocyte-derived dendritic cells activates an anti-inflammatory immunosuppressive program. Journal of Immunology. 2003;**171**(9):4552-4560. DOI: 10.4049/jimmunol.171.9.4552

[39] Astarie-Dequeker C, N'Diaye EN, Le Cabec V, Rittig MG, Prandi J, Maridonneau-Parini I. The mannose receptor mediates uptake of pathogenic and nonpathogenic mycobacteria and bypasses bactericidal responses in human macrophages. Infection and Immunity. 1999;**67**(2):469-477. DOI: 10.1128/IAI.67.2.469-477.1999

[40] Nigou J, Zelle-Rieser C, Gilleron M, Thurnher M, Puzo G. Mannosylated lipoarabinomannans inhibit IL-12 production by human dendritic cells: Evidence for a negative signal delivered through the mannose receptor. Journal of Immunology. 2001;**166**(12):7477-7485. DOI: 10.4049/jimmunol.166.12.7477

[41] Soilleux EJ, Morris LS, Leslie G, Chehimi J, Luo Q, Levroney E, et al. Constitutive and induced expression of DC-SIGN on dendritic cell and macrophage subpopulations in situ and in vitro. Journal of Leukocyte Biology. 2002;**71**(3):445-457

[42] Tailleux L, Pham-Thi N, Bergeron-Lafaurie A, Herrmann JL, Charles P, Schwartz O, et al. DC-SIGN induction in alveolar macrophages defines privileged target host cells for mycobacteria in patients with tuberculosis. PLoS Medicine. 2005;**12**:e381. DOI: 10.1371/journal.pmed.0020381

[43] Geijtenbeek TB, Van Vliet SJ, Koppel EA, Sanchez-Hernandez M, Vandenbroucke-Grauls CM, Appelmelk B, et al. Mycobacteria target DC-SIGN to suppress dendritic cell function. The Journal of Experimental Medicine. 2003;**197**(1):7-17. DOI: 10.1084/jem.20021229

[44] van Kooyk Y, Geijtenbeek TB. DC-SIGN: Escape mechanism for pathogens. Nature Reviews. Immunology. 2003;**3**(9):697-709. DOI: 10.1038/nri1182

[45] Wu T, Guo S, Wang J, Li L, Xu L, Liu P, et al. Interaction between mannosylated lipoarabinomannan and dendritic cell-specific intercellular adhesion molecule-3 grabbing nonintegrin influences dendritic cells maturation and T cell immunity. Cellular Immunology. 2011;**272**(1):94-101. DOI: 10.1016/j.cellimm.2011.09.001

[46] Taylor PR, Brown GD, Reid DM, Willment JA, Martinez-Pomares L, Gordon S, et al. The beta-glucan receptor, dectin-1, is predominantly expressed on the surface of cells of the monocyte/macrophage and neutrophil lineages. Journal of Immunology. 2002;**169**(7):3876-3882. DOI: 10.4049/jimmunol.169.7.3876

[47] Taylor PR, Reid DM, Heinsbroek SE, Brown GD, Gordon S, Wong SY. Dectin-2 is predominantly myeloid restricted and exhibits unique activation-dependent expression on maturing inflammatory monocytes elicited in vivo. European Journal of Immunology. 2005;**35**(7):2163-2174. DOI: 10.1002/eji.200425785

[48] Betz BE, Azad AK, Morris JD, Rajaram MVS, Schlesinger LS. β-Glucans inhibit intracellular growth of *Mycobacterium bovis* BCG but not virulent *Mycobacterium tuberculosis* in human macrophages. Microbes Pathogens. 2011;**51**(4):233-24274. DOI: 10.1016/j.micpath.2011.06.006

[49] Yadav M, Schorey JS. The beta-glucan receptor dectin-1 functions together with TLR2 to mediate macrophage activation by mycobacteria. Blood. 2006;**108**(9):3168-3175. DOI: 10.1182/blood-2006-05-024406

[50] Shin DM, Yang CS, Yuk JM, Lee JY, Kim KH, Shin SJ, et al. *Mycobacterium abscessus* activates the macrophage innate immune response via a physical and functional interaction between TLR2 and dectin-1. Cellular Microbiology. 2008;**10**(8):1608-1621. DOI: 10.1111/j.1462-5822.2008.01151.x

[51] van de Veerdonk FL, Teirlinck AC, Kleinnijenhuis J, Kullberg BJ, van Crevel R, van der Meer JW, et al. *Mycobacterium tuberculosis* induces IL-17A responses through TLR4 and dectin-1 and is critically dependent on

endogenous IL-1. Journal of Leukocyte Biology. 2010;**88**(2):227-232. DOI: 10.1189/jlb.0809550

[52] Rothfuchs AG, Bafica A, Feng CG, Egen JG, Williams DL, Brown GD, et al. Dectin-1 interaction with *Mycobacterium tuberculosis* leads to enhanced IL-12p40 production by splenic dendritic cells. Journal of Immunology. 2007;**179**(6):3463-3471. DOI: 10.4049/jimmunol.179.6.3463

[53] Matsumoto M, Tanaka T, Kaisho T, Sanjo H, Copeland NG, Gilbert DJ, et al. A novel LPS-inducible C-type lectin is a transcriptional target of NF-IL6 in macrophages. Journal of Immunology. 1999;**163**(9):5039-5048

[54] Schoenen H, Bodendorfer B, Hitchens K, Manzanero S, Werninghaus K, Nimmerjahn F, et al. Cutting edge: Mincle is essential for recognition and adjuvanticity of the mycobacterial cord factor and its synthetic analog trehalose-dibehenate. Journal of Immunology. 2010;**184**(6):2756-2760. DOI: 10.4049/jimmunol.0904013

[55] Ishikawa E, Ishikawa T, Morita YS, Toyonaga K, Yamada H, Takeuchi O, et al. Direct recognition of the mycobacterial glycolipid, trehalose dimycolate, by C-type lectin Mincle. Journal of Experimental Medicine. 2009;**206**(13):2879-2879. DOI: 10.1084/jem.20091750

[56] Behler F, Steinwede K, Balboa L, Ueberberg B, Maus R, Kirchhof G, et al. Role of Mincle in alveolar macrophage-dependent innate immunity against mycobacterial infections in mice. Journal of Immunology. 2012;**189**(6):3121-3129. DOI: 10.4049/jimmunol.1201399

[57] Heitmann L, Schoenen H, Ehlers S, Lang R, Hölscher C. Mincle is not essential for controlling *Mycobacterium tuberculosis* infection. Immunobiology. 2013;**218**(4):506-516. DOI: 10.1016/j.imbio.2012.06.005

[58] Krutzik SR, Modlin RL. The role of toll-like receptors in combating mycobacteria. Seminars in Immunology. 2004;**16**(1):35-41. DOI: 10.1016/j.smim.2003.10.005

[59] Hasan U, Chaffois C, Gaillard C, Saulnier V, Merck E, Tancredi S, et al. Human TLR10 is a functional receptor, expressed by B cells and plasmacytoid dendritic cells, which activates gene transcription through MyD88. Journal of Immunology. 2005;**174**(5):2942-2950. DOI: 10.4049/jimmunol.174.5.2942

[60] Liu PT, Stenger S, Li H, Wenzel L, Tan BH, Krutzik SR, et al. Toll-like receptor triggering of a vitamin D-mediated human antimicrobial response. Science. 2006;**311**(5768):1770-1773. DOI: 10.1126/science.1123933

[61] Quesniaux V, Fremond C, Jacobs M, Parida S, Nicolle D, Yeremeev V, et al. Toll-like receptor pathways in the immune responses to mycobacteria. Microbes and Infection. 2004;**6**(10):946-959. DOI: 10.1016/j.micinf.2004.04.016

[62] Jones BW, Means TK, Heldwein KA, Keen MA, Hill PJ, Belisle JT, et al. Different toll-like receptor agonists induce distinct macrophage responses. Journal of Leukocyte Biology. 2001;**69**(6):1036-1044

[63] Kindrachuk J, Potter J, Wilson HL, Griebel P, Babiuk LA, Napper S. Activation and regulation of toll-like receptor 9: CpGs and beyond. Mini Reviews in Medicinal Chemistry. 2008;**8**(6):590-600. DOI: 10.2174/138955708784534481

[64] Hölscher C, Reiling N, Schaible UE, Hölscher A, Bathmann C, Korbel D, et al. Containment of aerogenic *Mycobacterium*

tuberculosis infection in mice does not require MyD88 adaptor function for TLR2, −4 and −9. European Journal of Immunology. 2008;**38**(3):680-694. DOI: 10.1002/eji.200736458

[65] Peiser L, Mukhopadhyay S, Gordon S. Scavenger receptors in innate immunity. Current Opinion in Immunology. 2002;**14**(1):123-128. DOI: 10.1016/s0952-7915(01)00307-7

[66] Sever-Chroneos Z, Tvinnereim A, Hunter RL, Chroneos ZC. Prolonged survival of scavenger receptor class A-deficient mice from pulmonary *Mycobacterium tuberculosis* infection. Tuberculosis (Edinb). 2011;**91**(Suppl. 1): S69-S74. DOI: 10.1016/j.tube.2011.10.014

[67] Bowdish DM, Sakamoto K, Kim MJ, Kroos M, Mukhopadhyay S, Leifer CA, et al. TLR2, and CD14 are required for macrophage cytokine responses to mycobacterial trehalose dimycolate and *Mycobacterium tuberculosis*. PLoS Pathogens. 2009;**5**(6):e1000474. DOI: 10.1371/journal.ppat.1000474

[68] Court N, Vasseur V, Vacher R, Frémond C, Shebzukhov Y, Yeremeev VV, et al. Partial redundancy of the pattern recognition receptors, scavenger receptors, and C-type lectins for the long-term control of *Mycobacterium tuberculosis* infection. Journal of Immunology. 2010;**184**(12):7057-7070. DOI: 10.4049/jimmunol.1000164

[69] Bowdish DM, Sakamoto K, Lack NA, Hill PC, Sirugo G, Newport MJ, et al. Genetic variants of MARCO are associated with susceptibility to pulmonary tuberculosis in a Gambian population. BMC Medical Genetics. 2013;**14**:47. DOI: 10.1186/1471-2350-14-47

[70] Hawkes M, Li X, Crockett M, Diassiti A, Finney C, Min-Oo G, et al. CD36 deficiency attenuates experimental mycobacterial infection. BMC Infectious Diseases. 2010;**10**:299. DOI: 10.1186/1471-2334-10-299

[71] Cywes C, Hoppe HC, Daffé M, Ehlers MR. Nonopsonic binding of *Mycobacterium tuberculosis* to complement receptor type 3 is mediated by capsular polysaccharides and is strain dependent. Infection and Immunity. 1997;**10**:4258-4266. DOI: 10.1128/iai.65.10.4258-4266.1997

[72] Villeneuve C, Gilleron M, Maridonneau-Parini I, Daffé M, Astarie-Dequeker C, Etienne G. Mycobacteria use their surface-exposed glycolipids to infect human macrophages through a receptor-dependent process. Journal of Lipid Research. 2005;**46**(3):475-483. DOI: 10.1194/jlr.M400308-JLR200

[73] Hetland G, Wiker HG. Antigen 85C on *Mycobacterium bovis*, BCG and *M. tuberculosis* promotes monocyte-CR3-mediated uptake of microbeads coated with mycobacterial products. Immunology. 1994;**82**(3):445-449

[74] SchlesingerLS,Bellinger-KawaharaCG, Payne NR, Horwitz MA. Phagocytosis of *Mycobacterium tuberculosis* is mediated by human monocyte complement receptors and complement component C3. Journal of Immunology. 1990;**144**(7):2771-2780

[75] Vieira OV, Botelho RJ, Grinstein S. Phagosome maturation: Aging gracefully. The Biochemical Journal. 2002;**366**(Pt 3): 689-704. DOI: 10.1042/BJ20020691

[76] Gruenberg J, van der Goot FG. Mechanisms of pathogen entry through the endosomal compartments. Nature Reviews. Molecular Cell Biology. 2006;**7**(7):495-504. DOI: 10.1038/nrm1959

[77] Prashar A, Schnettger L, Bernard EM, Gutierrez MG. Rab GTPases in immunity and inflammation. Frontiers in Cellular and Infection Microbiology. 2017;7:435. DOI: 10.3389/fcimb.2017.00435

[78] Nguyen L, Pieters J. The Trojan horse: Survival tactics of pathogenic mycobacteria in macrophages. Trends in Cell Biology. 2005;**15**(5):269-276. DOI: 10.1016/j.tcb.2005.03.009

[79] Gutierrez MG. Functional role(s) of phagosomal Rab GTPases. Small GTPases. 2013;**4**(3):148-158. DOI: 10.4161/sgtp.25604

[80] Fratti RA, Backer JM, Gruenberg J, Corvera S, Deretic V. Role of phosphatidylinositol 3-kinase and Rab5 effectors in phagosomal biogenesis and mycobacterial phagosome maturation arrest. The Journal of Cell Biology. 2001;**154**(3):631-644. DOI: 10.1083/jcb.200106049

[81] Vergne I, Chua J, Deretic V. *Mycobacterium tuberculosis* phagosome maturation arrest: Selective targeting of PI3P-dependent membrane trafficking. Traffic. 2003;**4**(9):600-606. DOI: 10.1034/j.1600-0854.2003.00120.x

[82] Fratti RA, Chua J, Vergne I, Deretic V. *Mycobacterium tuberculosis* glycosylated phosphatidylinositol causes phagosome maturation arrest. Proceedings of the National Academy Science U S A. 2003;**100**(9):5437-5442. DOI: 10.1073/pnas.0737613100

[83] Tan T, Lee WL, Alexander DC, Grinstein S, Liu J. The ESAT-6/CFP-10 secretion system of *Mycobacterium marinum* modulates phagosome maturation. Cellular Microbiology. 2006;**8**(9):1417-1429. DOI: 10.1111/j.1462-5822.2006.00721.x

[84] Walburger A, Koul A, Ferrari G, Nguyen L, Prescianotto-Baschong C, Huygen K, et al. Protein kinase G from pathogenic mycobacteria promotes survival within macrophages. Science. 2004;**304**(5678):1800-1804. DOI: 10.1126/science.1099384

[85] Hou JM, D'Lima NG, Rigel NW, Gibbons HS, McCann JR, Braunstein M, et al. ATPase activity of *Mycobacterium tuberculosis* SecA1 and SecA2 proteins and its importance for SecA2 function in macrophages. Journal of Bacteriology. 2008;**190**(14):4880-4887

[86] Sturgill-Koszycki S, Schlesinger PH, Chakraborty P, Haddix PL, Collins HL, Fok AK, et al. Lack of acidification in Mycobacterium phagosomes produced by exclusion of the vesicular proton-ATPase. Science. 1994;**263**(5147):678-681. DOI: 10.1126/science.8303277

[87] Queval CJ, Song OR, Carralot JP, Saliou JM, Bongiovanni A, Deloison G, et al. *Mycobacterium tuberculosis* controls phagosomal acidification by targeting CISH-mediated signaling. Cell Reports. 2017;**20**(13):3188-3198. DOI: 10.1016/j.celrep.2017.08.101

[88] Patin EC, Geffken AC, Willcocks S, Leschczyk C, Haas A, Nimmerjahn F, et al. Trehalose dimycolate interferes with FcγR-mediated phagosome maturation through Mincle, SHP-1 and FcγRIIB signalling. PLoS One. 2017;**12**(4):e0174973

[89] Al-Shehri SS. Reactive oxygen and nitrogen species and innate immune response. Biochimie. 2021;**181**:52-64. DOI: 10.1016/j.biochi.2020.11.022

[90] Raman S, Song T, Puyang X, Bardarov S, Jacobs WR Jr, Husson RN. The alternative sigma factor SigH regulates major components of oxidative and heat stress responses in *Mycobacterium tuberculosis*. Journal of Bacteriology. 2001;**183**(20):6119-6125. DOI: 10.1128/JB.183.20.6119-6125.2001

[91] Dutta NK, Mehra S, Martinez AN, Alvarez X, Renner NA, Morici LA, et al. The stress-response factor SigH modulates the interaction between *Mycobacterium tuberculosis* and host phagocytes. PLoS One. 2012;7(1):e28958

[92] Sharp JD, Singh AK, Park ST, Lyubetskaya A, Peterson MW, Gomes AL, et al. Comprehensive definition of the SigH regulon of *Mycobacterium tuberculosis* reveals transcriptional control of diverse stress responses. PLoS One. 2016;**11**(3):e0152145. DOI: 10.1371/journal.pone.0152145

[93] Buchmeier NA, Newton GL, Koledin T, Fahey RC. Association of mycothiol with protection of *Mycobacterium tuberculosis* from toxic oxidants and antibiotics. Molecular Microbiology. 2003;**47**(6):1723-1732. DOI: 10.1046/j.1365-2958.2003.03416.x

[94] Buchmeier NA, Newton GL, Fahey RC. A mycothiol synthase mutant of *Mycobacterium tuberculosis* has an altered thiol-disulfide content and limited tolerance to stress. Journal of Bacteriology. 2006;**188**(17):6245-6252. DOI: 10.1128/JB.00393-06

[95] Piddington DL, Fang FC, Laessig T, Cooper AM, Orme IM, Buchmeier NA. Cu,Zn superoxide dismutase of *Mycobacterium tuberculosis* contributes to survival in activated macrophages that are generating an oxidative burst. Infection and Immunity. 2001;**69**(8):4980-4987. DOI: 10.1128/IAI.69.8.4980-4987.2001

[96] Bryk R, Lima CD, Erdjument-Bromage H, Tempst P, Nathan C. Metabolic enzymes of mycobacteria linked to antioxidant defense by a thioredoxin-like protein. Science. 2002;**295**(5557):1073-1077. DOI: 10.1126/science.1067798

[97] Yang CS, Yuk JM, Jo EK. The role of nitric oxide in mycobacterial infections. Immune Network. 2009;**9**(2):46-52. DOI: 10.4110/in.2009.9.2.46

[98] Mo S, Guo J, Ye T, Zhang X, Zeng J, Xu Y, et al. *Mycobacterium tuberculosis* utilizes host histamine receptor H1 to modulate reactive oxygen species production and phagosome maturation via the p38MAPK-NOX2 Axis. MBio. 2022;**13**(5):e0200422. DOI: 10.1128/mbio.02004-22

[99] Keane J, Remold HG, Kornfeld H. Virulent *Mycobacterium tuberculosis* strains evade apoptosis of infected alveolar macrophages. Journal of Immunology. 2000;**164**(4):2016-2020. DOI: 10.4049/jimmunol.164.4.2016

[100] Chen M, Gan H, Remold HG. A mechanism of virulence: Virulent *Mycobacterium tuberculosis* strain H37Rv, but not attenuated H37Ra, causes significant mitochondrial inner membrane disruption in macrophages leading to necrosis. Journal of Immunology. 2006;**176**(6):3707-3716. DOI: 10.4049/jimmunol.176.6.3707

[101] Gutierrez MG, Master SS, Singh SB, Taylor GA, Colombo MI, Deretic V. Autophagy is a defense mechanism inhibiting BCG and *Mycobacterium tuberculosis* survival in infected macrophages. Cell.

2004;**119**(6):753-766. DOI: 10.1016/j.cell.2004.11.038

[102] Singh V, Jamwal S, Jain R, Verma P, Gokhale R, Rao KV. *Mycobacterium tuberculosis*-driven targeted recalibration of macrophage lipid homeostasis promotes the foamy phenotype. Cell Host & Microbe. 2012;**12**(5):669-681. DOI: 10.1016/j.chom.2012.09.012

Chapter 4

Macrophage: From Recognition of Foreign Agents to Late Phagocytosis

Claudia I. Rivas Ortiz and Antonia Isabel Castillo Rodal

Abstract

The main line of defense that exists to eliminate foreign agents falls on phagocytic cells (neutrophils, dendritic cell, and macrophages), and it does so through phagocytosis, a complex cellular mechanism that occurs after the recognition and binding of the ligand by cellular receptors. Macrophages are part of a diverse lineage of innate immune cells. Once a macrophage receptor binds its ligand, a coordinated intracellular signaling cascade is activated to the clearance or otherwise of the foreign agent. Objects removed by macrophage phagocytosis include dead or dying host cells, cells opsonized with antibodies, and specific pathogens such as bacteria, fungi, parasites, and viruses. Currently, phagocytic macrophages have been shown to contribute to the killing of cancer cells, inflammatory bowel disease, atherosclerosis, Alzheimer's disease, and schizophrenia. For this reason, phagocytic macrophages are important in critical participation for health and disease.

Keywords: macrophages, phagocytosis, early phagosome, late phagosome, phagolysosome

1. Introduction

Macrophages are cells distributed in all body compartments under physiological conditions, presenting various forms and functions that depend on environmental stimuli. After their origin, macrophages are distributed to different tissues, taking the name of the tissue where they are maintained or circulate in the blood as monocytes until they face a foreign body, becoming macrophages [1, 2]. It is considered that the half-life of the macrophage is 70 h, and they make up 4–10% of the total leukocytes in peripheral blood, meaning that they constitute the second cell population of the immune system.

Macrophages are essential to innate immunity since they secrete more than 100 biologically active products and present diverse functions with different phenotypes, occupying dozens of extra and intracellular receptors. Owing to their versatility, macrophages actively participate in physiological and pathophysiological processes. As previously described, they have attributed three critical activities in the host: homeostasis, immune response, and phagocytosis [3].

In this chapter, we will focus on different parts of macrophage phagocytosis.

2. Background

Phagocytosis was first described by the Russian scientist Elia Metchnikoff, considered the father of cellular immunity. Between 1879 and 1882, he established a laboratory of marine biology and comparative embryology in Messina, Italy, where he observed and described this process. His description of "phagocytosis" (an evolutionarily conserved cellular process that recognizes and ingests particles larger than 0.5 microns within a vesicle derived from the plasma membrane) led to his being awarded the Nobel Prize in 1908 together with Paul Ehrlich [4].

Metchnikoff reported other macrophage functions such as resistance to infection, phagocytosis of cell debris, and tissue damage repair linking directly to immunology, gerontology, gut microbiome, and probiotics [4]. The macrophage has three distinct origins in development: tissue residents derived from the yolk sac, tissue residents from the fetal liver, and those derived from the bone marrow [5]. The macrophage is essential from the earliest stages in the development of life, performing various functions in development, growth, homeostasis, and remodeling [6].

Phagocytic cells are classified into professional phagocytes, such as neutrophils, monocytes, monocyte-derived macrophages, dendritic cells, and nonprofessional phagocytic cells, such as epithelial cells and fibroblasts [3]. Tissue macrophages are classified into subpopulations according to their location and phenotype:

- Microglia macrophages in the central nervous system (CNS)
- Osteoclasts in bone
- Alveolar macrophages in the lung
- Histiocytes in the spleen
- Interstitial connective tissue and cells
- Kupffer in the liver.

Monocytes are relatively inactive cells that are continuously monitoring their environment. When activated and become macrophages, they become involved in the processes of cellular homeostasis and the acute and chronic immune response. Macrophages recognize, ingest, and digest apoptotic particles, microbes, and cellular debris through phagocytosis. Its efficiency depends on the coordination of the physical characteristics of the macrophage and the particle to be phagocytosed [7]. Macrophages can phagocytose at the site where they are or migrate to the place that is required. Secondary to inflammation or tissue damage, they are attracted and activated by bacterial endotoxins, exotoxins, cytokines, and other biochemical and biological stimuli known as the pathogen-associated molecular pattern (PAMP) and damage-associated molecular pattern (DAMP).

This action allows them to transform into fully activated proinflammatory or anti-inflammatory macrophages for repair and homeostasis [8].

Macrophage migration occurs due to the attraction of the molecules released by pathogens (PAMPs) and the cells themselves (DAMPs). They migrate to the site by moving through podosomes, dynamic and unstable structures that temporarily adhere by pulling and pushing due to the force of traction and protrusion.

Podosomes present filaments rich in actin and a stable multiprotein complex of seven units, the Arp2/3 complex bound to membrane plaque proteins; the podosomes accumulate F-actin, Integrin beta1, and CD44 helps them to attach, detach, and penetrate into or through tissues, the endothelial barrier through the process of chemotaxis. The chemotaxis process in the macrophage is driven by small Rho GTPase and signaling through mitogen-activated protein kinase/extracellular signal kinase (MAP/ERK) and Phosphatidylinositol-3 kinase/serine/threonine protein kinase (P13K/Akt)[7].

The initiation of migration begins with the stimulation of the chemoattractant protein 1 (MCP-1). This chemokine is produced by different tissue cells secreted under the stimulation of the cytokines tumor necrosis factor alpha (TNF alpha), IL-6, IL-1beta, and is suppressed by IL-10 [9].

Before phagocytosis, the macrophage recognizes the white particle to rule out whether it is an invader or itself. The CD47 transmembrane protein is present in all host cells and is the signal they present to avoid being phagocytosed by macrophages. Receptors carry out phagocytosis on the plasma membrane, divided into opsonic and nonopsonic receptors. Nonopsonic receptors bind directly to PAMPs and induce phagocytosis. The nonopsonic receptors are lectin-like recognition molecules such as CD169, CD33, and Dectin 1, C-type lectins (MICL, Dectin 2, Mincle, and DNGR-1), as well as scavenger receptors (**Figure 1A**). These receptors are considered promiscuous and have a poorly defined intracellular signaling capacity. That is why the binding of various ligands and receptors is required to ingest the particle. The opsonic receptors are those that recognize the target particle surrounded by opsonins (proteins derived from the host, such as antibodies, complement factors, fibronectin, and mannose-linked lectin), within which we find the Fcy receptors (FcyRI, FcyRII, and

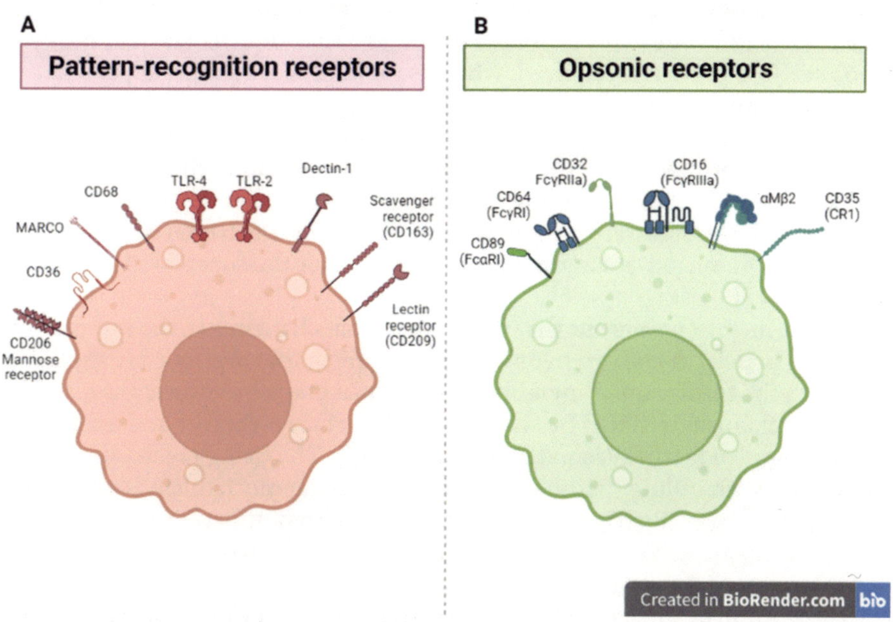

Figure 1.
Phagocytic receptors are present in the macrophage. A) Pattern recognition receptors (PRR): TLR, scavenger receptors, lectin receptors, mannose receptors, which recognize pathogen-associated molecular patterns (PAMPs) and damage-associated molecular patterns (DAM). B) Opsonic receptors: such as receptors for the crystallizable fraction of antibodies (FcR), complement receptors (CR), which recognize antibodies and C1 or C3b molecules that opsonize microorganisms and promote phagocytosis. Created with BioRender.com

FcγRIII) and glycoproteins that specifically bind to the Fc region of immunoglobulin G (IgG) forming a complex that is pooled on the membrane and phagocytosed by the macrophage. This phagocytosis is also known as antibody-dependent cellular phagocytosis (ADCP) [10]. In this group, we also have complement receptors (CR) such as CR1 (CD35) CR3 (CD11/CD18 or MAC-1), scavenger receptors, and C-type lectins (**Figure 1B**) [3]. Scavenger receptors, such as SR-A or CD36, recognize apoptotic and microbial polyanionic ligands [11]. The toll-like receptors (TLRs) [12] are detectors of PAMPs, but they do not function as phagocytic receptors. TLRs collaborate with nonopsonic receptors to stimulate ingestion [13].

3. Recognition of the target molecule by the macrophage

In the process of phagocytosis and the case of an infectious process, the binding of the ligand to the receptor, the dynamics of actin polymerization of the cytoskeleton of the pseudopods of the macrophage, and the mechanical stability of the fimbriae of the bacterium must be closely related and coordinated in a complex sequence of events to engulf the bacteria. Phagocytosis is initiated by the recognition of the target particle by multiple receptors, the identification of the particle's position, and the establishment of regular physical contact until the ingestion is processed. To date, more than 100 cell surface receptors have been described that participate in macrophage activation as well as various forms of phagocytosis. The initiation of phagosome formation, and the rate at which phagosome formation proceeds on the particle, is directly related to the membrane tension that counteracts that exerted on the growing ends of the actin filaments, and owing to the Rho family GTPase-controlled actin polymerization, phagosome rigidity increases as macrophages engulf prey.

For the formation of the phagosome and the particle's internalization, the cytoskeleton's scaffold protein is required, which is the GTPase1 activating protein that contains the IQ motif (IQGAP1) [7].

After the receptor's binding to the particle, the plasmatic membrane covers the microorganisms and closes at the distal end, forming a vacuole where the particles are internalized [14]. The duration of the ingestion of the particle, the formation of the phagosome, and its closure are proportional to the size of the bacterial filament, so if these times are prolonged, it has direct consequences for the survival of the pathogens inside the cells [7].

Jaumouille in 2019 points out that there are two mechanisms in the internalization of the target particle: a) activation or firing mechanism that occurs after signaling and results in the formation of membrane lifting plasmatic by actin action, and b) the zipper mechanism initiated by sequential cell surface receptors and ends with the particle surrounded by the plasmatic membrane [15]. The firing mechanism is associated with some intracellular pathogens, while the closing mechanism is associated with most pathogens. CRs trigger a distinct form of Rho family GTPase-dependent phagocytosis, characterized by a "sinking" of the particle into the cell without triggering proinflammatory mediators [16].

The recognition of the ligand by the phagocytic receptor of the macrophage is variable since there are differences according to the nature of its precursor and the signals sent by different factors, so depending on this, the response will be pro- or anti-inflammatory. Macrophages' response and phenotype are changeable due to their high plasticity. The action of phagocytosis by macrophages is not fully known, however. For an organism to survive an infection, a prompt response is required, eliminating the microorganisms; therefore, the phagocytosis rate will depend significantly on the speed with which the macrophages identify, trap, and eliminate the intruders. To begin phagocytosis, macrophages must locate the position of the microorganism and establish physical contact for phagocytosis to occur. Macrophages use chemotaxis and apply mechanical force through lamellipodium protuberances on the leading edge driven by actin polymerization, which allows them to migrate to the site of inflammation. The chemotaxis process in macrophages is carried out by small Rho GTPases and MAPK/ERK and PI3K/Akt signaling. Different chemokines regulate these signaling pathways in human macrophages [7].

In the phagocytosis process, various stages are involved:

1. Detection of the particle to be phagocytosed.

2. Activation of the internalization process.

3. Formation of the specialized vacuole called phagosome.

4. Maturation of the phagosome to transform itself.

The detection of PAMPs occurs through pattern recognition receptors (PRRs); these PRRs are phagocytized directly or through opsonins. The lectin-like family's nonopsonic receptors are Dectin-1, Mincle, MCL, and DC-SIGN, which bind to different PAMPs. Various target particles are surrounded by opsonins that bind to specific receptors, such as the FcγR receptor or complement receptors (CRs).

As previously mentioned, the phagocytosis process will have changes according to the ligand and the receptor; after the interaction between the receptors of the phagocytic cell with the target particle, signaling events occur to initiate phagocytosis. In the formation of the phagosome, there are changes in the lipid composition of the membrane, and significant changes occur in the remodeling of the membrane and the actin cytoskeleton leading to the formation of pseudopods that cover the microorganism due to the action of the enzymes coronin, cofilin, and gelsolin. To form pseudopods, Coronin 1 debranches F-actin, leaving it as loose fibers to be cut by cofilin and gelsolin, an action controlled by its binding to phosphoinositides. Actin filaments are knocked down or nucleated by the activity of the Arp2/3 protein complex to initiate F-actin polymerization and pseudopod formation.

The signaling pathways triggered by the best-studied phagocytic receptors are the FcRs and CRs. For FcR-mediated phagocytosis, Arp2/3 integrates into the new phagocytic cup, where its actin nucleation activity is stimulated by WASp and N-WASp [17], which are also activated by Cdc42-GTP, and PI [11, 18]. In the case of CR-mediated phagocytosis, actin polymerization is associated with RhoA. This GTPase recruits and stimulates mDia formins [19]; they also activate the Arp2/3 complex.

However, other GTPases, such as Rap, appear to play a role in CR-mediated phagocytosis, independent of RhoA [20]. Rap GTP also activates profilin, essential for actin polymerization via formins [21]. Rap GTP activates profilin, which is necessary for actin polymerization through formins [21]. Rap can also activate GTPase Rac [22].

At this point, lipids associate and dissociate from the phagosome membrane in an orderly fashion, and the GTPases Rho, Rac, and cell division cycle 42 (Cdc42), essential regulators of the actin cytoskeleton, are activated and recruited for phagosome formation. At the point of contact between the receptors and the microorganism, a depression in the membrane is formed, also called a phagocytic cup, followed by the polymerization of F-actin, triggering the pseudopod formation that surrounds the microorganism, and within minutes, they fuse at the distal end to seal and form the phagosome [14].

The action of myosin in the formation of the phagosome that is involved in its contractile activity is also known. Before the phagosome is complete, F-actin is removed from the phagocytic cup to facilitate phagosome closure by the enzyme PI 3-K. In FcγR-mediated phagocytosis, the WASP and N-WASP proteins (Wiskott-Aldrich syndrome protein) are activated to activate the Arp2/3 complex for actin polymerization at the base of the nascent phagocyte. The final part of the phagosome formation occurs when the membranes fuse in their distal portion. A moment before this step, F-actin disappears, helping to make the phagosome less rigid, an action that PI3-K is responsible for. The inhibition of this enzyme blocks the depolymerization of actin in the phagocytic cup, stopping the pseudopod extension [23].

We know that the activation of GTPases is necessary to stimulate the Arp2/3 complex during phagocytosis for actin polymerization [24]. However, PI [11, 25] P3, the PI3K product, can stimulate Rho family GTPase activation proteins (GAPs), which inactivate GTPases and prevent actin polymerization. PI3K inhibition has also increased GTPase activation in the phagocytic cup [24, 26]. PI3K activity decreases PI levels [11], P2. This phospholipid activates the Arp2/3 complex, via WASP and N-WASP [27]. Thus, the disappearance of the phagocytic cup promotes the extension of the pseudopod. As for myosins, they use their contractile activity to facilitate the formation of phagosomes [28]. In macrophages, that class II and IXb myosins were concentrated at the base of the phagocytic cups, with an increase in the phagocytic cup at its closure site. Myosin V appeared after phagosome closure [15]. In extension of the pseudopod, actin filaments move from the bottom to the top of the phagocytic cup, compressing the particle to be internalized [2]. This activity is dependent on myosin light chain kinase (MLCK). MLCK-activated myosin II is required for the contractile activity of phagocytic cups [29]. Because of this, the phagocytic cups push the fluid out of the phagosomes. Myosin X is PI3K-dependent and is essential for propagating pseudopods in phagocytosis [23]. The myosin I subclass, myosin Ic, is located at the tip of the phagocytic cup, which relates it to the generation of the force of contraction, which causes the opening of the phagocytic cup to close [23]. The myosin I subclass, myosin Ic, is located at the tip of the phagocytic cup, which relates it to the generation of the force of contraction, which causes the opening of the phagocytic cup to close [23]. Myosin IX appears in the phagocytic layers similarly to myosin II [30]. This myosin is involved in the contractile activity of phagocytic cups; it also functions as a signaling molecule for the reorganization of the actin cytoskeleton.

Myosins class IX contains a GTPase activation protein (GAP) domain that activates GTPase Rho [31] involved in actin remodeling. Myosin V appears in fully internalized phagosomes. It is involved in vesicular transport in other cells [32]; it is responsible for phagosome movement rather than phagosome formation [2].

4. Phagosome formation and binding to the lysosome

The newly formed phagosome will combine with early endosomes to form the phagolysosome [25, 33], involving membrane fusion events regulated by the Rab5 GTPase [34, 35]. Rab5 recruits early endosome antigen 1 (EEA1), a molecule that functions as a bridge between the early endosome and endocytic vesicles; it also induces the recruitment of Rab7. During phagosome maturation, Rab5 disappears, and Rab7 appears on the membrane [36]. Rab7 regulates phagosome fusion with late

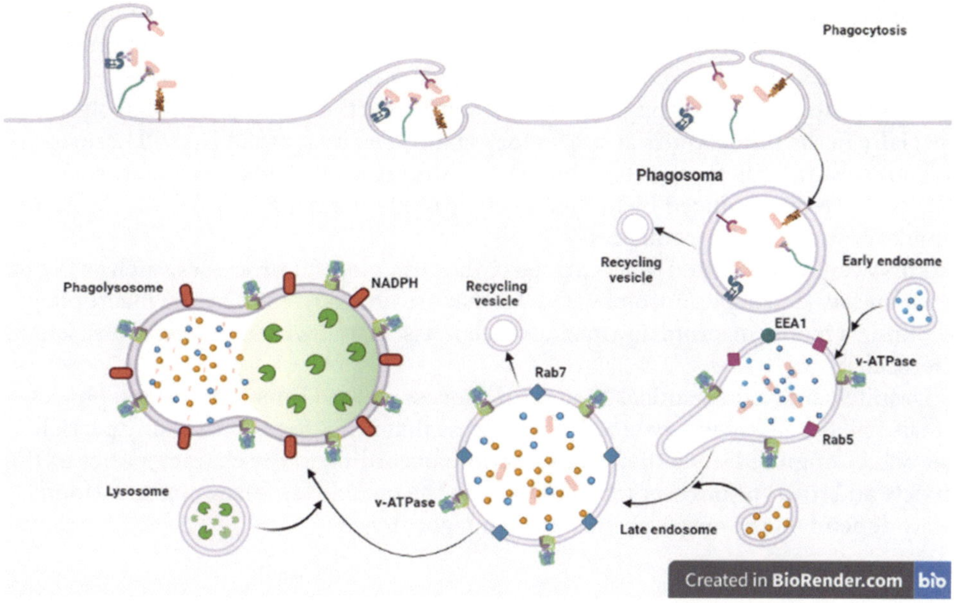

Figure 2.
Stages of phagosome maturation. The process is divided into several stages of maturation, phagosome formation, early phagosome, late phagosome, and phagolysosome formation. The process begins when the macrophage recognizes and captures a microorganism through exposed receptors on its membrane; a phagocytic cup is produced that culminates in the formation of the phagosome; the membrane includes molecules that control membrane fusion, such as Rab5 GTPases and Rab7. By joining the late phagosome with the lysosome, degrading enzymes, such as cathepsins, proteases, lysosomals, and lipases, are integrated that will cut the microorganism. The phagolysosome will become a very acidic site due to the action of V-ATPase, which pumps protons into the vesicle to kill the microorganism. EEA1: Early endosome antigen 1; NADPH: nicotinamide adenine dinucleotide phosphate oxidase. Created with BioRender.com

endosomes [37]. At this point, V-ATPase molecules accumulate on the phagosome membrane and acidify (pH 5.5–6.0) the interior of the phagosome by translocating protons (H+) into the phagosome lumen [36].

Lysosome-associated membrane proteins (LAMPs) and luminal proteases (cathepsin and hydrolases) are incorporated from fusion with late endosomes [38], culminating in the presence of hydrolytic enzymes that lead to the degradation of the microorganism, causing the breakdown of material into its essential components, and lipids, proteins, and carbohydrates are either recycled by the cell or excreted into the extracellular environment to be excreted from the body [39]. In macrophages, we find Fe2+ ions such as azurophilic granules that bind to chelators such as adenosine, myeloperoxidase (MPO) substitutes, and hydrolases and lysosomes that fuse in the phagosome and degrade microbial or apoptotic cells (**Figure 2**) [14].

5. The production of reactive oxygen species (ROS) and reactive nitrogen species (RNS) in the function of the macrophage

In an inflammatory process, the function of the macrophage is crucial since it is responsible for limiting that inflammation. After phagocytosis, in late phagosome, the phagosome binds with the lysosome presenting an acid pH due to the action of several V-ATPases and proteases with the stimulation of the foreign agent, the macrophage produces reactive oxygen species (ROS) and nitrogen (ON) (superoxide ion and hydrogen peroxide) secondary the catalytic activity of the nicotinamide adenine dinucleotide phosphate (NADPH) oxidase enzyme complex. This reaction is preferably intracellular through electron transfer reactions within the phagolysosome, especially in the mitochondrial respiratory chain. The increase in NADPH causes oxygen consumption (respiratory burst) and the creation of toxic products such as ROS, NO*. NO is produced by inducible nitric oxide synthase (iNOS), which, in turn, stimulates further NO production.

This event is associated with various pathophysiological processes, such as the oxidation of low-density lipoproteins (LDL) that are phagocytosed by the macrophage, becoming a foamy macrophage itself, which is associated with an increased risk of atherosclerosis [10].

Despite being a mechanical-biological process studied for several years, phagocytosis still has unknown events. It is a process that is not the same for any particle that will be engulfed since there are variations according to the characteristics of the particle and the type of receptor that binds to the ligand. The examples mentioned below depend on the target particle to be phagocytosed.

6. Phagocytosis in infectious diseases

Bacteria, viruses, fungi, and parasites present various PAMPs not detected by cellular receptors called pattern recognition receptors (PRRs). There is an extensive variety of PRRs that, according to the characteristics of the receptor, will identify and bind to a specific ligand. The phagocytosis of a PAMP occurs by binding to one or various receptors and one or different PAMPs of the same pathogen in a single event. There are several examples in this regard; the polysaccharides present on the surface of some yeasts bind to the mannose receptor or the dectin-1 receptor, while the lipopolysaccharide (LPS) of gram-negative bacteria is detected by the scavenger-A receptor (SR-A). The phagocytosis of mycobacteria occurs through complement receptors (opsonization of mycobacteria by complement) or by the mannose receptor that recognizes lipoarabinomannan (LAM), a structure that is part of the wall of mycobacteria; the coating of mycobacteria by surfactant protein A (Sp-A) has also been described [40]. Fungal phagocytosis is less studied; beta-glucans of the fungal cell wall bind to Dectin-1 receptors to initiate phagocytosis [41]. While the human serum amyloid protein (SAP) is considered a Trojan horse since some fungi and bacteria have a functional SAP on their wall that allows the fungus to bind to cells and be more invasive [42].

Interestingly, it has been reported how bacteria of the genus *Treponema pallidum* are phagocytosed when they are covered by opsonins or without opsonins [43]. Regarding the phagocytosis of the virus by the macrophage, we have the example of the person responsible for the current pandemic, the Coronavirus type 2 (severe acute respiratory syndrome coronavirus 2 [SARS-Cov-2]); the critical entry of the virus into the cell is the angiotensin 2 receptor (ACE-2). Different lectin-like receptors (CLRs) act as endocytic receptors for macrophages and are compromised when ingesting viruses or other pathogens [44].

The importance of removing apoptotic bodies through phagocytosis is known. Many cells die every day in healthy subjects, and phagocytes must remove their apoptotic bodies. Apoptotic cells display on their surface several molecules that distinguish them from healthy cells, such as phosphatidylserine (PS), a molecule restricted to the inner layer of the plasma membrane in healthy cells, which appears on the surface during the apoptosis process. In a sterile inflammation event produced by cells such as neutrophils that have been recruited to the site of inflammation and undergo cell death by apoptosis, they are phagocyted to decrease or eliminate tissue-damaging proinflammatory factors and ROS. This process called spherocytosis is the part of the interaction of a complex network involving binding molecules, molecules that signal the cell through PS that helps tissue homeostasis [45]. It is a complex mechanism by which various interactions are related as ligand-receptor and signals. Cells undergoing apoptosis release multiple molecules such as ATP, lysophosphatidylcholine, fractalkine, and sphingosine 1-phosphate. These molecules act as chemotactic factors that recruit phagocytes to the site of cell death. Multiple phagocytic receptors bind PS. Direct binding to PS is mediated by receptors such as TIM1, brain-specific angiogenesis inhibitor 1 (BAI1), and stabilin-2 [30]. In other cases, the molecules can bind to PS and to surface receptors forming a bridge; an example of this is MFG-E8 that links PS to $\alpha V\beta 3$ integrins, which are effective phagocytic receptors.

Another example is Gas6 and protein S molecules that are between PS and phagocytic receptors, such as TAMs (Tyro3, Axl, Mer) [46]. Derivatives of PS metabolism may also contribute to the recognition of apoptotic bodies. PS appears to undergo oxidation, and some phagocytic receptors, such as CD36 and CD68, bind modified lipids, including oxidized PS [30].

7. Macrophage response in phagocytosis

The macrophage presents high metabolic plasticity, which is associated with the polarization of the macrophage and the molecules and factors they produce, so their response will be unique in each case. The macrophage response can be controlled by the target particle inducing specific signaling pathways directed by receptors that recognize the target particle and by overlapping signaling pathways.

An example is phagocytosis secondary to antibodies recognition that is controlled by protein kinase C (KPC) without stimulating phosphatidylinositol 3-kinase or extracellular signal regulated kinases (ERK). However, antibody phagocytosis stimulates these last two molecules through cytokines and depending on these multiple factors, we have the macrophages 0 (M0), which are naïve macrophages, M1 characterized by proinflammatory and accompanied by IL-6, IL-12, and TNF alpha, M2, which are anti-inflammatory and produce IL-10, TGF-beta, and Arginase; Mreg are regulatory macrophages with anti-inflammatory characteristics and IL-10 producers. Other recently reported macrophages, such as M-mox and M4, are mentioned, but less is known about them. The M2 group is classified into M2a, M2b, M2c, and M2d.

This classification, carried out practically for a better understanding, is based on the expressed transcription factors and the signaling pathways used by macrophages. However, these macrophages display high plasticity and change their status depending on the medium and environmental signals. Despite the plasticity of macrophages, three responses are recognized, two of which are well characterized. The description of the macrophage's immune response is diverse and changing since it depends on the characteristics of the target particle, especially if it is a pathogen, the receptors responsible for binding to that particle, and whether or not it is opsonized and the capacity of the macrophage to remove the foreign agent.

One of many examples is the binding of polysaccharide from fungi to mannose or Dectin-1 receptors, the binding of lipopolysaccharide from a gram negative bacterium to TLRs, or the binding of bacteria to SR-A or framework. Each of these events will stimulate transcription factors and stimulus-dependent signaling pathways. Even with this diversity, we can state in general that there is an immune response that is characterized by the production of various molecules such as lipases, nucleases, proteases, glycosidases, and phosphatases responsible for degrading the target particle, the expression of NADPH oxidase (Nox2), and oxide synthase 2 (Nos2) responsible to produce reactive oxygen and nitrogen species. In infections, the macrophage activates proteins that sequester iron (Fe) and Mn, essential elements for microorganisms.

8. Conclusions

In this chapter, we show the complexity of phagocytosis from the clue particle recognition going through physicochemical characteristics between macrophage and the target particle to the development of the phagolysosome. Phagocytosis is not as simple as it sounds, even though we know the types of immune responses promoted by the macrophage; recent research shows that the variability may be wider. That is why more research is required to broaden the knowledge of phagocytosis, which will help improve patient's clinical conditions.

Conflict of interest

The authors declare no conflict of interest.

Author details

Claudia I. Rivas Ortiz and Antonia Isabel Castillo Rodal*
Medicine Faculty, Microbiology and Parasitology Department, Universidad Nacional Autónoma de Mexico México

*Address all correspondence to: castillorodal@gmail.com

References

[1] Nelson MC, O'Connell RM. MicroRNAs: At the Interface of metabolic pathways and inflammatory responses by macrophages. Frontiers in Immunology. 2020;**11**:1797. DOI: 10.3389/fimmu.2020.01797

[2] Yu Y, Zhang Z, Walpole GFW. Kinetics of phagosome maturation is coupled to their intracellular motility. Commune Biology. 2022;**5**(1):1014. DOI: 10.1038/s42003-022-03988-4

[3] Lim JJ, Grinstein S, Roth Z. Diversity and versatility of phagocytosis: Roles in innate immunity, tissue Remodeling, and homeostasis. Frontiers in Cellular and Infection Microbiology. 2017;**7**:191. DOI: 10.3389/fcimb.2017.00191

[4] Gordon S. Elie Metchnikoff, the man and the myth. Journal of Innate Immunity. 2016;**8**(3):223-227. DOI: 10.1159/000443331

[5] Niedergang F. In: Bradshaw RA, editor. Phagocytosis, in Encyclopedia of Cell Biology. Academic Press; 2016. pp. 751-757. Available from: https://www.sciencedirect.com/science/article/pii/B9780123944474200734?via%3Dihub

[6] Theret M, Mounier R, Rossi F. The origins and non-canonical functions of macrophages in development and regeneration. Development. 2019;**146**(9). DOI: 10.1242/dev.156000

[7] Jain N, Moeller J, Vogel V. Mechanobiology of macrophages: How physical factors Coregulate macrophage plasticity and phagocytosis. Annual Review of Biomedical Engineering. 2019;**21**:267-297. DOI: 10.1146/annurev-bioeng-062117-121224

[8] Hirayama D, Iida T, Nakase H. The phagocytic function of macrophage-enforcing innate immunity and tissue homeostasis. International Journal of Molecular Sciences. 2017;**19**(1). DOI: 10.3390/ijms19010092

[9] Shapouri-Moghaddam A et al. Macrophage plasticity, polarization, and function in health and disease. Journal of Cellular Physiology. 2018;**233**(9):6425-6440. DOI: 10.1002/jcp.26429

[10] Lendeckel U, Venz S, Wolke C. Macrophages: Shapes and functions. ChemTexts. 2022;**8**(2):12. DOI: 10.1007/s40828-022-00163-4

[11] Canton J, Neculai D, Grinstein S. Scavenger receptors in homeostasis and immunity. Nature Reviews. Immunology. 2013;**13**(9):621-634. DOI: 10.1038/nri3515

[12] Kawai T, Akira S. Toll-like receptors and their crosstalk with other innate receptors in infection and immunity. Immunity. 2011;**34**(5):637-650. DOI: 10.1016/j.immuni.2011.05.006

[13] Iwasaki A, Medzhitov R. Control of adaptive immunity by the innate immune system. Nature Immunology. 2015;**16**(4):343-353. DOI: 10.1038/ni.3123

[14] Uribe-Querol E, Rosales C. Control of phagocytosis by microbial pathogens. Frontiers in Immunology. 2017;**8**:1368. DOI: 10.3389/fimmu.2017.01368

[15] Jaumouille V, Waterman CM. Physical constraints and forces involved in phagocytosis. Frontiers in Immunology. 2020;**11**:1097. DOI: 10.3389/fimmu.2020.01097

[16] Stuart LM, Ezekowitz RA. Phagocytosis: Elegant complexity. Immunity. 2005;**22**(5):539-550. DOI: 10.1016/j.immuni.2005.05.002

[17] Rusanov AL et al. Proteome profiling of PMJ2-R and primary peritoneal macrophages. International Journal of Molecular Sciences. 2021;**22**(12). DOI: 10.3390/ijms22126323

[18] Gordon S. Phagocytosis: An Immunobiologic process. Immunity. 2016;**44**(3):463-475. DOI: 10.1016/j.immuni.2016.02.026

[19] Ahangar P, Cowin AJ. Reforming the barrier: The role of Formins in wound repair. Cell. 2022;**11**(18). DOI: 10.3390/cells11182779

[20] Kim JG et al. Ras-related GTPases Rap1 and RhoA collectively induce the phagocytosis of serum-opsonized zymosan particles in macrophages. The Journal of Biological Chemistry. 2012;**287**(7):5145-5155. DOI: 10.1074/jbc.M111.257634

[21] Schutt CE, Karlen M, Karlsson R. A structural model of the profilin-formin pacemaker system for actin filament elongation. Scientific Reports. 2022;**12**(1):20515. DOI: 10.1038/s41598-022-25011-w

[22] Boero E et al. Purified complement C3b triggers phagocytosis and activation of human neutrophils via complement receptor 1. Scientific Reports. 2023;**13**(1):274. DOI: 10.1038/s41598-022-27279-4

[23] Montano-Rendon F et al. PtdIns(3,4)P2, Lamellipodin, and VASP coordinate actin dynamics during phagocytosis in macrophages. The Journal of Cell Biology. 2022;**221**(11). DOI: 10.1083/jcb.202207042

[24] Herron JC et al. Spatial models of pattern formation during phagocytosis. PLoS Computational Biology. 2022;**18**(10):e1010092. DOI: 10.1371/journal.pcbi.1010092

[25] Levin R, Grinstein S, Canton J. The life cycle of phagosomes: Formation, maturation, and resolution. Immunological Reviews. 2016;**273**(1):156-179. DOI: 10.1111/imr.12439

[26] Seta Y et al. Morphological evidence for novel roles of microtubules in macrophage phagocytosis. International Journal of Molecular Sciences. 2023;**24**(2). DOI: 10.3390/ijms24021373

[27] Ding B et al. Structures reveal a key mechanism of WAVE regulatory complex activation by Rac1 GTPase. Nature Communications. 2022;**13**(1):5444. DOI: 10.1038/s41467-022-33174-3

[28] Masters TA, Kendrick-Jones J, Buss F. Myosins: Domain organisation, motor properties, physiological roles and cellular functions. Handbook of Experimental Pharmacology. 2017;**235**:77-122. DOI: 10.1007/164_2016_29

[29] Maekawa M, Natsume R, Arita M. Functional significance of ion channels during macropinosome resolution in immune cells. Frontiers in Physiology. 2022;**13**:1037758. DOI: 10.3389/fphys.2022.1037758

[30] Vorselen D. Dynamics of phagocytosis mediated by phosphatidylserine. Biochemical Society Transactions. 2022;**50**(5):1281-1291. DOI: 10.1042/BST20211254

[31] Comer SP. Turning platelets off and on: Role of RhoGAPs and RhoGEFs in platelet activity. Frontier in Cardiovascular Medicine. 2021;**8**:820945. DOI: 10.3389/fcvm.2021.820945

[32] Langford GM. Inclusivity in cell biology: Cultural identity and the power of authenticity. Molecular Biology of the

Cell. 2022;**33**(14):ae5. DOI: 10.1091/mbc.E22-08-0378

[33] Uribe-Querol E, Rosales C. Phagocytosis: Our current understanding of a universal biological process. Frontiers in Immunology. 2020;**11**:1066. DOI: 10.3389/fimmu.2020.01066

[34] Gutierrez MG. Functional role(s) of phagosomal Rab GTPases. Small GTPases. 2013;**4**(3):148-158. DOI: 10.4161/sgtp.25604

[35] Kitano M et al. Imaging of Rab5 activity identifies essential regulators for phagosome maturation. Nature. 2008;**453**(7192):241-245. DOI: 10.1038/nature06857

[36] Kondethimmanahalli C, Ganta RR. Proteome analysis of Ehrlichia chaffeensis containing phagosome membranes revealed the presence of numerous bacterial and host proteins. Frontiers in Cellular and Infection Microbiology. 2022;**12**:1070356. DOI: 10.3389/fcimb.2022.1070356

[37] Jin Y, Deng Z, Zhu T. Membrane protein trafficking in the anti-tumor immune response: Work of endosomal-lysosomal system. Cancer Cell International. 2022;**22**(1):413. DOI: 10.1186/s12935-022-02805-6

[38] Fairn GD, Grinstein S. How nascent phagosomes mature to become phagolysosomes. Trends in Immunology. 2012;**33**(8):397-405. DOI: 10.1016/j.it.2012.03.003

[39] Nunes-Hasler P, Demaurex N. The ER phagosome connection in the era of membrane contact sites. Biochimica Biophysica Acta Molecular Cell Research. 2017;**1864**(9):1513-1524. DOI: 10.1016/j.bbamcr.2017.04.007

[40] BoseDasgupta S, Pieters J. Macrophage-microbe interaction: Lessons learned from the pathogen mycobacterium tuberculosis. Seminars in Immunopathology. 2018;**40**(6):577-591. DOI: 10.1007/s00281-018-0710-0

[41] Patin EC, Thompson A, Orr SJ. Pattern recognition receptors in fungal immunity. Seminars in Cell & Developmental Biology. 2019;**89**:24-33. DOI: 10.1016/j.semcdb.2018.03.003

[42] Behrens NE et al. Serum amyloid P component binds fungal surface amyloid and decreases human macrophage phagocytosis and secretion of inflammatory cytokines. mBio. 2019;**10**(2). DOI: 10.1128/mBio.00218-19

[43] Chen H et al. The whole process of macrophage-Treponema pallidum interactions: Opsonic phagocytosis, nonopsonic phagocytosis and active invasion. International Immunopharmacology. 2022;**107**:108657. DOI: 10.1016/j.intimp.2022.108657

[44] Monteiro JT, Lepenies B. Myeloid C-type lectin receptors in viral recognition and antiviral immunity. Viruses. 2017;**9**(3). DOI: 10.3390/v9030059

[45] Kourtzelis I, Hajishengallis G, Chavakis T. Phagocytosis of apoptotic cells in resolution of inflammation. Frontiers in Immunology. 2020;**11**:553. DOI: 10.3389/fimmu.2020.00553

[46] Burstyn-Cohen T, Maimon A. TAM receptors, phosphatidylserine, inflammation, and cancer. Cell Communication and Signaling: CCS. 2019;**17**(1):156. DOI: 10.1186/s12964-019-0461-0

Chapter 5

Regulation of Phagocytosis in Macrophages

Victory Ibigo Poloamina

Abstract

When the first line of defence—the integumentary system fails, the immune system protects us from infections by pathogens. Macrophages are crucial for mediating effects in the innate immune system by eliminating impaired cells and harmful micro-organisms through phagocytosis. Although other cells undergo phagocytosis, the cellular processes that regulate phagocytosis may vary from cell to cell. These include metabolic changes, signal transduction, and changes in molecular expression or post-translational modifications. This chapter will comprehensively review biological processes that regulate phagocytosis in macrophages, including; changes in metabolic processes, signal transduction, molecular expression, and post-translational modifications.

Keywords: macrophage, innate immunity, phagocytosis, regulation, receptors

1. Introduction

There are millions of human pathogens grouped into about 1400 species [1]. The integumentary system serves as the first line of defence against infection; however, when the integumentary system fails, the immune system defends us against infectious pathogens [2, 3]. It consists of physical barriers such as the dermis, epidermis, and associated glands [4]. Innate immunity describes the initial reaction of the immune system to invasion by microbial pathogens by controlling tissue damage and coordinates the activation of the adaptive immune system [5–8]. When the integuments fail, innate immune cells like macrophages recognise pathogen-associated molecular patterns (PAMP) through pathogen recognition receptors (PRR) and are activated [9]. Macrophage responses involve phagocytosis of the PAMP and the release of inflammatory cytokines resulting in inflammation [10]. Inflammation is a natural reaction that can prevent tissue injury and heal wounded tissues. The strength of inflammation is proportionate to the severity of tissue injury [8, 11]. A normal inflammatory response is structured and involves; vasodilation, higher permeability of blood capillaries, blood clotting, an influx of many granulocytes and monocytes, and tissue swelling [8].

This review chapter will discuss various biomolecules and biochemical processes that regulate phagocytosis in macrophages.

2. The macrophage: functions and phenotypes

Macrophages are crucial for mediating EFFECTS in the innate immune system [12]. Elie Metchnikoff first identified phagocytic cells in the 1900s and observed that macrophages effectively phagocytosed bacteria. Since then, there has been more research on macrophages—their types, function, polarisation, origin, and how they are regulated. Macrophage phagocytosis can be affected by its type, phenotype, and source. In addition, macrophages phagocytose other pathogens, such as viruses, fungi, and parasites [13]. They originate either from yolk-sac erythromyeloid progenitors or haematopoietic progenitors, thus generating monocyte-derived macrophages and tissue-resident macrophages. However, researchers have suggested heterogeneity in the origin of tissue-resident macrophages, as monocyte-derived macrophages can replace embryonic macrophages [8, 12, 14]. In addition, metabolic stimuli can regulate macrophage differentiation. For instance, haem and retinoic acid activate red pulp and peritoneal macrophage differentiation, respectively. Furthermore, tissue-resident macrophages contribute significantly to the heterogeneous functions of macrophages as they have specialised functions according to the tissue environment. Some examples of tissue-resident macrophages include alveolar macrophages, microglia, kupffer cells, and peritoneal macrophages [15].

2.1 Function of macrophages

The classical functions of macrophages include; cytokine secretion, the release of reactive oxygen species and reactive nitrogen species, removal of impaired cells and harmful micro-organisms, tissue surveillance, antigen presentation, T-cell activation, cytotoxicity and fibrosis [8, 16–18]. Tissue-resident macrophages carry out extra functions contingent upon the tissue requirements. For instance, alveolar macrophages clear away lung surfactants [19, 20]. Various stimuli coordinate macrophage fundamental functions and responses to tissue warning signals, including the presence of elements of microbial organisms [21].

In addition, macrophages participate in several pathologies that involve inflammation. For instance, macrophages regulate neuropathic and inflammatory pain by releasing cytokines and interacting with neurons [22]. In cancer, macrophages phagocytose tumour cells and participate in tumour immunosurveillance [23, 24]. In their research, Yang et al., 2021 [25] showed that macrophages could promote cartilage regeneration in mice where macrophage depletion hindered cartilage regeneration. Furthermore, macrophages encourage fibroblast proliferation. As a result, it regulates wound healing [26, 27]. Finally, poor differentiation of microglia during foetal development can cause neuropsychiatric disorders [28].

2.2 Macrophage phenotypes

There are three known macrophage phenotypes; M0 defines the macrophage in an inactive state, M1 defines a phenotype that promotes inflammation, and M2 defines a phenotype that resolves inflammation and promotes wound healing. In addition, M2 macrophages have four sub-phenotypes (M2a, M2b, M2c, M2d), which can affect the extent of phagocytosis [29, 30].

Lipopolysaccharide (LPS) and interferon-gamma (IFNγ), granulocyte-macrophage colony-stimulating factor (GMCSF), and PAMPs are conventional stimulators of the M1 macrophage phenotype. In contrast, macrophage colony-stimulating factors (MCSF), IL4,

IL10, and IL13 are stimulators of the M2 macrophage phenotype [8, 31, 32]. Macrophages show phenotypic characteristics based on an environmental stimulus. Epigenetic factors, including non-coding RNAs, histone modifications, and DNA methylation, can reprogram macrophages to switch between M1 and M2 phenotypes [24, 33–35]. Likewise, macrophage metabolic pathways participate in polarisation into different phenotypes. Lipid metabolism plays a significant role in macrophage phenotype formation. There are metabolic pathways specific to the M1 and M2 macrophage phenotype [36, 37].

3. Regulation of phagocytosis In macrophages

3.1 Pathogen-associated molecular patterns

Various microbial pathogens exist; therefore, PAMPs vary accordingly [11, 38].

LPS is the toxin element of the exterior membrane of gram-negative bacteria. It primarily consists of three components: the variable O-antigen, the core oligosaccharide, covalently bound to the third component—a hydrophobic "anchor" termed lipid A, which commonly contains acyl tails attached to a phosphorylated β-1′, 6-linked glucosamine disaccharide head group. The lipid A component of LPS is highly potent; however, the structural variance of lipid A can influence its potency [8, 39]. In addition, some bacteria retain genetic mutation that hinders the expression of some components of LPS resulting in smooth, semi-rough and rough LPS chemotypes. Smooth LPS refers typically to the prevalent LPS containing the O-antigen. Smooth and Rough LPS may have differential mechanisms for regulating inflammation; rough LPS may be less CD14-dependent than smooth LPS [40]. In the same vein, rough LPS from B. abortus strains of bacteria are more potent in inducing the release of pro-inflammatory cytokines than smooth LPS [41]. Even amongst different species, there are dissimilarities in the strengths of LPS; for instance, the rough chemotype of E. coli LPS is more potent than the rough chemotype of B. abortus LPS [42]. LPS-induced activation of TLR4 activates signals that cause an increase in NFκβ and IRF3 activity hence the secretion of pro-inflammatory and pro-resolving cytokines [43].

Lipopeptides are on the cell walls of gram-positive bacteria, some species of gram-negative bacteria, and fungi. The structure of lipopeptides could be either cyclical peptides attached to an acyl chain, tri-palmitoyl peptides, or dipalmitoyl peptides. Tri-palmitoyl peptides activate TLR2/1 or TLR1/6 receptor heterodimers to induce inflammation. For example, Pam3CysK4 activates cytotoxic T lymphocytes against influenza-virus-infected cells [44, 45]. On the other hand, dipalmitoyl peptides activate TLR2/6 receptor heterodimers, activating the MyD88-dependent pathway and promoting the production of pro-inflammatory cytokines through NFκβ activation [46, 47].

Bacterial and viral DNA are potent macrophage stimulators. They have a repeated series of unmethylated CpG motifs that bind to TLR9 homodimers. Microbial DNA increases the synthesis and secretion of nitric oxide and pro-inflammatory cytokines. Unlike microbial DNA, mammalian DNA has low-frequency CpG dinucleotides, mostly methylated. Therefore, typical mammalian DNA would not cause inflammation [38, 48–52].

On the other hand, viral RNA exist in either a single-stranded or a double-stranded form resulting in differential inflammatory responses. For example, TLR7 and TLR8 commonly recognise single-stranded RNA [53, 54] and form homodimers after activation. However, some scientific evidence [55, 56] has suggested that TLR3, which commonly recognises double-stranded RNA, can also recognise single-stranded RNA.

Microbial RNA induces the secretion of type I interferons and tumoricidal activity in macrophages. They also activate the synthesis of NFκβ-dependent cytokines [57]. Although IRF3 is the primary transcription factor activated by the TRIF-dependent signalling pathway, a study showed that IFNβ could be significantly induced in the absence of detectable IRF3 activation by double-stranded RNA through an unknown mechanism. These studies indicate the necessity for a better understanding of microbial RNA's interactions with its receptors [58–63].

The cell walls of bacteria [64] and fungi [65] contain microbial polysaccharides such as glucans, mannans, and peptidoglycans. A broad variety of receptors, including; toll-like receptors TLR4, TLR2, and TLR6 [11], mannose receptors, DC-SIGN, complement receptors, and dectin receptors recognise microbial polysaccharides and peptidoglycans [66]. Nonetheless, they have differential mechanisms for mediating inflammation [67, 68].

Flagellin from gram-negative bacteria, profilin from T. gondii, and hemozoin from P. Falciparum are examples of microbial proteins that cause inflammation. Knockout of TLR5 weakens flagellin-induced inflammation, implying that TLR5 is crucial for recognising flagellin [69, 70]. Flagellin also binds to the inflammasome receptor NLRC4 resulting in the cleaving of pro-IL1β by caspase 1 to IL1β [71]. Moreso, TLR11 recognises profilin; however, this is limited to mice as human TLR11 is nonfunctional due to a stop codon in its gene [72]. Finally, hemozoin indirectly induces an inflammatory response by enhancing TLR9 responses to DNA from malaria parasites [73, 74].

3.2 Opsonins

Immunoglobulins are well-characterised molecules that recognise foreign micro-organisms or bodies [75]. The basic structure of immunoglobulin comprises two heavy chains and two light chains. The Fab fragment, known to bind and crosslink antigens, and the Fc fragment, which binds to pathogen recognition receptors on phagocytes, are also sub-structures of immunoglobulins [76]. In addition, Immunoglobulin G (IgG) plays a crucial role in immunity by binding invading pathogens and consequently activating the classical pathway of the complement system in macrophages [77]. Furthermore, the interaction of immunoglobulin A (IgA) with Fc alpha receptors (FcαRs) mediates macrophage phagocytosis [49].

Pentraxins refer to a group of serum proteins with a pentameric structure that binds and opsonises microbial pathogens or cellular debris during infection and inflammation. Their pentameric design allows high stability and resistance to enzymatic activity [78]. Both complement receptors and Fc receptors recognise pentraxins. Serum amyloid P (SAP) and C-reactive protein (CRP) are notable pentraxins. SAP recognises phosphoethanolamine, DNA, chromatin, heparin, apoptotic cells and amyloid fibrils in a calcium-dependent manner. On the other hand, CRP recognises phosphocholine, snRNP, histones, apoptotic cells, and oxidised low-density lipoproteins (LDL) [78, 79].

The recognition of microbial pathogens initiates the complement system. Complement proteins involved in recognising microbial pathogens also function as opsonins. Such complement proteins include C1q, mannose-binding lectin (MBL), ficolins, C3b, and C4b [80]. As the cell requires, C3 is cleaved to produce C3a, an anaphylatoxin and C3b, an opsonin [81]. The complement system has three pathways; C1q is involved with the classical pathway, MBLs and ficolins participate in the lectin pathway, and C3b and C4b are concerned with the alternative pathway [80]. In addition, complement proteins tend to promote the secretion of anti-inflammatory cytokines [80, 82].

3.3 Pathogen recognition receptors

Non-opsonic pathogen recognition receptors consist of Toll-Like receptors, RIG-I-Like receptors, Nod-Like receptors, and C-Type Lectin receptors.

Nod-Like and RIG-I-Like receptors localise in the cell cytoplasm. RIG-I, MDA5, and LGP2 helicases recognise single- and double-stranded microbial RNA in the cytosol. They cause a substantial secretion of type I interferons to fight viral infection [83]. On the other hand, over 20 subtypes of Nod-Like receptors exist. Nod-like receptors have four categories according to their functions: autophagy, inflammasome assembly, transcription activation, and signal transduction. They recognise a variety of pathogens, including flagellin, viral RNA, and peptidoglycan. Activation of Nod-Like receptors results in the secretion of IL1β through the inflammasome pathway, and it activates other transcription factors such as NFκβ and CREBBP [84–86].

C-type lectin receptors bind to mannans and peptidoglycans from microbes and primarily facilitate phagocytosis [87–89].

At least nine subtypes of TLRs exist, and they have LRR motifs and TIR domains. TLRs bind to components of microbial pathogens and interact with TIR-containing adapter proteins such as MyD88, Mal, TRIF, and TRAM. The signalling cascade interacts with transcription factors, producing inflammatory cytokines [90–95].

Macrophages have Fc receptors (FcR) and complement receptors that recognise opsonins such as immunoglobulins, CRP, SAP, and complement proteins.

As the name implies, Fc receptors are 60kD glycoproteins that recognise and bind to immunoglobulins to mediate phagocytosis [96]. FcγR recognises and binds to IgG, whereas FcαR recognises and binds to IgA [78]. FcR also recognises and binds to other opsonins, such as SAP and CRP. FcR-mediated phagocytosis leads to internalisation in clathrin-coated pits and vesicles, delivery to endosomes and acid hydrolase-rich lysosomes [97]. Not all FcR transmit signals; however, signalling FcR require either ITAM or ITIM domains for signal transduction. The ITAM pathway is pro-inflammatory, and the ITIM pathway is anti-inflammatory [98]. FcR also requires ubiquitination to mediate phagocytosis [99]. Research has shown that the FcR-ITAM-Syk signalling pathway is similar to the Dectin-1 signalling pathway [100], and there is a crosstalk with the TLR-MyD88 pathway [101].

On the other hand, complement receptors are members of the integral family that primarily recognise and bind to complement proteins [102]. Although there are several complement receptors, scientific research has only shown CR3, CR4, and CRIg on macrophages. CR3 and CR4 are involved in phagocytosis, leukocyte trafficking and migration, synapse formation and co-stimulation. Furthermore, CRIg is part of the immunoglobulin superfamily [103]. There are species-specific differences in complement receptor activation [104]. Although early phagocytosis studies concluded that complement receptor-mediated phagocytosis was less pro-inflammatory in macrophages, recent research found significant up-regulation of pro-inflammatory mediators during complement receptor-mediated phagocytosis [105]. As is the case for many receptors, other biomolecules can affect the expression or function of complement receptors. For example, Pyk2 is essential for CR3-mediated phagocytosis as it significantly contributes to the coordination of phagocytosis-promoting signals downstream of CR3 [102]. Likewise, Vitamin D upregulates the expression of CRIg and its phagocytic activity [106].

3.4 Biochemical processes that regulate receptor function

Ubiquitination describes post-translational modification with small conserved peptides known as ubiquitin. Ubiquitin covalently attaches to the amino group of lysine residues of target proteins. Amongst other functions, protein ubiquitination enables the internalisation and formation of early endosomes [99].

Three major classes of ubiquitinating enzymes mediate ubiquitination: the E1 ubiquitin-activating enzymes, the E2 ubiquitin-conjugating enzymes, and the E3 ubiquitin ligases. Two genes encode for the E1 ubiquitin-activating enzymes, about 100 genes encode the E2 ubiquitin-conjugating proteins, and over 1000 genes encode for the E3 ubiquitin ligases. E2 ubiquitin-conjugating enzymes and E3 ubiquitin ligases work together to create high specificity of protein ubiquitination [107, 108]. E3 ubiquitin ligases regulate TLR signalling; Nrdp1 ubiquitylates MyD88 and targets it for degradation [109]; TRAF6 is also essential for MyD88-dependent, and TRIF-dependent TLR signalling [110], Triad3A and Pelle-interacting proteins also participate in TLR signalling [111, 112]. In addition, the translocation of NFκβ to the nucleus in response to TLR activation highly depends on the ubiquitination of IKK proteins bound to NFκβ to keep it in the cytosol [107, 113]. Monoubiquitylation may indirectly influence PRR function by; initiating the internalisation of cell surface receptors by phagocytosis, sourcing amino acids for protein synthesis, negatively regulating RIG-I helicases and affecting antigen presentation by MHC class I molecules [107, 114, 115].

Phosphorylation describes the attachment of phosphate groups to amino acid residues such as tyrosine, serine, and threonine by protein kinases. TLR Phosphorylation occurs on tyrosine residues and activates interaction with adapter proteins. LPS causes IRAK1-mediated phosphorylation; consequently, IRAK1 phosphorylates Tollip–a negative regulator of TLR-MyD88 signalling, enabling TRAF6 activity essential for the downstream TLR-MyD88 signalling. Moreso, IRAKs interact with the MyD88 death domain [116, 117]. The Serine/Threonine kinase PI3 is vital for activating transcription factors downstream of the TLR signalling pathway [116, 118]. Furthermore, knockout of MyD88 enhanced phosphorylation of IRF3, resulting in significant secretion of IFNβ. Finally, inhibition of MNK kinases decreased macrophage TNFα secretion [119, 120].

The phospholipid remodelling pathway describes the release and esterification of fatty acids in phospholipid pools. Phospholipid remodelling is an efficient energy source, generates membrane diversity and asymmetry, regulates protein lipidation, and the synthesis of PAF, leukotrienes, and eicosanoids [121, 122]. The quantity of arachidonic acid during inflammation in macrophages relies on the reacylation and deacylation of phospholipids. Macrophage TLR activation also alters the phospholipid composition of the macrophage membrane by activating phospholipid remodelling enzymes [123–125].

Lipid rafts function as platforms for internalisation and early endosomal sorting functions. They are nano-sized dynamic liquid-ordered plasma membrane domains enriched with cholesterol and sphingolipids and resistant to extraction with non-ionic detergents [126–130]. Lipid rafts participate in membrane transport [130] and signal transduction. They are also essential for receptor-mediated endocytosis [128] and control signal transduction by averting protein-protein interactions and inherent protein activities [129].

3.5 Regulators of phagosomes, and lysosomes

The cellular mechanism of phagocytosis involves the formation of phagosomes, phagosome maturation and the fusion of phagosomes with lysosomes [18, 131]. Phagosomes are cellular vesicles formed to contain the ingested pathogen [132]. There are early and late phagosomes; early phagosomes fuse with early endosomes, whereas phagosome maturation results in late phagosomes. Profound rearrangements of the actin cytoskeleton occur to extend the plasma membrane into a phagocytic cup that internalises the pathogen [133]. Several biomolecules influence this process. For example, dynamin-2 participates in phagosome closure in macrophages. It co-localises with actin during phagosome formation [134].

Furthermore, converting PIP2 to PIP3 is essential for pseudopod extension and phagosome closure. Although PIP2 participates in clathrin-mediated endocytosis, research has shown that clathrin-mediated endocytosis does not influence phagosome formation or maturation [134, 135]. Phagosomal development occurs when phagosomes acquire microbicidal and lytic enzymes after fusion with various endolysosomal compartments. During phagosomal maturation, the phagosome lumen increases its acidification levels [136].

The Nod-like receptor (NLRP3), critical for inflammasome activation, also affects phagosome maturation. Knockout of NLRP3 from macrophages impaired phagosome acidification and phagolysosome formation [137].

SNAP23, a membrane SNARE protein, caused a significant delay in phagosome maturation after its knockdown. On the hand, overexpression of SNAP23 enhances phagosome acidification in J774 macrophages [138].

During FcγR-mediated phagocytosis, actin polymerisation and reorganisation occur, which drives the formation of a phagocytic cup. Rho GTPases promote the polymerisation of F-Actin, thereby regulating cytoskeletal dynamics and affecting cell polarity and motility. As phagolysosome formation requires the disappearance of the F-Actin structure surrounding the phagosome, Rho GTPases participate in this process. Scientific evidence shows that RhoC modulates phagosome formation by modifying actin cytoskeletal remodelling [133]. Furthermore, Syk, which mediates FcgammaR signalling, interrupts the reconstruction of F-Actin around phagosomes, thereby accelerating the fusion of phagosomes with lysosomes [132].

Rab GTPases are proteins that play crucial roles in phagosome maturation [136, 139]. They constitute the most prominent family of small monomeric GTPases that function as molecular switches by cycling between their GDP and GTP-bound forms and regulating membrane trafficking [140]. Rab5 participates in early phagosome maturation by regulating fusion with sorting endosomes, and Rab 7 allows late phagosomes leading to the formation of phagolysosomes [136, 140]. Rab20 regulates phagosome maturation during FcγR-mediated phagocytosis [140].

Lysosomes are membrane-bound acidic compartments formed by lipid bilayers containing proteins such as LAMPs, Rab GTPases, LIMP, CD63, and over 60 hydrolases [141–143]. Lysosome function is heavily dependent on its fusogenic and acidic properties. The cytosolic tails of LAMP proteins interact with microtubules, thus having an essential role in lysosome function. Moreso, the lack of Rab14 slowed the addition of LAMP1 and lysosomal cathepsin, implying a slower formation of completely bioactive lysosomes [136].

In conclusion, the complex process of phagocytosis is crucial in macrophages as they are professional phagocytes. Numerous biomolecules participate directly or indirectly in macrophage phagocytosis, hence the complexity. This chapter has described some of these biomolecules and biochemical processes that regulate macrophage phagocytosis.

3.6 Conclusion

In conclusion, macrophages play an important role as early responders to infection through their primary phagocytic function. This primary function is upheld by the synergy of pathogen associated molecular patterns and macrophage recognition molecules (opsonins and pattern recognition receptors) leads to downstream effects such as phagosome formation, lysosome formation, ubiquitination, phosphorylation, and phospholipid remodelling. Macrophage regulation is still being studied and there are recent discoveries of how macrophages can be regulated. Therefore, in spite of ample information about the regulation of phagocytosis in macrophages, there is more to learn. A better understanding of the regulation of phagocytosis can aid the use macrophages for therapeutic purposes (**Figure 1**).

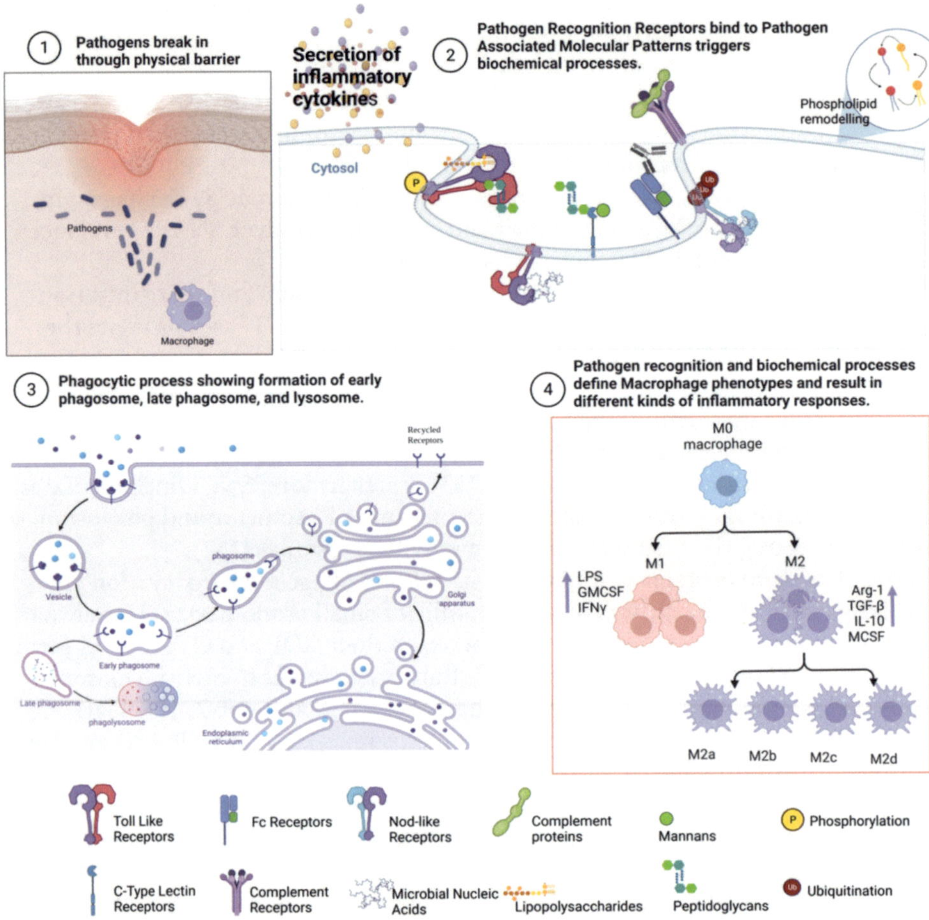

Figure 1.
Graphical summary.

Author details

Victory Ibigo Poloamina
School of Biomedical Sciences, University of Plymouth, England

*Address all correspondence to: dr.vipoloamina@outlook.com

References

[1] Microbiology NR. Microbiology by numbers. Nature Reviews Microbiology. 2011;**9**:628-628

[2] Lee H-J, Kim M. Skin barrier function and the microbiome. International Journal of Molecular Sciences. 2022;**23**:13071

[3] Nicholson LB. The immune system. Essays in Biochemistry. 2016;**60**:275-301

[4] Mauldin EA, Peters-Kennedy J. Chapter 6 - integumentary system. In: Maxie MG, editor. Jubb, Kennedy Palmer's Pathology of Domestic Animals. Sixth ed. Pennsylvania, United States of America: W.B. Saunders; 2016. pp. 509-736. Available from: https://www.sciencedirect.com/science/article/pii/B9780702053177000060

[5] Blaser H, Dostert C, Mak TW, Brenner D. TNF and ROS crosstalk in inflamma- tion. Trends in Cell Biology. 2016;**26**:249-261

[6] Colaço HG, Moita LF. Initiation of innate immune responses by surveillance of homeostasis perturbations. The FEBS Journal. 2016;**283**:2448-2457

[7] Zheng X-F et al. Lipopolysaccharide-induced m2 to m1 macrophage transformation for IL-12p70 production is blocked by candida albicans mediated up-regulation of EBI3 expression. PLoS One. 2013;**8**:e63967

[8] Poloamina VI. Regulation of the Expression and Lysine Acetylation of pro-Inflammatory Molecules by Lipid-Modifying Enzyme (LPCAT2) in RAW264.7 Cells. England: University of Plymouth; 2021

[9] Lerm M, Netea MG. Trained immunity: A new avenue for tuberculosis vaccine development. Journal of Internal Medicine. 2015;**279**:337-346

[10] Romo MR, Pérez-Martínez D, Ferrer CC. Innate immunity in vertebrates: An overview. Immunology. 2016;**148**:125-139

[11] Owen JA, Punt J, Stranford SA, Jones PP. Kuby Immunology. New York: WH Freeman; 2013. pp. 52-75

[12] Italiani P, Boraschi D. New insights into tissue macrophages: From their origin to the development of memory. Immune Network. 2015;**15**:167

[13] Liu Y-S et al. The pattern-recognition molecule mindin binds integrin mac-1 to promote macrophage phagocytosis via syk activation and nf-b p65 translocation. Journal of Cellular and Molecular Medicine. 2019;**23**:3402-3416

[14] Hoeffel G, Ginhoux F. Ontogeny of tissue-resident macrophages. Frontiers in Immunology. 2015;**6**:486

[15] Gordon S, Plüddemann A. Tissue macrophages: Heterogeneity and functions. BMC Biology. 2017;**15**(1):1-18

[16] Watanabe S, Alexander M, Misharin AV, Budinger GRS. The role of macrophages in the resolution of inflammation. The Journal of Clinical Investigation. 2019;**129**:2619-2628

[17] Lendeckel U, Venz S, Wolke C. Macrophages: Shapes and functions. ChemTexts. 2022;**8**:12

[18] Lovewell RR, Patankar YR, Berwin B. Mechanisms of phagocytosis and host clearance of pseudomonas aeruginosa. American Journal of Physiology. Lung Cellular and Molecular Physiology. 2014;**306**:L591-L603

[19] Mass E et al. Specification of tissue-resident macrophages during organogenesis. Science. 2016;**353**(6304):aaf4238

[20] Okabe Y, Medzhitov R. Tissue biology perspective on macrophages. Nature Immunology. 2015;**17**:9-17

[21] Glass CK, Natoli G. Molecular control of activation and priming in macrophages. Nature Immunology. 2015;**17**:26-33

[22] Domoto R, Sekiguchi F, Tsubota M, Kawabata A. Macrophage as a peripheral pain regulator. Cell. 2021;**10**:1881

[23] Jaiswal S, Chao MP, Majeti R, Weissman IL. Macrophages as mediators of tumor immunosurveillance. Trends in Immunology. 2010;**31**:212-219

[24] Chen S, Lai SWT, Brown CE, Feng M. Harnessing and enhancing macrophage phagocytosis for cancer therapy. Frontiers in Immunology. 2021;**12**:635173

[25] Yang J et al. Macrophages promote cartilage regeneration in a time- and phenotype- dependent manner. Journal of Cellular Physiology. 2022;**237**:2258-2270

[26] Hesketh M, Sahin KB, West ZE, Murray RZ. Macrophage phenotypes regulate scar formation and chronic wound healing. International Journal of Molecular Sciences. 2017;**18**:1545

[27] Kloc M et al. Macrophage functions in wound healing. Journal of Tissue Engineering and Regenerative Medicine. 2018;**2018**:99-109

[28] Ginhoux F, Schultze JL, Murray PJ, Ochando J, Biswas SK. New insights into the multidimensional concept of macrophage ontogeny, activation and function. Nature Immunology. 2015;**17**:34-40

[29] Orekhov AN et al. Role of phagocytosis in the pro-inflammatory response in LDL- induced foam cell formation a transcriptome analysis. International Journal of Molecular Sciences. 2020;**21**:817

[30] Schulz D, Severin Y, Zanotelli VRT, Bodenmiller B. In-depth characterization of monocyte-derived macrophages using a mass cytometry-based phagocytosis assay. Scientific Reports. 2019;**9**:1925

[31] Hamilton TA, Zhao C, Pavicic PG, Datta S. Myeloid colony-stimulating factors as regulators of macrophage polarization. Frontiers in Immunology. 2014;**5**:554

[32] Günthner R, Anders H-J. Interferon-regulatory factors determine macrophage pheno- type polarization. Mediators of Inflammation. 2013;**2013**:1-8

[33] Niu X, Schulert GS. Functional regulation of macrophage phenotypes by MicroRNAs in inflammatory arthritis. Frontiers in Immunology. 2019;**10**:2217

[34] Graff JW, Dickson AM, Clay G, McCaffrey AP, Wilson ME. Identifying functional MicroRNAs in macrophages with polarized phenotypes. Journal of Biological Chemistry. 2012;**287**:21816-21825

[35] Self-Fordham JB, Naqvi AR, Uttamani JR, Kulkarni V, Nares S. MicroRNA: Dynamic regulators of macrophage polarization and plasticity. Frontiers in Immunology. 2017;**8**:1062

[36] Galván-Peña S, O'Neill LAJ. Metabolic reprograming in macrophage polarization. Frontiers in Immunology. 2014;**5**:420

[37] He C, Carter AB. The metabolic prospective and redox regulation of macrophage polarization. Journal of Clinical & Cellular Immunology. 2015;**6**(6)

[38] Atianand MK, Fitzgerald KA. Molecular basis of DNA recognition in the immune system. The Journal of Immunology. 2013;**190**:1911-1918

[39] Paramo T, Tomasio SM, Irvine KL, Bryant CE, Bond PJ. Energetics of endotoxin recognition in the toll-like receptor 4 innate immune response. Scientific Reports. 2015;**5**:17997

[40] Zanoni I et al. Similarities and differences of innate immune responses elicited by smooth and rough LPS. Immunology Letters. 2012;**142**:41-47

[41] Rittig MG et al. Smooth and rough lipopolysaccharide phenotypes ofibrucella/iinduce different intracellular trafficking and cytokine/chemokine release in human monocytes. Journal of Leukocyte Biology. 2003;**74**:1045-1055

[42] Jarvis BW, Harris TH, Qureshi N, Splitter GA. Rough lipopolysaccharide from ibrucella abortus/i and iescherichia coli/i differentially activates the same mitogen-activated protein kinase signaling pathways for tumor necrosis factor alpha in RAW 264.7 macrophage-like cells. Infection and Immunity. 2002;**70**:7165-7168

[43] Chen S, Yang J, Wei Y, Wei X. Epigenetic regulation of macrophages: From homeostasis maintenance to host defense. Cellular & Molecular Immunology. 2019;**17**:36-49

[44] Hamley IW. Lipopeptides: From self-assembly to bioactivity. Chemical Communications. 2015;**51**:8574-8583

[45] Raaijmakers JM, De Bruijn I, Nybroe O, Ongena M. Natural functions of lipopeptides from bacillus and pseudomonas: More than surfactants and antibiotics. FEMS Microbiol Review. 2010;**34**:1037-1062

[46] Kiura K et al. The synthetic analogue of mycoplasmal lipoprotein FSL-1 induces dendritic cell maturation through toll-like receptor 2. FEMS Immunology &amp Medical Microbiology. 2006;**46**:78-84

[47] Kurkjian CJ et al. The toll–like receptor 2/6 agonist, FSL–1 lipopeptide, therapeutically mitigates acute radiation syndrome. Scientific Reports. 2017;**7**:17355

[48] Elkon KB. Review: Cell death, nucleic acids, and immunity. Arthritis & Rheumatology. 2018;**70**:805-816

[49] Francés R et al. Intracellular cytokine expression in peritoneal monocyte/ macrophages obtained from patients with cirrhosis and presence of bacterial DNA. European Journal of Gastroenterology & Hepatology. 2005;**17**:45-51

[50] Hemmi H et al. A toll-like receptor recognizes bacterial DNA. Nature. 2000;**408**:740-745

[51] Kawai T, Akira S. The role of pattern-recognition receptors in innate immunity: Update on toll-like receptors. Nature Immunology. 2010;**11**:373-384

[52] Talati A, Kim H, Kim Y, Yi A, English B. Role of bacterial DNA in macrophage activation by group b streptococci73. Microbes and Infection. 2008;**10**:1106-1113

[53] Diebold S. Recognition of viral single-stranded RNA by toll-like receptors73. Advanced Drug Delivery Reviews. 2008;**60**:813-823

[54] Lund JM et al. Recognition of single-stranded RNA viruses by toll-like receptor 7. Proceedings of the National Academy of Sciences. 2004;**101**:5598-5603

[55] Allen IC et al. The NLRP3 inflammasome mediates in vivo innate

immunity to influenza a virus through recognition of viral RNA. Immunity. 2009;**30**:556-565

[56] Tatematsu M, Nishikawa F, Seya T, Matsumoto M. Toll-like receptor 3 recognizes incomplete stem structures in single-stranded viral RNA. Nature Communications. 2013;**4**:1833

[57] Alexopoulou L, Holt AC, Medzhitov R, Flavell RA. Recognition of double- stranded RNA and activation of NF-b by toll-like receptor 3. Nature. 2001;**413**:732-738

[58] Djeu JY, Heinbaugh JA, Holden HT, Herberman RB. Role of macrophages in the augementation of mouse natural killer cell activity by poly i:c and interferon. Journal of Immunology. 1979;**122**:182-188

[59] Kato H, Oh S-W, Fujita T. RIG-i-like receptors and type i interferonopathies. Journal of Interferon & Cytokine Research. 2017;**37**:207-213

[60] Matsumoto M, Seya T. TLR3: Interferon induction by double-stranded RNA including poly(i:c)73. Advanced Drug Delivery Reviews. 2008;**60**:805-812

[61] Reimer T, Brcic M, Schweizer M, Jungi TW. Poly(i:c) and LPS induce distinct IRF3 and NF-b signaling during type-i IFN and TNF responses in human macrophages. Journal of Leukocyte Biology. 2008;**83**:1249-1257

[62] Taramelli D, Varesio L. Activation of murine macrophages. i. Different pattern of activation by poly i:c than by lymphokine or lps. Journal of Immunology. 1981;**127**:58-63

[63] Yoneyama M, Fujita T. Structural mechanism of RNA recognition by the RIG-i-like receptors. Immunity. 2008;**29**:178-181

[64] Sahly H, Keisari Y, Crouch E, Sharon N, Ofek I. Recognition of bacterial surface polysaccharides by lectins of the innate immune system and its contribution to defense against infection: The case of pulmonary pathogens. Infection and Immunity. 2008;**76**:1322-1332

[65] Hollmig ST, Ariizumi K, Cruz PD. Recognition of non-self-polysaccharides by c-type lectin receptors dectin-1 and dectin-2. Glycobiology. 2009;**19**:568-575

[66] Snarr B, Qureshi S, Sheppard D. Immune recognition of fungal polysaccharides. Journal of Fungi. 2017;**3**:47

[67] Silva-Martín N et al. Structural basis for selective recognition of endogenous and microbial polysaccharides by macrophage receptor SIGN-r1. Structure. 2014;**22**:1595-1606

[68] Wesener DA et al. Recognition of microbial glycans by human intelectin-1. Nature Structural & Molecular Biology. 2015;**22**:603-610

[69] Hayashi F et al. The innate immune response to bacterial flagellin is mediated by toll-like receptor 5. Nature. 2001;**410**:1099-1103

[70] Mizel SB, Bates JT. Flagellin as an adjuvant: Cellular mechanisms and potential. The Journal of Immunology. 2010;**185**:5677-5682

[71] Zhao Y et al. The NLRC4 inflammasome receptors for bacterial flagellin and type III secretion apparatus. Nature. 2011;**477**:596-600

[72] Yarovinsky F et al. TLR11 activation of dendritic cells by a protozoan profilin-like protein. Science. 2005;**308**:1626-1629

[73] Coban C et al. Toll-like receptor 9 mediates innate immune activation by the malaria pigment hemozoin. Journal of Experimental Medicine. 2005;**201**:19-25

[74] Parroche P et al. Malaria hemozoin is immunologically inert but radically enhances innate responses by presenting malaria DNA to toll-like receptor 9. Proceedings of the National Academy of Sciences. 2007;**104**:1919-1924

[75] den Hartog G et al. Specificity and effector functions of human RSV-specific IgG from bovine milk. PLoS One. 2014;**9**:e112047

[76] Schroeder HW, Cavacini L. Structure and function of immunoglobulins. Journal of Allergy and Clinical Immunology. 2010;**125**:S41-S52

[77] Vincents B et al. Cleavage of IgGsub1/suband IgGsub3/subby gingipain k fromiporphyromonas gingivalis/imay compromise host defense in progressive periodontitis. The FASEB Journal. 2011;**25**:3741-3750

[78] Lu J, Mold C, Clos TWD, Sun PD. Pentraxins and fc receptor-mediated immune responses. Frontiers in Immunology. 2018;**9**:2607

[79] Clos TWD. Pentraxins: Structure, function, and role in inflammation. ISRN Inflammation. 2013;**2013**:1-22

[80] Bohlson SS, O'Conner SD, Hulsebus HJ, Ho MM, Fraser DA. Complement, c1q, and c1q-related molecules regulate macrophage polarization. Frontiers in Immunology. 2014;**5**:402

[81] Dunkelberger JR, Song W-C. Complement and its role in innate and adaptive immune responses. Cell Research. 2009;**20**:34-50

[82] Takeda Y et al. Inhibition of CXCL10 release by monomeric c3bi and c4b. Clinical and Experimental Immunology. 2011;**167**:149-157

[83] Brisse M, Ly H. Comparative structure and function analysis of the RIG-i-like receptors: RIG-i and MDA5. Frontiers in Immunology. 2019;**10**:1586

[84] Ekman A-K, Cardell LO. The expression and function of nod-like receptors in neutrophils. Immunology. 2010;**130**:55-63

[85] Kim YK, Shin J-S, Nahm MH. NOD-like receptors in infection, immunity, and diseases. Yonsei Medical Journal. 2016;**57**:5

[86] Mavrogiorgos N, Mekasha S, Yang Y, Kelliher MA, Ingalls RR. Activation of NOD receptors byineisseria gonorrhoeae/imodulates the innate immune response. Innate Immunity. 2013;**20**:377-389

[87] Bermejo-Jambrina M et al. C-type lectin receptors in antiviral immunity and viral escape. Frontiers in Immunology. 2018;**9**:590

[88] Geijtenbeek TBH, Gringhuis SI. Signalling through c-type lectin receptors: Shaping immune responses. Nature Reviews Immunology. 2009;**9**:465-479

[89] Hadebe S, Brombacher F, Brown GD. C-type lectin receptors in asthma. Frontiers in Immunology. 2018;**9**:733

[90] Arrese M, Cabrera D, Kalergis AM, Feldstein AE. Innate immunity and in-flammation in NAFLD/NASH. Digestive Diseases and Sciences. 2016;**61**:1294-1303

[91] Blasius AL, Beutler B. Intracellular toll-like receptors. Immunity. 2010;**32**:305-315

[92] Mukherjee S et al. Lipopolysaccharide-driven th2 cytokine production in macrophages is regulated by both MyD88 and TRAM. Journal of Biological Chemistry. 2009;**284**:29391-29398

[93] Papageorgiou IE et al. TLR4-activated microglia require IFN- to induce severe neuronal dysfunction and

death in situ. Proceedings of the National Academy of Sciences. 2015;**113**:212-217

[94] Perkins DJ, Vogel SN. Species-specific TLR signalling — Insight into human disease. Nature Reviews Rheumatology. 2016;**12**:198-200

[95] Radoshevich L, Dussurget O. Cytosolic innate immune sensing and signaling upon infection. Frontiers in Microbiology. 2016;**7**:313

[96] Ravetch JV, Kinet JP. Fc receptors. Annual Review of Immunology. 1991;**9**:457-492

[97] Ukkonen P, Lewis V, Marsh M, Helenius A, Mellman I. Transport of macrophage fc receptors and fc receptor-bound ligands to lysosomes. Journal of Experimental Medicine. 1986;**163**:952-971

[98] Guilliams M, Bruhns P, Saeys Y, Hammad H, Lambrecht BN. The function of fc receptors in dendritic cells and macrophages. Nature Reviews Immunology. 2014;**14**:94-108

[99] Molfetta R et al. Regulation of fc receptor endocytic trafficking by ubiquitination. Frontiers in Immunology. 2014;**5**:449

[100] Goodridge HS, Underhill DM, Touret N. Mechanisms of fc receptor and dectin-1 activation for phagocytosis. Traffic. 2012;**13**:1062-1071

[101] Lennartz M, Drake J. Molecular mechanisms of macrophage toll-like receptor–fc receptor synergy. F1000Research. 2018;**7**:21

[102] Paone C et al. The tyrosine kinase pyk2 contributes to complement-mediated phagocytosis in murine macrophages. Journal of Innate Immunity. 2016;**8**:437-451

[103] van Lookeren Campagne M, Wiesmann C, Brown EJ. Macrophage complement receptors and pathogen clearance. Cellular Microbiology. 2007;**9**:2095-2102

[104] Ray TD et al. Species-specific differences in regulation of macrophage inflammation by the c3a–c3a receptor axis. Innate Immunity. 2018;**24**:66-78

[105] Acharya D, Li XRL, Heineman RE-S, Harrison RE. Complement receptor-mediated phagocytosis induces proinflammatory cytokine production in murine macrophages. Frontiers in Immunology. 2022;**10**:770969

[106] Small AG et al. Vitamin d upregulates the macrophage complement receptor immunoglobulin in innate immunity to microbial pathogens. Communications Biology. 2021;**4**:401

[107] Lecker SH, Goldberg AL, Mitch WE. Protein degradation by the ubiquitin–proteasome pathway in normal and disease states. Journal of the American Society of Nephrology. 2006;**17**:1807-1819

[108] Kulkarni M, Smith HE. E1 ubiquitin-activating enzyme uba-1 plays multiple roles throughout c. elegans development. PLoS Genetics. 2008;**4**:e1000131

[109] Wang C et al. The e3 ubiquitin ligase nrdp1 'preferentially' promotes TLR-mediated production of type i interferon. Nature Immunology. 2009;**10**:744-752

[110] Shi C-S, Kehrl JH. Traf6 and a20 regulate lysine 63-linked ubiquitination of beclin-1 to control tlr4-induced autophagy. Science Signaling. 2010;**3**:ra42

[111] Chuang T-H, Ulevitch RJ. Triad3a, an e3 ubiquitin-protein ligase regulating toll-like receptors. Nature Immunology. 2004;**5**:495-502

[112] Jin W, Chang M, Sun S-C. Peli: A family of signal-responsive e3 ubiquitin

ligases mediating TLR signaling and t-cell tolerance. Cellular & Molecular Immunology. 2012;**9**:113-122

[113] Carmody RJ, Ruan Q, Palmer S, Hilliard B, Chen YH. Negative regulation of toll-like receptor signaling by NF-b p50 ubiquitination blockade. Science. 2007;**317**:675-678

[114] Ciechanover A. The ubiquitin-proteasome pathway: On protein death and cell life. The EMBO Journal. 1998;**17**:7151-7160

[115] Ichiro Arimoto K et al. Negative regulation of the RIG-i signaling by the ubiquitin ligase RNF125. Proceedings of the National Academy of Sciences. 2007;**104**:7500-7505

[116] Chattopadhyay S, Sen GC. Tyrosine phosphorylation in toll-like recep- tor signaling. Cytokine Growth Factor Reviews. 2014;**25**:533-541

[117] Miggin SM. New insights into the regulation of TLR signaling. Journal of Leukocyte Biology. 2006;**80**:220-226

[118] Fukao T, Koyasu S. PI3k and negative regulation of TLR signaling. Trends in Immunology. 2003;**24**:358-363

[119] Rowlett RM et al. MNK kinases regulate multiple TLR pathways and innate proin- flammatory cytokines in macrophages. American Journal of Physiology-Gastrointestinal and Liver Physiology. 2008;**294**:G452-G459

[120] Siednienko J, Gajanayake T, Fitzgerald KA, Moynagh P, Miggin SM. Absence of MyD88 results in enhanced TLR3-dependent phosphorylation of IRF3 and increased IFN- and RANTES production. The Journal of Immunology. 2011;**186**:2514-2522

[121] Shindou H, Shimizu T. Acyl-CoA: Lysophospholipid acyltransferases. Journal of Biological Chemistry. 2009;**284**:1-5

[122] Hutchins PM, Murphy RC. Cholesteryl ester acyl oxidation and remodeling in murine macrophages: Formation of oxidized phosphatidylcholine. Journal of Lipid Research. 2012;**53**:1588-1597

[123] Shindou H, Hishikawa D, Harayama T, Eto M, Shimizu T. Generation of membrane diversity by lysophospholipid acyltransferases. Journal of Biochemistry. 2013;**154**:21-28

[124] Astudillo AM et al. Altered arachidonate distribution in macrophages from caveolin-1 null mice leading to reduced eicosanoid synthesis. Journal of Biological Chemistry. 2011;**286**:35299-35307

[125] Kröner E, Peskar B, Fischer H, Ferber E. Control of arachi- donic acid accumulation in bone marrow-derived macrophages by acyltrans- ferases. Journal of Biological Chemistry. 1981;**256**:3690-3697

[126] Simons K, Toomre D. Lipid rafts and signal transduction. Nature Reviews Molecular Cell Biology. 2000;**1**:31-39

[127] Pathak P, London E. The effect of membrane lipid composition on the formation of lipid ultrananodomains. Biophysical Journal. 2015;**109**:1630-1638

[128] Suzuki T, Suzuki Y. Virus infection and lipid rafts. Biological and Pharmaceutical Bulletin. 2006;**29**:1538-1541

[129] Pike LJ. Lipid rafts: Bringing order to chaos. Journal of Lipid Research. 2003;**44**:655-667

[130] Ikonen E. Roles of lipid rafts in membrane transport. Current Opinion in Cell Biology. 2001;**13**:470-477

[131] Uribe-Querol E, Rosales C. Phagocytosis: Our current understanding of a universal biological process. Frontiers in Immunology. 2020;**11**:1066

[132] Tabata H, Morita H, Kaji H, Tohyama K, Tohyama Y. Syk facilitates phagosome- lysosome fusion by regulating actin-remodeling in complement-mediated phagocytosis. Scientific Reports. 2020;**10**:1-16

[133] Egami Y, Kawai K, Araki N. RhoC regulates actin remodeling to form phagosomes during fcr-mediated phagocytosis. Journal of Cell Science. 2017;**2017**:4168-4179

[134] Marie-Anaïs F, Mazzolini J, Herit F, Niedergang F. Dynaminactin cross talk contributes to phagosome formation and closure. Traffic. 2016;**17**:487-499

[135] Walpole GFW, Grinstein S. Endocytosis and the internalization of pathogenic organisms: Focus on phosphoinositides. F1000Research. 2020;**9**:368

[136] Okai B, Lyall N, Gow NAR, Bain JM, Erwig L-P. Rab14 regulates maturation of macrophage phagosomes containing the fungal pathogen candida albicans and outcome of the host-pathogen interaction. Infection and Immunity. 2015;**83**:1523-1535

[137] Huang X-H et al. NLRP3 and mTOR reciprocally regulate macrophage phagolysosome formation and acidification against vibrio vulnificus infection. Frontiers in Cell and Developmental Biology. 2020;**8**:587961

[138] Sakurai C et al. SNAP-23 regulates phagosome formation and maturation in macrophages. Molecular Biology of the Cell. 2012;**23**:4849-4863

[139] Prashar A, Schnettger L, Bernard EM, Gutierrez MG. Rab GTPases in immunity and inflammation. Frontiers in Cellular and Infection Microbiology. 2017;**7**:435

[140] Egami Y, Araki N. Rab20 regulates phagosome maturation in RAW264 macrophages during fc gamma receptor-mediated phagocytosis. PLoS One. 2012;**7**:e35663

[141] Xu H, Ren D. Lysosomal physiology. Annual Review of Physiology. 2015;**77**:57-80

[142] Matte U, Pasqualim G. Lysosome. Journal of Inborn Errors of Metabolism and Screening. 2016;**4**:232

[143] Li P, Ma C, Li J, You S, Dang L, Wu J, et al. Proteomic characterization of four subtypes of M2 macrophages derived from human THP-1 cells. Journal of Zhejiang University-science B. 2022;**23**(5):407-422. DOI: 10.1631/jzus.b2100930

Section 2

Phagocytosis in Diseases

Chapter 6

Muscularis Macrophages in Healthy and Diseased Gut

Magdalini Mischopoulou and Gianluca Cipriani

Abstract

Muscularis macrophages are a newly discovered population of macrophages distributed within the smooth muscle layers of the gastrointestinal tract. Muscularis macrophages are emerging as essential cell keepers of homeostatic gastrointestinal function, and when affected, can lead to functional gastrointestinal disorders. In this chapter, we briefly introduce the phenotype, the distribution of muscularis macrophages, and the difference compared with other tissue-resident macrophages. We next describe how they contribute to normal gastrointestinal function by interacting with cells required for gastrointestinal motility, such as enteric neurons. Finally, we highlight the increasing pieces of evidence suggesting the contribution of muscularis macrophages to gastrointestinal function diseases, such as gastrointestinal inflammation, gastroparesis and post operative ileus.

Keywords: macrophages, muscularis propria, gastrointestinal tract, enteric neurons, gastrointestinal motility

1. Introduction

Macrophages are specialized immune cells found in all body organs, whose role is to phagocytose antigens, foreign material, cancer cells, and cellular debris [1]. In addition to their primary role in regulating the innate immune response, tissue macrophages keep tissue homeostasis and niche-specific functions. The first report describing the presence of macrophages in the gut muscularis propria (MMs) was performed [2, 3] by Mikkelsen in 1980. This report identified MMs as "macrophage-like cells" based on their peculiar morphologic features [4]. The same authors concluded later that MMs, with their irregular stellate shape, represent a specialized type of macrophages, distinct from most resident tissue macrophages [5]. The gastrointestinal (GI) tract contains a heterogeneous population of tissue macrophages, most of which lie within the mucosa, where they phagocytose bacterial antigens [6] and constitute the first layer of defense against external pathogens. MMs are localized within the smooth muscle layers and are closely associated with cells essential for GI motility [7]. Due to this spatial relationship, MMs can regulate gut peristalsis by secreting chemokines, partially in response to microbial stimulation [8, 9]. This chapter will highlight the complex role of MMs in regulating GI homeostasis and functional diseases.

2. Anatomic localization of MMs

Histologically the GI tract is a complex organ consisting of different layers: the mucosa, the submucosal layer, the muscularis propria, and the serosa (**Figure 1**).

The mucosa, which consists of epithelium, the lamina propria, and the muscularis mucosa, is the innermost layer, and consequently, it is continuously exposed to digested food and microbiota. On the opposite side, the serosa is associated with the peritoneum and constitutes the gate for extrinsic fibers engraftment onto the GI tract from the central nervous system (CNS). The submucosa layer presents large blood vessels, lymphatics, and connective tissue.

Underneath, the muscularis propria consists of two muscle layers with different orientations separated by the myenteric plexus region, which houses enteric neurons' (ENs) cell bodies [10]. The primary function of the muscularis propria is to regulate the GI contraction needed for a proper movement of food.

Gut tissue-resident macrophages are encountered in all the different layers of the GI tract. However, most gut tissue macrophages are localized in the lamina propria, below the epithelial lining. These macrophages are in a close anatomical relationship with adult tissue stem cells of intestinal crypts, as well as Paneth cells, a specialized cellular population secreting antimicrobial substances to the gut lumen [11]. A second discrete population of macrophages is associated with the submucosal nervous plexus [7]. Because of the massive presence of blood vessels, this anatomical region also represents the door for circulating monocyte entrance onto the underneath muscularis propria.

MMs have a different distribution and morphology within the regions of the muscularis propria. MMs lying in the two muscular layers share an elongated morphology following the muscle orientation. Most MMs are distributed within the myenteric plexus, where they are closely associated with ENs. This population of MMs shares a characteristic morphology with multiple branches originating from the same cell body.

In comparison to the macrophages present in the mucosa, MMs have an overall anti-inflammatory, protective phenotype, as they express CD163, IL10, Mrc1, and Hmox1, all anti-inflammatory genes [7]. In addition, these cells have phagocytic properties and a distinct $CD11c^{low}$ / $MHCII^{high}$ / $CSF\text{-}1R^{high}$ phenotype [8]. In line with other tissue-resident macrophages, colony-stimulating factor-1 (Csf1–1) is critical for their survival and maintenance. In experimental mice models lacking CSF-1R, MMs with $CD11c^{low}$ / $MHCII^{high}$ phenotype is virtually absent, supporting a primary role of CSF-1R in maintaining this macrophage population [12].

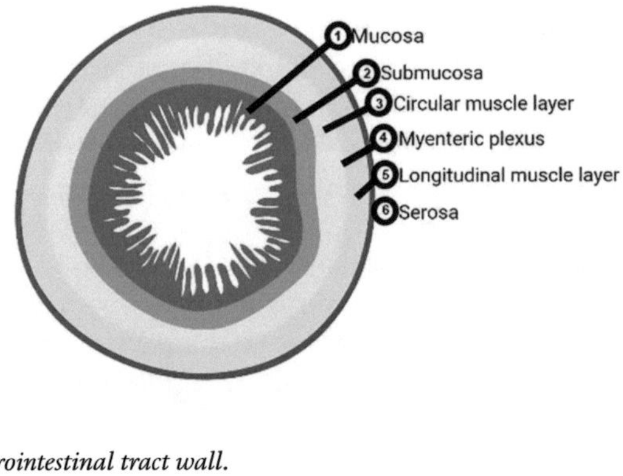

Figure 1.
Different layers of the gastrointestinal tract wall.

Macrophages can also be found in the capillary-rich subserosal connective tissue [13], as well as the mucosa-associated lymphoid tissue (MALT), which includes Peyer's patches [14]. Finally, a layer of macrophages is present within the serosal layer. We have little information regarding these cells' role and function; further studies are needed to elucidate their function in GI homeostasis and diseases. New technologies, such as spatial transcriptomic, will fill the knowledge gap in understanding the phenotypic differences between MMs distributed within the different muscularis propria regions. This information will uncover the specific role of niche-specific macrophages on GI dysfunction and their possible contributions to functional diseases.

3. Origins and natural history of MMs

Like many other tissue-resident macrophages, MMs are heterogeneous. Multiple sequencing approaches identified populations that share a distinct phenotype and function. One of the main factors contributing to such diversity is represented by their origin [2]. The classic hypothesis of macrophages originating from blood monocytes has been recently challenged by the so-called theory of "resident macrophages" [15]. The initial unified hypothesis about tissue macrophages was that monocytes freely circulate in the blood and transmigrate to the tissues under a suitable stimulus, where they acquire a macrophage phenotype [16]. However, we now know that part of tissue-resident macrophages also derives directly from progenitor cells in the fetal liver and yolk sac [2]. For this reason, in most organs, tissue-resident macrophages consist of both embryonic- and monocyte-derived cells. Embryonic macrophages engraft into the tissue during the development phase, and throughout life, these cells are maintained by self-renewing. The latter have a shorter life and continuously invade the tissue to maintain tissue-resident macrophages. The first information regarding a possible alternative origin to circulating monocytes was acquired in the CNS, showing that the tissue-resident macrophages of the CNS originate from precursors presumably located in the yolk sac. These precursors express the CSF-1 receptor and migrate to the liver during embryogenesis. Unlike other tissue macrophage populations [17, 18], the microglial population shares an embryonic origin exclusively.

With the progression of technologies, other studies have shown that in opposition to microglia, the whole pool of tissue-resident macrophages are characterized by the coexistence of monocyte- and embryonic-derived macrophages in other organs, such as the heart, liver, and dermis [19]. Only recently, studies shed light on the dual origin of MMs. Like microglia in the CNS, MMs highly expressed CX3CR1, a tissue-resident cell marker [20]. Using a lineage tracing mouse model, CX3CR1 MMs were followed during the evolutive stages (from embryonic to adulthood) [21]. This population represents tissue-resident MMs at the embryonic stage but rapidly decline in the first weeks after birth. With age, embryonic cells that remain in the tissue are named long-lived MMs and, in concert with circulating monocytes, form tissue-resident MMs [22]. Although a decline in this population during development was observed, the total number of MMs throughout the years is maintained due to the ongoing circulating monocytes' ingress.

It comes without surprise that embryonic and monocyte-derived MMs have different molecular transcriptional profiles. They have two distinct subsets, as demonstrated based on the expression of CX3CR1. The first subset is CX3CR1 high, and the second is CX3CR1 low. The latter also expresses C-C chemokine receptor 2 (CCR2), which significantly regulates monocytic inflammatory response [23]. Also, the close anatomical relationship of MMs with ENs is sustained by the expression of multiple genes related to cellular adhesion, anchoring the cytoskeleton and neuronal development. Not surprisingly, these genes are not expressed by other MMs populations but are also enriched by microglia that are also closely communicating with neurons in the CNS. A non-exhaustive list of these genes includes Apolipoprotein E (ApoE), Fc receptor-like scavenger (FCRLS), Platelet factor 4 (PF4), Cystatin C (CST3), and Disabled-2 (Dab2) [24]. MMs are located within dedicated niches of the muscularis propria. The close interaction of MMs with ENs can be demonstrated by depleting MMs and observing the resulting depletion of ENs [25]. The same can be observed not only in animals but also in human subjects. Bajko et al. investigated the transcriptional molecular profile of macrophages, pointing towards two distinct populations of macrophages, the former deriving from the yolk sac and the latter from monocytes [26]. Those macrophages that survived after embryonic life showed localization into anatomical niches in the same way it had previously been demonstrated in mice [27]. Moreover, several investigators demonstrated tissue-resident macrophages in patients with monocyte deficiency, as in congenital monocytopenia [28].

4. Role of MM-enteric neuron communication in GI motility

4.1 Intrinsic innervation and MMs

The intrinsic and extrinsic sympathetic and parasympathetic neurons innervate the GI tract. The enteric nervous system (ENS) contains more than 100 million neurons and more than 400 million glial cells distributed in thousands of small ganglia that cooperate with the CNS, controlling digestive function [29]. However, the ENS can also control digestive function independently from the CNS. MMs share the space with cells contributing to GI motility, such as interstitial cells of Cajal (ICC), ENs, smooth muscle cells, PDGFRα-expressing cells, and glial cells [30]. In the last 5 years, multiple studies shed light on the functional interactions between MMs with all those different cell types to regulate GI motility. Here, we will describe the novel insights into the intimate communication MMs establish with ENs to control GI motility in health and disease.

From their first discovery, few morphological studies clearly showed the close anatomical association between MMs and ENs. Muller et al. described for the first time the interaction between MMs and ENs functionally [8]. Since then, multiple studies have been performed to elucidate the impact of this interaction on health and disease. This study showed that MMs express morphogenetic protein 2 (BMP2), while ENs express the BMP2 receptor (BMP2r). Functional interaction between BMP2 and BMP2r led to molecular pathway activations via the pSMAB1/5/8 pathway. Microbiome in this type of interaction was also playing a role. It was demonstrated that applying BMP2 to GI tissue in vitro promotes GI motility acceleration. In addition, the depletion of MMs led to colonic dysmotility in both ex vivo and in vivo models [8].

Neurohypophysis, known as the posterior portion of the pituitary gland, releases oxytocin into circulation. This hormone is essential during labor for inducing uterine contractions [31]. In addition, pro-inflammatory MMs can regulate the expression of oxytocin and its receptor. This has been shown in cell cultures of ENs, and the interaction is made possible via the STAT3 or NF-κB pathways. On the other side, anti-inflammatory MMs cause upregulation of oxytocin and its receptor via a TGF-β related mechanism [32]. Interestingly, lower concentrations of oxytocin and its receptor have been associated with more pro-inflammatory cytokines in mouse models of dextran sulfate sodium (DSS) associated colitis [33].

A small population of MMs within the ganglia of the intestines was recently reported. These cells, also known as intra-ganglionic macrophages (IGMs), seem to have phagocytic properties [34]. Although IGMs interact with ENs in the same way as CX3CR1^{high} MMs, there is not enough evidence to support critical phenotypic differences between these two cellular populations. In addition, experimental mice models of induced colitis have demonstrated loss of IGMs in association with increased pro-inflammatory MMs and enteric neural inflammation [35].

An interesting mouse model for the indirect study of MMs-ENs functional communication is Csf1$^{op/op}$. These mice have a genetic lack mutation in the Csf1 gene that results in the absence of tissue macrophages [36]. This mouse model had an abnormal myenteric nervous plexus and more ENs than controls. Interestingly abnormal cellular changes are not confirmed for the other cell types, as both ICC and smooth muscle cells are not changed in the same animal model. MMs potentially also regulate ENs subtypes. For this reason, cholinergic neurons remained unchanged despite the increased numbers of nitrergic ENs [37]. This finding suggested that MMs may be capable of inducing different phenotypes of ENs. Furthermore, we used the same mouse model to find increased neuronal cells with shared cholinergic and nitrergic phenotypes, pointing to a more primitive population of ENs preserved in the adult muscularis propria [38]. Interestingly, this population is enriched during development in wild-type mice but is almost absent in adults. More studies are needed to show the possible contribution of MMs in the maturation of ENs to a specific adult subtype.

In the brain, microglia create an anatomical specialized somatic connection with neurons that facilitate their functional interaction. A concentration of organelles is associated with this connection, favoring the production of substances responsible for the functional interaction via the P2Y1R receptor. Recently a study has shown for the first time the presence of the same receptor on gut MMs and enteric glia, which must be studied further in the future. In addition, similar specialized anatomical connections between MMs, smooth muscle cells, and fibroblast-like cells have been described.

Although most of the studies were focused on the regulation of ENs by MMs, a few reports showed that also macrophage phenotype is shaped by ENs. For example, evidence from the study by Muller et al. showed that ENs supply Csf1 into the anatomic location of the muscularis propria, which in turn has an active role in the homeostasis of MMs, particularly in inducing an anti-inflammatory phenotype [8].

In the CNS, the microglia–neuron interaction happens early during development and is instrumental in setting up the adult brain. Recently, some studies have highlighted a possible role of MMs in the organization of ENS during development. A common finding is the independent intestine colonization by these two distinct cellular populations. In addition, MMs are directed towards specific niches, a particular localization that facilitates connection with the neural processes of ENs [21]. In addition, although Csf1r is mainly expressed in adulthood by ENs, it is primarily expressed by ICC and PDGF receptor alpha-positive cells during development. This result shows that during development, MMs may establish functional interactions with ENs independently of the Csf1 mechanism. Recent findings in a zebrafish irf8-deficient model showed that a lack of irf8 gene expression, typically expressed in MMs, can lead to MMs depletion and impaired gut motility [39].

By regulating membrane properties and ion exchange, ion channels respond to external changes with intracellular biochemical responses. Mounting evidence suggested the central role of ion channels in regulating tissue-resident macrophage functions. For example, in a variety of organs, ion channels contribute to macrophage phenotype, differentiation, and circulating monocyte extravasation. Although mounting evidence suggests the implication of those channels in regulating macrophage homeostasis and function in multiple organs, little is known about their contribution to MMs function.

TRP channels constitute a superfamily of Ca^{2+}-permeable, nonselective cation channels [40]. These channels can respond to temperature, pain, sound, and taste stimuli. Recent studies have highlighted an exciting novel role for these channels in regulating immune cells [41–43].

TRPV4 is expressed preferentially by MMs, and its activation leads to changes in GI motility by producing prostaglandin E2. The release of prostaglandin-2 from activated MMs produced a colonic contraction independently of neuronal activation. This channel may play a role in functional disease conditions. For example, an increase in TRPV4 expression has been reported in the colon of TNBS-treated mice, underlying a possible contribution of this channel to trigger inflammatory mediate the immune response. Notably, administering a selective channel antagonist reduces the severity of the inflammation. In line with this discovery, applying an agonist promotes the severity of inflammation. All this information about the TRPV4 channel is solid evidence of its implication in regulating homeostasis and inflammatory response. Although the mechanism by which this channel is implicated in regulating GI motility has been elucidated, further studies are needed to understand the mechanisms underlying TRPV4 implication in inflammation. The block of the P2X2 receptor channel reduced inflammation-related cellular damage in an IBD mouse model. Recently a study provided the expression of these channels on MMs and enteric glia. P2X2 MMs appeared to be mostly distributed within the myenteric plexus, where they anatomically establish a connection with ENs. Future studies are required to validate these studies and determine the role of this channel in immune-mediated GI function.

4.2 Extrinsic innervation and MMs

Gut-brain axis is made possible through the anatomic framework of visceral sensory (extrinsic afferent), sympathetic, and parasympathetic (efferent/autonomous) innervation. Visceral sensory nerve fibers do not directly regulate intestinal motility. However, they are extremely important for the gut-brain axis connection and regulation of several cells encountered within the ENS [44]. Several studies have suggested a possible physiologic relationship between MMs and peripheral nerves. One example is represented by CX3CR1-positive macrophages, which can be found in close association with nerve fibers of the sympathetic nervous system [45].

The interaction between MMs and visceral sensory fibers has recently been the subject of intensive investigations. More specifically, MMs affect catecholaminergic sympathetic signaling and its impact on systemic immunomodulation [46]. Recently, Gabanyi et al. proposed a role of β-adrenergic receptor 2 (β2AR) in this interaction. MMs expressing β2AR can be found in close anatomical relationship to the cell bodies of ENs. Indeed, MMs express higher levels of this receptor than other types of macrophages, including those of the lamina propria [7]. Furthermore, an effect of post-infectious neuronal loss mediated through adrenergic signaling by β2AR has also been demonstrated [47].

The primary neurotransmitter secreted by the vagus nerve, specifically from its preganglionic fibers, is acetylcholine (ACh). Besides its neurotransmitting role, ACh has essential parts in the inflammation process. This has been demonstrated by experimental models of endotoxin administration, where the subjects showed a reduced inflammatory response after ACh stimulation [48]. In addition, stimulation of the vagus nerve, which is a primary source of ACh signaling increase, has a positive impact on reducing inflammation by promoting an anti-inflammatory MMs activation through the alpha-7-nACh receptor (α7nAChR) [49]. Vagal nerve stimulation is important in the pathophysiology of gastroparesis, enhancing a pro-inflammatory response [50]. The vagus nerve, also known as the tenth cranial nerve, or cranial nerve X, is the longest nerve in the body and one of the major suppliers of parasympathetic innervation to the gut. The vagus nerve originates from two distinct regions of the CNS: the ambiguous nucleus and the dorsal motor nucleus [51]. The multiple effects of vagal innervation on the gut have been well investigated in various studies.

Stimulation of the vagal nerve induces an anti-inflammatory phenotype in MMs. This has been studied in an experimental model of mechanical mucosal stimulation, which reduces overall inflammation. This effect is independent of splenic vagal stimulation since vagal splenic denervation does not hinder MMs activation. It seems that α7nAChR is extremely important in this process since MMs extracted from mice deficient in α7nAChR are unresponsive to vagal nerve stimulation [52–54].

In addition, extrinsic vagus nerve innervation participates in gastric motility regulation. According to preclinical studies, the vagus nerve plays a significant role in ameliorating inflammatory response in Inflammatory Bowel Disease (IBD). Mice with resected vagal nerves can develop a severe form of colitis, resulting in a surge of pro-inflammatory cytokines such as TNF-α, interleukin-1β, and interleukin-6 [55]. MMs from experimental models of genetic or pharmacological sympathetic nerve deprivation display pro-inflammatory phenotype. This MMs phenotypic activation in sympathetic innervation-deprived mice depends partially on monocyte transmigration into the intestinal muscularis propria [56].

As a consequence of an overall increase in inflammation, the same mouse models experienced an acceleration of GI transit. As discussed below, manual manipulation of the gut during surgery is implicated in the induction of postoperative ileus, a condition associated with increased levels of macrophages with anti-inflammatory phenotype [57]. It seems that severe forms of IBD frequently arise in patients with clinical depression or a setting of severe psychological stress. Although most research has been performed in humans, experimental animal models of depression exist, and it has been shown that they are more susceptible to developing severe colitis [58]. Notably, a post-vagotomy status can diminish any benefit from administering antidepressant medications. Through an unclear mechanism, transferring macrophages from experimental animal models of depression induces a trait in the recipient mice, which can become much more susceptible to severe forms of colitis [59].

Stimulation of the vagal nerve has important implications in gastroparesis, a disease we will discuss in detail below. Briefly, gastroparesis is characterized by reduced gastric motility and an enhanced pro-inflammatory phenotype in MMs. In addition, vagal nerve stimulation induces anti-inflammatory MMs activation, which improves overall clinical symptoms [60].

The induction of anti-inflammatory MMs underlines the preventive role of vagal nerve stimulation in gastroparesis by the STAT3-JAK2 molecular signaling pathway [61]. In contrast, pro-inflammatory MMs induction occurs during and after abdominal surgery, leading to increased inflammation of muscularis propria and reduced gastric and intestinal mobility. This situation can be regulated by performing vagal nerve stimulation [50]. Furthermore, optogenetic manipulation of colonic sympathetic nerves reduces leukocyte recruitment, favoring a recovery from induced experimental colitis.

5. MMs and GI diseases

Because of the intimate interaction which MMs establish with ENs and other cells required for GI motility, it comes without surprise that these cells are implicated in various pathologic conditions impairing GI motility. Therefore, we will describe below different pathological conditions where an implication of MMs has been described.

5.1 Gastrointestinal inflammation

Inflammatory bowel disease (IBD) is a disorder characterized by inflammation of the GI tract. Because of this inflammation, the muscularis propria undergoes tissue changes, such as smooth muscle hypertrophy and plexitis of the ENs. The gut microbiota functions as a continuous reserve of bacterial antigens. Due to their anatomical association, these microorganisms continuously activate lamina propria macrophages, preventing them from becoming tolerant during sustained inflammatory conditions [62]. MMs activation depends on pathogen-associate molecular patterns (PAMPs) in the post-operated gut [63]. Although Toll-like receptors usually recognize PAMPs, an event which is crucial in further mediation of the innate immune response [64], postoperative gut hypomotility, also known as postoperative ileus, does not directly depend on Toll-like receptor pathways, but on interleukin-1 upstream receptor (IL-1R1) [65].

In experimental mouse models, expression of IL-1R1 by enteric glial cells is associated with co-expression, among others, of the proinflammatory cytokine interleukin-6. Therefore, it is not surprising that the administration of anakinra, a potent IL-1R1 antagonist, reduced inflammation and the occurrence of postoperative ileus in these animals [65]. Given that interleukin-17 positively regulates inducible nitric oxide synthase (iNOS) expression by MMs, it seems reasonable that gut motility can be impaired following an interleukin-17 surplus in the gut microenvironment [66]. A resulting hypomotility contrasts with clinical symptoms of bacterial GI infections, which normally are intestinal hypermotility and episodes of diarrhea. In rat animal models of IBD, MMs within the myenteric nervous plexus are responsible for the persistent inflammatory condition underlying the pathogenesis of the disease [67].

Inflammation is generally associated with increased monocyte recruitment onto the muscularis propria. In one recent study, during inflammation, monocyte recruitment is promoted by enteric glia that expresses multiple genes potentially responsible for monocyte engraftment onto the muscularis. In addition, in the presence of enteric glia supernatant, bone marrow-derived macrophages induce macrophage activation to an anti-inflammatory phenotype. This finding was confirmed in-vivo, where tamoxifen-induced enteric glial removal reduced monocyte recruitment responsible for the anti-inflammatory protective CD206 MMs. However, this leads to an increased overall level of inflammation in the tissue. Also, a functional interaction in the opposite direction seems true. IL1B, a proinflammatory marker, induces the activation of enteric glia to an "activated state" called gliosis. Importantly conditional removal of Il1BR in ECC prevents MMs activation in POI.

Interestingly, this is in line with similar observations on astrocytes in the CNS, cells that have a similar function to EGC. Recently, another group proposed a new route for monocyte recruitment during inflammation. After damage, large peritoneal macrophages are recruited from the serosal side and participate in tissue repair via ATP. Until now, the immediate and unique access for monocytes onto the muscularis propria was considered the submucosa region where big blood vessels are present.

5.2 Gastroparesis

Gastroparesis is a significant motility GI disorder characterized by delayed emptying without obvious etiopathogenic factors [13]. Gastroparesis is commonly seen in patients with diabetes mellitus (DM), with a prevalence of approximately 40% in type 1 DM and 20% in type 2 DM. Given the prevalence of DM in the general population, gastroparesis is a prevalent condition, leading to increased patient morbidity and socioeconomic costs [68]. Other conditions predisposing to the development of gastroparesis are surgical operations of the stomach or esophagus. However, in a significant subset of patients, the condition can be idiopathic, meaning no apparent predisposing factor can be identified [13].

The clinical signs and symptoms of gastroparesis vary. Patients often present with GI symptoms such as bloating, postprandial fullness, reduced food intake, nausea and vomiting, and weight loss, which can be evident at later stages [69]. The condition is frustrating for patients, severely affecting their quality of life, and is associated with concomitant anxiety or clinical depression symptoms in as many as half of them [70]. Gastroparesis has also been associated with reduced survival of patients. In a significant cohort of patients with gastroparesis, the 5-year overall survival of patients with DG, adjusted for age and gender, was 67%, in contrast to 81% in the non-gastroparesis population [70]. Patients with idiopathic gastroparesis had slightly better outcomes than patients with diabetic gastroparesis (DG). This finding can be explained by the increased co-morbidities that can be seen in patients suffering from DM [70].

The underlying mechanisms responsible for DG have long been unclear until recent evidence suggested a significant role of MMs in the pathophysiology of this condition. In mouse models and patients with DG, a reduction of CD206, anti-inflammatory MMs has been observed compared to controls. In addition to reduced anti-inflammatory MMs, DG has been associated with more pro-inflammatory markers, normally absent in controls. Therefore, this series of studies highlighted the possible role of MMs activation in the pathophysiology of DG. It is crucial to notice that in vitro experiments identified MMs activation via oxidative stress as one of the possible causes. Increased oxidative stress levels, generally associated with DG-induced activation of MMs to a pro-inflammatory phenotype and combination of IL6 and TNF-alpha, lead to ICC reduction in vitro.

Further studies are required to understand the underlying mechanisms driving immune-mediated ICC loss in DG, which represent the main cellular changes observed in DG. Neshatian et al. showed that the phenotype of MMs could be altered in response to DM-induced tissue oxidative stress [68]. More specifically, activated MMs produce heme oxygenase-1 (HO1), which has an important anti-oxidative role, protecting against the development of gastroparesis in experimental models of diabetic mice. In contrast, neuromuscular depletion can occur secondary to the activation of those MMs that cannot produce HO1 [68]. This can severely impact gastric motility, acting as a prerequisite for developing gastroparesis [68]. Further evidence has shown that in an experimental model of diabetic mice, the depletion of MMs reduced the incidence of the development of DG [71].

5.3 Post operative ileus

Post operative ileus (POI) is a very common condition, which can be described as a transient decreased GI motility condition following abdominal surgery. This results in prolonged hospitalization and recovery time, reducing patient quality of life and increasing healthcare expenditure. Although the pathophysiology of POI is complex, it seems to be arising in a background of neurogenic and inflammatory deregulation, mediated by corticotropin-releasing factor, which promotes central and autonomic nervous system response [72]. The resulting inflammatory response is characterized by sustained expression of intercellular adhesion molecule-1 (ICAM-1) and P-selectin, which both facilitate circulating monocyte extravasation [73]. This is further supported by experimental evidence, demonstrating that targeting of the adhesion molecules by monoclonal antibodies leads to reduction of transmigrating white blood cells and attenuating muscle contractility dysfunction [74]. Neurogenic dysregulation can be experimentally prevented by activation of 5-hydroxytryptamine receptor-4 (5HT4R) and reduction of nicotinic receptor activation. This happens mostly during vagus nerve stimulation, since activation of cannabinoid receptors (CB) in cholinergic neurons inhibits acetylcholine release and reduces gut motility, leading to delayed gastric emptying. These findings are supported by experimental findings using CB1 −/− mice. Although POI and systemic inflammation were noted both in wild-type and CB1 −/− mice, the latter had higher plasma levels of interleukin-6 (IL-6) and cytokine-induced neutrophil chemoattractant-1 (KC/CINC1) in gut mucosal and submucosal tissues [75]. Mast cells also contribute to the development of POI with a variety of mechanisms, including degranulation induced by neurotransmitters released in response to gut surgical manipulation and mechanical stretch. The exacerbation of gastroparesis by mast cell degranulation can be partially alleviated by mast-cell stabilizing treatments [76]. As mast cells express Kit, experiments in mast cell deficient Kit / Kitv mice showed that gut manipulation did not result in significant increase in transmigration of white blood cells [77]. Moreover, mice with abnormal Kit also have deficits in the ICC, which explains the impaired gut mobility even without surgical manipulation [78]. The above findings demonstrate the multifactorial background of development of POI, warranting further investigation on the role of MPMs in POI.

5.4 Aging-associated dysmotility

Life expectancy is increasing progressively, and some GI diseases are more prevalent in the elderly. Old people have a slower gastric emptying that can affect appetite regulation. This usually represents an underrecognized clinical problem that may lead to adverse life quality and increased mortality. Most GI dysmotility problems in the elderly happen in the colon, where region-specific changes to enteric neuron numbers have been observed in both mice and humans. This is in line with changes observed in neuronal-mediated smooth muscle contractility. Since a smooth muscle contractility pattern is required for an effective GI transit, those changes may reflect gastrointestinal motility disorders in the elderly. Like many other different cell types, macrophages are affected by time by changing their transcriptome, functions, and phenotype. Changes to the macrophage population observed in aging may underline the tissue changes associated with diseases. For example, multiple reports show the central role of microglia in brain tissue changes related to Alzheimer's disease and other aging associated brain diseases [79]. Also, in the gut, recent changes to MMs have been reported in humans and mice that could be underlying GI motility changes in the elderly. A recent characterization of MMs phenotype in old mice showed an increased MMs subpopulation that expresses pro-inflammatory genes [80]. Notably, the accumulation of this population is contracted within the myenteric plexus, where they co-localized with the A-Synuclein marker, suggesting that they may play a role in phagocyting. Lineage tracing experiments to study the origin of tissue-resident MMs revealed that also, with age, the number of protective CX3CR1 MMs are reduced. The remaining CX3CR1 are accumulated within the myenteric plexus where they continue to interact with ENs. Further studies are needed to understand the underlying mechanism responsible for this type of reduction, given the role of embryonic MMs in preserving GI homeostasis.

6. Concluding remarks

This chapter highlights the role of MMs in health and disease. In summary, MMs are part of tissue-resident macrophages in the gut, having a dual origin from monocytes and embryonic macrophages, that colonize tissues and persist after birth [22]. MMs are localized in close anatomical relationship to the ICC, which form part of the enteric ENS [30]. The interaction between MMs and ENs is important in regulating gut peristalsis in health and disease [8]. An inflammatory component also mediates the interaction mentioned above, as proven by experimental evidence, which shows that loss of MMs can induce a neuroinflammatory response in the gut [35]. Extrinsic innervation by the vagus nerve plays an important role in regulating acetylcholine signaling [44] and counterbalancing sympathetic neuro-inflammatory interaction [42]. Finally, recent experimental evidence has illustrated the paramount importance of MMs as intermediate factors in motility disorders of the gastrointestinal tract, such as gastroparesis [13], post-operative ileus [72] and intestinal ischemia–reperfusion injury [13], leading to interesting etiopathogenic and treatment-implicative considerations.

Author details

Magdalini Mischopoulou and Gianluca Cipriani*
Department of Medicine, Division of Gastroenterology, Enteric Neuroscience Program, Mayo Clinic, United States of America

*Address all correspondence to: gianluca.cipriani@mayo.edu

References

[1] Ovchinnikov DA. Macrophages in the embryo and beyond: Much more than just giant phagocytes. Genesis. 2008;**46**:447-462

[2] Ginhoux F, Jung S. Monocytes and macrophages: Developmental pathways and tissue homeostasis. Nature Reviews. Immunology. 2014;**14**:392-404

[3] Rumessen JJ, Thuneberg L, Mikkelsen HB. Plexus muscularis profundus and associated interstitial cells. II. Ultrastructural studies of mouse small intestine. The Anatomical Record. 1982;**203**:129-146

[4] Mikkelsen HB, Thuneberg L, Rumessen JJ, Thorball N. Macrophage-like cells in the muscularis externa of mouse small intestine. The Anatomical Record. 1985;**213**:77-86

[5] Mikkelsen HB. Macrophages in the external muscle layers of mammalian intestines. Histology and Histopathology. 1995;**10**:719-736

[6] Bain CC, Mowat AM. Macrophages in intestinal homeostasis and inflammation. Immunological Reviews. 2014;**260**:102-117

[7] Gabanyi I, Muller PA, Feighery L, Oliveira TY, Costa-Pinto FA, Mucida D. Neuro-immune interactions drive tissue programming in intestinal macrophages. Cell. 2016;**164**:378-391

[8] Muller PA, Koscsó B, Rajani GM, Stevanovic K, Berres ML, Hashimoto D, et al. Crosstalk between muscularis macrophages and enteric neurons regulates gastrointestinal motility. Cell. 2014;**158**:300-313

[9] Gordon S, Plüddemann A, Martinez EF. Macrophage heterogeneity in tissues: Phenotypic diversity and functions. Immunological Reviews. 2014;**262**:36-55

[10] Mescher AL. Junqueira's Basic Histology Text & Atlas. Fifteenth ed. New York City: McGraw-Hill Education; 2018

[11] Peterson LW, Artis D. Intestinal epithelial cells: Regulators of barrier function and immune homeostasis. Nature Reviews. Immunology. 2014;**14**:141-153

[12] Koscsó B, Gowda K, Schell TD, Bogunovic M. Purification of dendritic cell and macrophage subsets from the normal mouse small intestine. Journal of Immunological Methods. 2015;**421**:1-13

[13] De Schepper S, Stakenborg N, Matteoli G, Verheijden S, Boeckxstaens GE. Muscularis macrophages: Key players in intestinal homeostasis and disease. Cellular Immunology. 2018;**330**:142-150

[14] Bonnardel J, Da Silva C, Henri S, Tamoutounour S, Chasson L, Montañana-Sanchis F, et al. Innate and adaptive immune functions of peyer's patch monocyte-derived cells. Cell Reports. 2015;**11**:770-784

[15] Cerovic V, Bain CC, Mowat AM, Milling SW. Intestinal macrophages and dendritic cells: what's the difference? Trends in Immunology. 2014;**35**:270-277

[16] Yáñez A, Bono C, Goodridge HS. Heterogeneity and origins of myeloid cells. Current Opinion in Hematology. 2022;**29**:201-208

[17] Gomez Perdiguero E, Schulz C, Geissmann F. Development and homeostasis of “resident” myeloid

cells: The case of the microglia. Glia. 2013;**61**:112-120

[18] Kaur C, Hao AJ, Wu CH, Ling EA. Origin of microglia. Microscopy Research and Technique. 2001;**54**:2-9

[19] Gomez Perdiguero E, Klapproth K, Schulz C, Busch K, Azzoni E, Crozet L, et al. Tissue-resident macrophages originate from yolk-sac-derived erythro-myeloid progenitors. Nature. 2015;**518**:547-551

[20] Waisman A, Ginhoux F, Greter M, Bruttger J. Homeostasis of microglia in the adult brain: Review of novel microglia depletion systems. Trends in Immunology. 2015;**36**:625-636

[21] Verheijden S, De Schepper S, Boeckxstaens GE. Neuron-macrophage crosstalk in the intestine: A "microglia" perspective. Frontiers in Cellular Neuroscience. 2015;**9**:403

[22] De Schepper S, Verheijden S, Aguilera-Lizarraga J, Viola MF, Boesmans W, Stakenborg N, et al. Self-maintaining gut macrophages are essential for intestinal homeostasis. Cell. 2018;**175**:400-15.e13

[23] Bain CC, Scott CL, Uronen-Hansson H, Gudjonsson S, Jansson O, Grip O, et al. Resident and pro-inflammatory macrophages in the colon represent alternative context-dependent fates of the same Ly6Chi monocyte precursors. Mucosal Immunology. 2013;**6**:498-510

[24] Domanska D, Majid U, Karlsen VT, Merok MA, Beitnes AR, Yaqub S, et al. Single-cell transcriptomic analysis of human colonic macrophages reveals niche-specific subsets. The Journal of Experimental Medicine. 2022;**219**:e20211846

[25] Meroni E, Stakenborg N, Viola MF, Boeckxstaens GE. Intestinal macrophages and their interaction with the enteric nervous system in health and inflammatory bowel disease. Acta Physiologica (Oxford, England). 2019;**225**:e13163

[26] Bujko A, Atlasy N, Landsverk OJB, Richter L, Yaqub S, Horneland R, et al. Transcriptional and functional profiling defines human small intestinal macrophage subsets. The Journal of Experimental Medicine. 2018;**215**:441-458

[27] Sreejit G, Fleetwood AJ, Murphy AJ, Nagareddy PR. Origins and diversity of macrophages in health and disease. Clinical Translational Immunology. 2020;**9**:e1222

[28] Bigley V, Haniffa M, Doulatov S, Wang XN, Dickinson R, McGovern N, et al. The human syndrome of dendritic cell, monocyte, B and NK lymphoid deficiency. The Journal of Experimental Medicine. 2011;**208**:227-234

[29] Dowling LR, Strazzari MR, Keely S, Kaiko GE. Enteric nervous system and intestinal epithelial regulation of the gut-brain axis. The Journal of Allergy and Clinical Immunology. 2022;**150**:513-522

[30] Chanpong A, Borrelli O, Thapar N. Recent advances in understanding the roles of the enteric nervous system. Factory Review. 2022;**11**:7

[31] Hall JE. Guyton and Hall Textbook of Medical Physiology. Thirteenth ed. Amsterdam: Elsevier Health Sciences; 2015

[32] Shi Y, Li S, Zhang H, Zhu J, Che T, Yan B, et al. The effect of macrophage polarization on the expression of the oxytocin signalling system in enteric neurons. Journal of Neuroinflammation. 2021;**18**:261

[33] Welch MG, Tamir H, Gross KJ, Chen J, Anwar M, Gershon MD.

Expression and developmental regulation of oxytocin (OT) and oxytocin receptors (OTR) in the enteric nervous system (ENS) and intestinal epithelium. The Journal of Comparative Neurology. 2009;**512**:256-270

[34] Dora D, Arciero E, Hotta R, Barad C, Bhave S, Kovacs T, et al. Intraganglionic macrophages: A new population of cells in the enteric ganglia. Journal of Anatomy. 2018;**233**:401-410

[35] Dora D, Ferenczi S, Stavely R, Toth VE, Varga ZV, Kovacs T, et al. Evidence of a myenteric plexus barrier and its macrophage-dependent degradation during murine colitis: Implications in enteric Neuroinflammation. Cellular and Molecular Gastroenterology and Hepatology. 2021;**12**:1617-1641

[36] Banaei-Bouchareb L, Gouon-Evans V, Samara-Boustani D, Castellotti MC, Czernichow P, Pollard JW, et al. Insulin cell mass is altered in Csf1op/Csf1op macrophage-deficient mice. Journal of Leukocyte Biology. 2004;**76**:359-367

[37] Cipriani G, Gibbons SJ, Miller KE, Yang DS, Terhaar ML, Eisenman ST, et al. Change in populations of macrophages promotes development of delayed gastric emptying in mice. Gastroenterology. 2018;**154**:2122-36.e12

[38] Cipriani G, Terhaar ML, Eisenman ST, Ji S, Linden DR, Wright AM, et al. Muscularis Propria macrophages Alter the proportion of Nitrergic but not cholinergic gastric myenteric neurons. Cellular and Molecular Gastroenterology and Hepatology. 2019;7:689-91.e4

[39] Graves CL, Chen A, Kwon V, Shiau CE. Zebrafish harbor diverse intestinal macrophage populations including a subset intimately associated with enteric neural processes. iScience. 2021;**24**:102496

[40] Wu LJ, Sweet TB, Clapham DE. International Union of Basic and Clinical Pharmacology. LXXVI. Current progress in the mammalian TRP ion channel family. Pharmacological Reviews. 2010;**62**:381-404. DOI: 10.1124/pr.110.002725

[41] Inada H, Iida T, Tominaga M. Different expression patterns of TRP genes in murine B and T lymphocytes. Biochemical and Biophysical Research Communications. 2006;**350**:762-767

[42] Parenti A, De Logu F, Geppetti P, Benemei S. What is the evidence for the role of TRP channels in inflammatory and immune cells? British Journal of Pharmacology. 2016;**173**:953-969

[43] Froghi S, Grant CR, Tandon R, Quaglia A, Davidson B, Fuller B. New insights on the role of TRP channels in calciumsignallingandimmunomodulation: Review of pathways and implications for clinical practice. Clinical Reviews in Allergy and Immunology. 2021;**60**:271-292

[44] Schneider KM, Kim J, Bahnsen K, Heuckeroth RO, Thaiss CA. Environmental perception and control of gastrointestinal immunity by the enteric nervous system. Trends in Molecular Medicine. 2022;**28**:989-1005

[45] Blaszkiewicz M, Gunsch G, Willows JW, Gardner ML, Sepeda JA, Sas AR, et al. Adipose tissue myeloid-lineage Neuroimmune cells express genes important for neural plasticity and regulate adipose innervation. Frontiers in Endocrinology (Lausanne). 2022;**13**:864925

[46] Mallesh S, Ten Hove AS, Schneider R, Schneiker B, Efferz P, Kalff JC, et al. Sympathetic innervation modulates mucosal immune homeostasis and epithelial host Defense. Cell. 2022;**11**:2606

[47] Matheis F, Muller PA, Graves CL, Gabanyi I, Kerner ZJ, Costa-Borges D, et al. Adrenergic Signaling in Muscularis macrophages limits infection-induced neuronal loss. Cell. 2020;**180**:64-78.e16

[48] Hoover DB. Cholinergic modulation of the immune system presents new approaches for treating inflammation. Pharmacology & Therapeutics. 2017;**179**:1-16

[49] Zhou L, Zheng LF, Zhang XL, Wang ZY, Yao YS, Xiu XL, et al. Activation of α7nAChR protects against gastric inflammation and Dysmotility in Parkinson's disease rats. Frontiers in Pharmacology. 2021;**12**:793374

[50] Yuan PQ, Taché Y. Abdominal surgery induced gastric ileus and activation of M1-like macrophages in the gastric myenteric plexus: Prevention by central vagal activation in rats. American Journal of Physiology. Gastrointestinal and Liver Physiology. 2017;**313**:G320-G3g9

[51] Standring S, Ellis H, Healy J, Johnson D, Williams A, Collins P, et al. Gray's anatomy: The anatomical basis of clinical practice. American Journal of Neuroradiology. 2005;**26**:2703

[52] Matteoli G, Boeckxstaens GE. The vagal innervation of the gut and immune homeostasis. Gut. 2013;**62**:1214-1222

[53] Matteoli G, Gomez-Pinilla PJ, Nemethova A, Di Giovangiulio M, Cailotto C, van Bree SH, et al. A distinct vagal anti-inflammatory pathway modulates intestinal muscularis resident macrophages independent of the spleen. Gut. 2014;**63**:938-948

[54] Mischopoulou M, D'Ambrosio M, Bigagli E, Luceri C, Farrugia G, Cipriani G. Role of macrophages and mast cells as key players in the maintenance of gastrointestinal smooth muscle homeostasis and disease. Cellular and Molecular Gastroenterology and Hepatology. 2022;**13**:1849-1862

[55] Ghia JE, Blennerhassett P, Collins SM. Vagus nerve integrity and experimental colitis. American Journal of Physiology. Gastrointestinal and Liver Physiology. 2007;**293**:G560-G567

[56] Willemze RA, Welting O, van Hamersveld P, Verseijden C, Nijhuis LE, Hilbers FW, et al. Loss of intestinal sympathetic innervation elicits an innate immune driven colitis. Molecular Medicine. 2019;**25**:1

[57] Kalff JC, Schraut WH, Simmons RL, Bauer AJ. Surgical manipulation of the gut elicits an intestinal muscularis inflammatory response resulting in postsurgical ileus. Annals of Surgery. 1998;**228**:652-663

[58] Ghia JE, Blennerhassett P, Deng Y, Verdu EF, Khan WI, Collins SM. Reactivation of inflammatory bowel disease in a mouse model of depression. Gastroenterology 2009;136:2280-8.e1-4.

[59] Ghia JE, Park AJ, Blennerhassett P, Khan WI, Collins SM. Adoptive transfer of macrophage from mice with depression-like behavior enhances susceptibility to colitis. Inflammatory Bowel Diseases. 2011;**17**:1474-1489

[60] Goyal RK, Cristofaro V, Sullivan MP. Rapid gastric emptying in diabetes mellitus: Pathophysiology and clinical importance. Journal of Diabetes and its Complications. 2019;**33**:107414

[61] de Jonge WJ, van der Zanden EP, The FO, Bijlsma MF, van Westerloo DJ, Bennink RJ, et al. Stimulation of the vagus nerve attenuates macrophage activation by activating the Jak2-STAT3 signaling pathway. Nature Immunology. 2005;**6**:844-851

[62] Wehner S, Engel DR. Resident macrophages in the healthy and inflamed intestinal muscularis externa. Pflügers Archiv. 2017;**469**:541-552

[63] Kim OY, Monsel A, Bertrand M, Cavaillon JM, Coriat P, Adib-Conquy M. Translocation of bacterial NOD2 agonist and its link with inflammation. Critical Care. 2009;**13**:R124

[64] Kawasaki T, Kawai T. Toll-like receptor signaling pathways. Frontiers in Immunology. 2014;**5**:461

[65] Stoffels B, Hupa KJ, Snoek SA, van Bree S, Stein K, Schwandt T, et al. Postoperative ileus involves interleukin-1 receptor signaling in enteric glia. Gastroenterology. 2014;**146**:176-87.e1

[66] Mori D, Watanabe N, Kaminuma O, Murata T, Hiroi T, Ozaki H, et al. IL-17A induces hypo-contraction of intestinal smooth muscle via induction of iNOS in muscularis macrophages. Journal of Pharmacological Sciences. 2014;**125**:394-405

[67] Kinoshita K, Horiguchi K, Fujisawa M, Kobirumaki F, Yamato S, Hori M, et al. Possible involvement of muscularis resident macrophages in impairment of interstitial cells of Cajal and myenteric nerve systems in rat models of TNBS-induced colitis. Histochemistry and Cell Biology. 2007;**127**:41-53

[68] Neshatian L, Gibbons SJ, Farrugia G. Macrophages in diabetic gastroparesis--the missing link? Neurogastroenterology and Motility. 2015;**27**:7-18

[69] Bharucha AE, Kudva YC, Prichard DO. Diabetic gastroparesis. Endocrine Reviews. 2019;**40**:1318-1352

[70] Jung HK, Choung RS, Locke GR 3rd, Schleck CD, Zinsmeister AR, Szarka LA, et al. The incidence, prevalence, and outcomes of patients with gastroparesis in Olmsted County, Minnesota, from 1996 to 2006. Gastroenterology. 2009;**136**:1225-1233

[71] Cipriani G, Gibbons SJ, Verhulst PJ, Choi KM, Eisenman ST, Hein SS, et al. Diabetic Csf1(op/op) mice lacking macrophages are protected against the development of delayed gastric emptying. Cellular and Molecular Gastroenterology and Hepatology. 2016;**2**:40-47

[72] Wells CI, Milne TGE, Seo SHB, Chapman SJ, Vather R, Bissett IP, et al. Post-operative ileus: Definitions, mechanisms and controversies. ANZ Journal of Surgery. 2022;**92**:62-68

[73] Hussain Z, Park H. Inflammation and impaired gut physiology in post-operative ileus: Mechanisms and the treatment options. Journal of Neurogastroenterology Motility. 2022;**28**:517-530

[74] Dustin ML. Integrins and their role in immune cell adhesion. Cell. 2019;**177**:499-501

[75] Kalff JC, Carlos TM, Schraut WH, Billiar TR, Simmons RL, Bauer AJ. Surgically induced leukocytic infiltrates within the rat intestinal muscularis mediate postoperative ileus. Gastroenterology. 1999;**117**:378-387

[76] Li YY, Cao MH, Goetz B, Chen CQ, Feng YJ, Chen CJ, et al. The dual effect of cannabinoid receptor-1 deficiency on the murine postoperative ileus. PLoS One. 2013;**8**:e67427

[77] de Jonge WJ, The FO, van der Coelen D, Bennink RJ, Reitsma PH, van Deventer SJ, et al. Mast cell degranulation during abdominal surgery initiates postoperative ileus in mice. Gastroenterology. 2004;**127**:535-545

[78] Gomez-Pinilla PJ, Farro G, Di Giovangiulio M, Stakenborg N, Némethova A, de Vries A, et al. Mast cells play no role in the pathogenesis of postoperative ileus induced by intestinal manipulation. PLoS One. 2014;**9**:e85304

[79] Shimojima N, Nakaki T, Morikawa Y, Hoshino K, Ozaki H, Hori M, et al. Interstitial cells of Cajal in dysmotility in intestinal ischemia and reperfusion injury in rats. The Journal of Surgical Research. 2006;**135**:255-261

[80] Yoo HJ, Kwon MS. Aged microglia in neurodegenerative diseases: Microglia lifespan and culture methods. Frontiers in Aging Neuroscience. 2022;**13**:766267

Chapter 7

Non-Myeloid Cell Phagocytosis

Ben A. Calvert and Amy L. Ryan

Abstract

As professional phagocytes, myeloid cells, including macrophages, dendritic cells, and neutrophils, are often the targets for investigation and analysis of phagocytosis. Phagocytosis, however, has also been observed in nonmyeloid cells, including epithelium, mesenchymal, and smooth muscle cells. Colloquially known as nonprofessional phagocytes, these nonmyeloid cells are capable of phagocytosis of pathogenic material and efferocytosis of apoptotic bodies. Cells, such as those found in the epithelium, are often the primary site for viral and bacterial infection and have evolved to possess strong anti-pathogenic machinery of their own. The processes by which nonmyeloid cells can engage in phagocytic functions have wide implications for tissue homeostasis and disease pathogenesis, including infection and colonization. This chapter will review the phagocytosis capabilities in these nonmyeloid cells.

Keywords: efferocytosis, epithelial cells, internalization, barrier, nonprofessional, opsonization, trigger phagocytosis, zipper phagocytosis

1. Introduction

As professional phagocytes, myeloid cells, including neutrophils, macrophages, monocytes, mast cells, and dendritic cells, are actively recruited to sites of tissue damage, infection, and inflammation playing a key role in host defense [1]. Of these, neutrophils and macrophages are perhaps the most widely studied in terms of their roles in phagocytosis [2–4]. However, there is increasing evidence that nonmyeloid cells, including epithelial [5, 6] endothelial [7–9], mesenchymal [7, 10–12], and smooth muscle cells [13–16], can also engage in phagocytosis, or phagocytic-like mechanisms when phagocytosis is not their principal function. Phagocytosis by nonprofessional phagocytes is often referred to as internalization or even cannibalism, especially in the case of efferocytosis of apoptotic neighboring cells [17]. Nonprofessional phagocytes were first distinguished from professional phagocytes as early as 1970 after Rabinovitch demonstrated particulate uptake in fibroblasts [18, 19], although reports had demonstrated particulate uptake in nonmyeloid cells almost 40 years prior [20]. Since this initial observation, many nonprofessional phagocytes have been identified to have the phagocytic capacity and the capacity to clear potentially dangerous pathogens [21]. **Table 1** includes a summary of these cell types and the roles that they have been observed to play in phagocytosis. Compared to professional phagocytes, nonmyeloid cells engage in distinctively different

Nonmyeloid cell	Cell subtype	Phagocytosis	Key findings	Ref'
Epithelial	Hu. respiratory	Pathogen clearance	*P.aeruginosa* internalization is independent of CFTR expression.	[22]
	Hu. bladder, lung, ileocecal	Pathogen clearance	Involvement of an N-glycosylated protein receptor required for internalization.	[23]
	Hu. T84 monkey kidney	Pathogen clearance	Ineffective phagolysosome maturation in epithelium.	[24]
	MDCK, Hu. 16HBE14o-	Pathogen clearance *via* efferocytosis	*P.aeruginosa* internalized *via* efferocytosis of apoptotic cells.	[25]
	Hu. A549	Pathogen clearance	Containment of pathogen colonization by epithelium.	[26]
	Hu. A549	Pathogen clearance	Less efficient than professional phagocytes.	[27]
	CHO cells	Pathogen clearance	Heparin/Heparan-dependent internalization of pathogen.	[28]
	Ms. mammary	Efferocytosis	Receptor mediated engulfment *via* PSR, CD36, vitronectin receptor alpha vbeta3, and CD91.	[29]
	Hu. BEAS-2B Ms. HBEC Ms. MLE-12	Efferocytosis	Uptake induces anti-inflammatory cytokine release *via* Rac1.	[30]
	Hu. Thymus	Efferocytosis	Uptake relies on PSR and SR-B1.	[31]
	Rt. bladder	Efferocytosis	Epithelial clearance of erythrocytes	[32]
	Hu. hepatic biliary	Efferocytosis	PSR-mediated clearance results in chemokine increase.	[33]
	Hu. A549	Efferocytosis	Receptor-mediated recognition of apoptotic bodies.	[34]
	Rt. Kidney	Efferocytosis	KIM-1 recognition internalizes apoptotic bodies.	[35]
	CHO cells	Efferocytosis	LOX-1 recognition of apoptotic bodies.	[36]
	Ms. retinal pigment	Efferocytosis	Role of ABCF1 recognition in apoptotic bodies.	[37]
	Ms. HBEC	Efferocytosis	Efferocytosis by epithelium avoids IL-33-mediated inflammation.	[38]
	Hu. ARPE-19	Efferocytosis	Increased efficiency over macrophages in apoptotic clearance.	[39]
	Ms. follicular	Efferocytosis	Clearance of apoptotic neighboring cells.	[40]
	Ms. colonic	Efferocytosis	Role for BAI-1 mediated uptake in controlling inflammation.	[41]
	Ms. retinal	Phagocytosis (Photo receptor material)	Gas6 & Protein S ligands for TAM-mediated phagocytosis.	[42]

DOI: http://dx.doi.org/10.5772/intechopen.110583

Nonmyeloid cell	Cell subtype	Phagocytosis	Key findings	Ref'
Endothelial	Hu. vascular	Pathogen clearance	Rho kinase in endothelial cells bind listeria and internalization mediated by formins.	[43]
	Ms. Hepatic sinusoidal	Efferocytosis	IL-1 enhanced scavenging of apoptotic bodies.	[44]
	Ms. Endothelium	Efferocytosis	SCARF1 mediated clearance of apoptotic bodies.	[45]
	Bovine Aortic	Efferocytosis	LOX-1 recognition of apoptotic bodies.	[36]
	Hu. umbilical vein	Phagocytosis platelet clearance	PS recognition on platelets-mediated phagocytosis.	[46]
	Ms. (brain) microvascular	Phagocytosis myelin clearance	IgG opsonization is required for endothelial cell clearance, inducing endothelial-mesenchymal transition.	[47]
Mesenchymal	Hu. MRC5 cells	Pathogen clearance	Actin-dependent uptake. LAMP-1 mediated phagolysosome maturation.	[27]
	Hamster embryonic fibroblasts	Pathogen clearance Efferocytosis	ConA-dependent zipper phagocytosis.	[48]
	Ms. ESCs	Efferocytosis	Inefficient (relative to macrophages) but effective clearance of apoptotic bodies.	[11]
	Hu. BM-MSCs	Efferocytosis	Observation of mesenchymal stem cell efferocytosis enhancing inflammation.	[10]
Smooth muscle	Hu. vascular	Efferocytosis	PS-PSR mediated phagocytosis.	[16]
	Pigeon vascular	Phagocytosis (cholesterol)	First identification of smooth muscle cell-derived foam cells.	[49]
	Ms. aortic	Phagocytosis (cholesterol)	Smooth muscle cells differentiate to a macrophage phenotype after cholesterol loading.	[50]
Hepatic	Hu. primary Stellate cells Hu. Hep G2 cells	Efferocytosis	Apoptotic clearance causes fibrogenic response.	[51]
	Rt. hepatocytes	Phagocytosis (lecithin-coated particles)	Exogenous substance uptake by hepatocytes.	[52]

Nonmyeloid cell	Cell subtype	Phagocytosis	Key findings	Ref'
Other	Rt. Sertoli cells	Efferocytosis	PS mediated clearance.	[53]
	Hu. Mesangial Kidney	Efferocytosis	CD36 independent clearance of apoptotic bodies.	[54]
	Ms. neuronal progenitor	Efferocytosis	Identifies neuronal precursors as nonprofessional phagocyte.	[55]
	Rt. chondrocytes	Phagocytosis (cartilage fragments)	CD163+ chondrocytes have phagocytic role in arthritis.	[56]

Hu.: Human, CFTR: Cystic Fibrosis Transmembrane Conductance Regulator, Ms.: Mouse, PSR: Phosphatidylserine Receptor, CD: Cluster of Differentiation, HBEC: Human Bronchial Epithelial Cells, Rac1: Ras-related C3 botulinum toxin substrate 1, SR-B1: The scavenger receptor, class B type 1, Rt.: Rat, KIM-1: Kidney Injury Molecule-1, LOX-1: lectin-like oxLDL [oxidized low-density lipoprotein] receptor 1, ABCF1: ATP-binding cassette sub-family F member 1, IL: Interleukin, BAI-1: Brain-specific angiogenesis inhibitor, Gas6: Growth arrest-specific 6, SCARF1: Scavenger receptor class F member 1, IgG: Immunoglobulin G, LAMP-1: Lysosomal-associated membrane protein 1, PS: Phosphatidylserine, ESCs: Embryonic Stem Cells, BM-MSCs: Bone Marrow Mesenchymal Stem Cells.

Table 1.
Key studies in nonmyeloid cell phagocytosis.

mechanisms to recognize, engulf, and destroy pathogens through phagocytosis. Nonprofessional phagocytes are demonstrably less efficient and lack factors such as Pattern Recognition Receptors (PRRs) capable of recognizing Pathogen Associated Molecular Patterns (PAMPs), as well as reactive oxygen species (ROS) and degradation enzymes required for effective clearance and degradation [19]. Nonmyeloid cells, however, provide a significant contribution toward the clearance of exogenous pathogens, cellular debris, and apoptotic bodies *via* phagocytosis, and what they lack in efficiency, can make up for in cell number [5, 57]. This chapter will focus on the specific functions of nonprofessional phagocytes, highlighting their differences from professional phagocytes and their specific and important contribution to tissue homeostasis.

2. Pathogen-induced phagocytosis

The active role of the host cell in the process of pathogen internalization, involving cytoskeletal rearrangements after pathogen recognition, ultimately distinguishes nonprofessional phagocytosis from infection [7, 19, 57]. There may be a few exceptions to this rule, such as Rotaviruses, known to gain infectious entry into the cell using the zipper mechanism, described below [58]. Internalization of the pathogen is, however, only the initial stage in the bigger mechanism of phagocytosis. The pathogen-containing internalized vesicle, otherwise known as the early phagosome, requires subsequent fusion with lysosomes in order to achieve pathogen killing [59]. The early phagosome matures by fusion with internal endocytic vesicles [59], recruiting factors, such as Rab5 [60], a small GTPase important for the maturation of the phagosome, and early endosome antigen 1 (EEA1) [61]. Rab5 remains transiently expressed in the early phagosome, directing the fusion of early endosomes [62, 63]. The schematic in **Figure 1** depicts the process of endosome formation, maturation, and role of Rab proteins in phagocytosis. Rab5 has been extensively studied and understood in myeloid cells during professional phagocytosis and has also been shown to be constitutively expressed in nonmyeloid cells, including epithelial cells [64–66], fibroblasts [66], and smooth muscle cells [67], controlling the phagocytic processes. Rab5 is considered a master regulator of early endosome formation and trafficking to the early phagosome. Rab5 expressing early phagosomes initiates the process of pathogen killing or apoptotic recycling by creating a mildly acidic microenvironment (pH 6.1) within the phagosome and engaging in relatively low levels of hydrolysis [68]. Rab conversion is a term used to convey phagosome maturation beyond the early phagosome. Maturation involves the recruitment of Rab7, functionally replacing Rab5 in the phagosome [69]. Rab7, like Rab5, is a member of the GTPase family that manages the maturation of phagosomes and recruits other factors, such as the RAB7 interacting lysosomal protein (RILP), necessary for later phagosome fusion with lysosomes [70]. Formation of a late-stage phagosome also requires the recruitment of Lysosomal-Associated Membrane Process-1(LAMP-1), necessary for lysosomal fusion [27, 71] Rab7 functionally interacts with RILP [70, 72], resulting in lysosomal fusion with the late-stage phagosome. Consequently, the phagolysosome structure is formed, creating a more acidic environment (pH 5.5) and generating a cocktail of degradation enzymes and ROS in effort to kill invading pathogens or break down apoptotic bodies [57]. While the process leading to the formation of the phagolysosome is similar, the recognition of the pathogen by nonmyeloid cells and internalization can occur through one of several known pathways. These pathways,

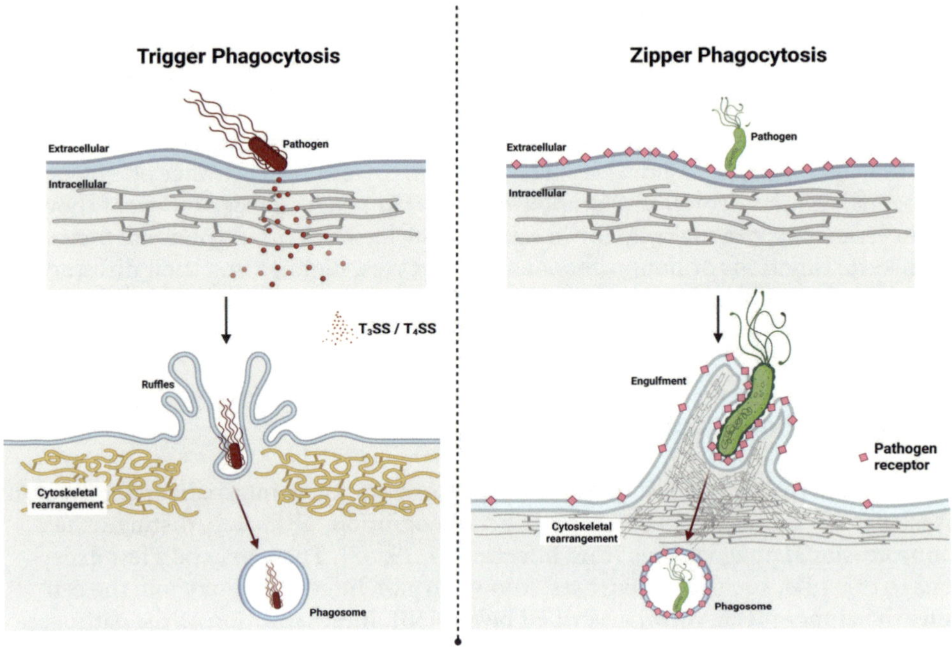

Figure 1.
Internalization models for pathogen-induced phagocytosis. For nonprofessional phagocytes, phagocytosis is induced by the pathogen. Two primary models are proposed: 1) trigger phagocytosis, caused when type 3 / type 4 secretion systems (T_3SS/T_4SS) cause cytoskeletal rearrangement, resulting in "ruffles" of the host cell membrane that engulfs and internalizes the pathogen and 2) zipper phagocytosis where the pathogen engages with a receptor complementary to ligands expressed on the pathogen. Following cytoskeletal rearrangement, further receptors engage with the pathogen in a "zipper" or "ratchet" like fashion, engulfing the pathogen into the phagosome. This figure was created with BioRender.com.

including efferocytosis, zipper phagocytosis, trigger phagocytosis, and opsonization, are discussed in more detail below.

2.1 Efferocytosis

Efferocytosis of apoptotic cells is the primary phagocytosis mechanism utilized by nonmyeloid cells. Recognition of apoptotic bodies is, therefore, critical for the clearance of apoptotic cells, and tissues have evolved ligand-receptor-based recognition as part of the initial engagement ultimately triggering efferocytosis of the apoptotic cell [7, 73, 74]. The primary component of this mechanism is the recognition of phosphatidylserine expressed in apoptotic cells [75]. During early apoptosis, phosphatidylserine molecules translocate to the cells' surface, anchoring to the membrane, where they act as an "eat-me" signal to localized phagocytes, both professional and nonprofessional [76]. Phosphatidylserine can be recognized by several receptors, including integrins $\alpha_V\beta_3$ and $\alpha_V\beta_5$ [9, 29, 34]. CD36 [29, 34], CD91 [29], and even bio-specific phosphatidylserine receptors [16, 77]. Other ligands have been proposed to induce receptor-mediated efferocytosis of apoptotic cells by neighboring nonprofessional phagocytes, including Apoptosis Inhibitor of Macrophage (AIM) recognition by Kidney Injury Molecule-1 (KIM-1) [78] and milk fat globule-epidermal growth factor 8 (MFG-E8) by integrin $\alpha v\beta 3$ [79].

2.2 "Zipper" phagocytosis

In the initial stages of nonmyeloid cell phagocytosis, one of the primary processes is the "Zipper" mechanism [6, 80, 81]. The zipper mechanism was first coined in 1975 by Griffin *et. al* to describe the phenomena of attachment of opsonized erythrocytes and macrophages [82, 83]. Essentially, the structure is opsonized by immunoglobulins and becomes engulfed by a sequential recognition by Fcγ receptors in a "zipper" like fashion [80, 81]. Since this initial observation, similar phagocytic mechanisms have been noted that do not require opsonin-Fcγ receptor-mediated recognition, including mechanisms of phagocytosis by nonmyeloid cells. Instead, the pathogen engages with a component of the target cells' external structure. Such structures are typically cell surface integrins, adhesins, or invasins [4, 6, 34, 84]. This interaction initiates microtubule and actin rearrangements within the host cell. Following engagement, a continuous and sequential binding of the host cells "target structures" to the corresponding structures on the pathogen, leads to the complete engulfing and internalization of the pathogen by the cell in a phagosome-like vesicle, similar to that observed with opsonized mediated phagocytosis (**Figure 2**, [7, 81]).

2.3 "Trigger" phagocytosis

In contrast to zipper phagocytosis, the "trigger mechanism" is a process where engagement of the pathogen with a pathogen recognition receptor is not a critical component of the process. Some engagement with cell surface ligands may occur to secure the pathogen to the cell [80]; however, the distinguishable difference in trigger phagocytosis is that the pathogen "injects" effectors into the host cell. The injected components known as type-III (T3SS) [85] and type-IV (T4SS) [86] secretion systems result in host cell cytoskeletal rearrangements localized to the site of pathogen contact. Rearrangement generates "ruffles" along the cell surface, which then fold over the pathogen and fuse, internalizing the pathogen (**Figure 2**) [80].

2.4 Antibody opsonization

Emerging data suggest a potential role for opsonin-mediated phagocytosis in nonmyeloid cells [87–93]. Classical membrane-bound Fcγ receptors, namely FcγRI, FcγRII, and FcγRIII, and their capacity to recognize immunoglobulins are more typically associated with myeloid cell-based professional phagocytosis [57]. A more poorly understood, and somewhat atypical, class of immunoglobulin receptor, known as the neonatal Fc receptor (FcRn), is expressed ubiquitously throughout multiple tissue types, including pulmonary epithelium [92], intestinal epithelium [87], microvascular endothelium [91], and the placenta [89]. It was initially thought that FcRn is expressed in fetal and neonatal tissues; however, it has since been demonstrated that expression is sustained throughout life [90]. The FcRn has a strong affinity for albumin [90] and IgG antibodies [88]. IgG-mediated phagocytosis *via* FcRn has been noted in myeloid cells [93], but evidence for phagocytosis in nonmyeloid cells *via* this receptor is lacking. FcRn expression in nonmyeloid cells appears to be intracellular, thus lacking the capacity for extracellular surveillance [94]. Instead, it is thought that the primary function for FcRn is transcytosis of IgGs across endothelial and epithelial membranes, as opposed to opsonin-mediated phagocytosis. The fundamental machinery is, however, present in nonmyeloid tissues and models have even been proposed based on studies demonstrating IgG-mediated phagocytosis of extracellular myelin debris [7, 47].

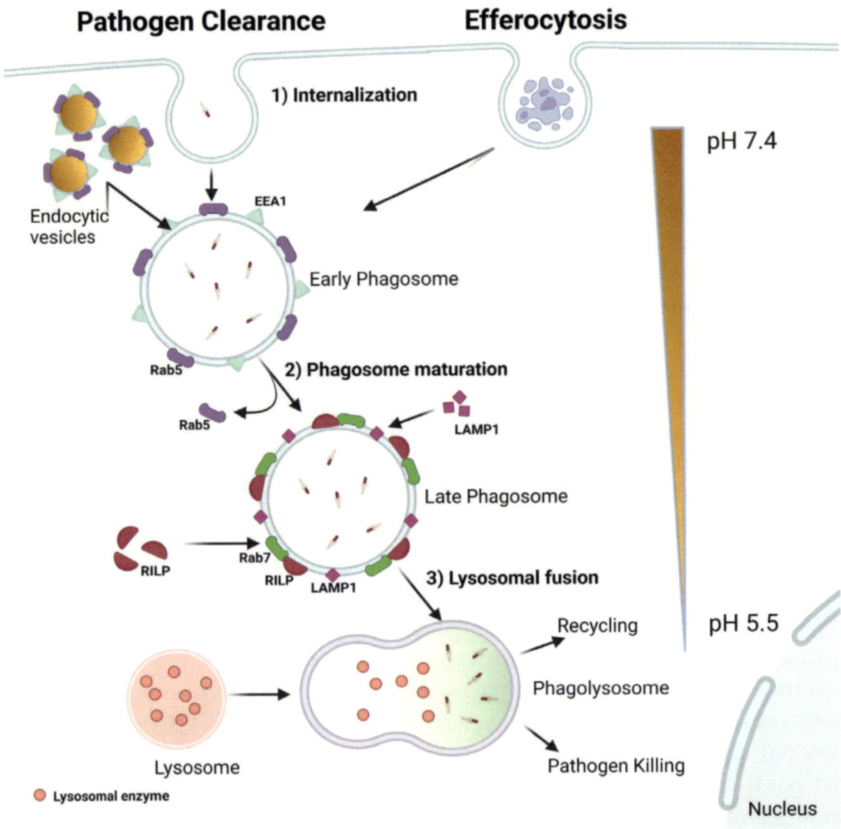

Figure 2.
Phagosome maturation. Phagosome maturation in nonmyeloid cells is like that of professional phagocytes, however less efficient. The phagocytosis process is outlined as; 1) internalization, resulting in the formation of the early phagosome, recruiting components such as Rab5 and EEA1. 2) Phagosome maturation, where Rab5 is replaced with Rab7 and factors such as RILP and LAMP 1 are recruited. 3) Lysosomal fusion, releasing factors such as degradation enzymes within the phagosome, which can result in pathogen killing and recycling of degraded products. This figure was created with BioRender.com.

3. Epithelial cell phagocytosis

The primary function of epithelial cells is to form a barrier between the internal organs and the external environment. As such these tissues have evolved to be relatively efficient in anti-pathogenic mechanisms, including the secretion of antimicrobial peptides, functional mucociliary clearance, and phagocytosis [6, 7]. The integumentary skin layer is perhaps the most obvious epithelial cell layer; however, the epithelium also lines internal organs and mucosal surface tissues, such as the respiratory tract, digestive system, genitourinary organs, and neuronal tissues, among others [95]. The physiological organization and structure of the epithelium can vary, even within the same organ system, for example, the pseudostratified epithelium that lines the proximal airways progressively changes to a simple squamous epithelium that lines the alveolar airspace [96, 97]. Despite the multiple structural phenotypes, the primary function of any epithelium is to form a barrier, a protective layer of epithelial cells connected by tight junctions [98]. Tissue-resident myeloid cells, such as macrophages, are often labeled as the first line of defense when it comes to invading pathogens; however, it could be argued that epithelial cells provide that initial functional defense [6].

Efferocytosis appears to be a function of practically all tissues and cell types [7, 73]. Relative to professional phagocytes. The removal of damaged or dying cells can leave the barrier exposed and prone to further damage or infection. As such epithelial tissues have a remarkable capacity for repair to maintain barrier integrity and homeostasis [98]. It is well established that the primary mechanism to eliminate apoptotic epithelial cells is through extrusion into the external apical lumen [6, 99]; however, epithelial cells also engage in efferocytosis [7]. Efferocytosis is particularly important for subapical apoptotic bodies or if the epithelial lumen does not have a functional system for debris removal such as mucociliary clearance in the airways.

Apoptotic epithelia can express a wide array of "eat me" signals with the most common being phosphatidylserine [21, 29, 34]. Recognition of apoptotic cells by epithelia is somewhat less understood; however, uptake of apoptotic bodies and recognition by phosphatidylserine receptors on the epithelial cells are acknowledged to be an integral part of this process [34]. Some studies provide evidence that the process of efferocytosis observed in epithelia is distinct from that of professional phagocytes and even from other phagocytic processes [74]. Epithelial cells have a relatively strong expression of PRRs with innate capabilities of recognizing exogenous PAMPs [5, 6, 100, 101]. Activation of PRRs can induce strong inflammatory responses including cytokine release [102], however mucosal epithelial cells must maintain a bio-symbiotic relationship with natural bacterial flora and control the potential for excessive inflammatory stimulation [103]. To achieve this, many of the PRRs are either intracellular [103–106] to recognize pathogens in the process of infecting the epithelium or on the surface of a polarized epithelium restricted to the basolateral surface [101, 107] to detect pathogens that have breached the epithelial barrier. PRRs expressed on epithelial cells include the Toll-Like Receptors (TLRs), the C-type Lectin Receptors (CLRs), the NOD-like Receptors (NLRs), and the RIG-I-like receptors (RLRs) [6, 108, 109]. It has also been proposed that PRRs can also engage in zipper phagocytosis, as integral parts of internalizing pathogenic stimuli, in addition to internalization of the receptor itself to control excessive inflammatory responses [110–112]; however, it is unclear if this pathogen-induced internalization is consistent with zipper phagocytosis or even conserved in nonmyeloid cells, in principle it is a possibility. Often the overarching inflammatory response is studied in isolation from that of any possible phagocytosis response. However, it is important to recognize that there is significant overlap and control of one by the other. Indeed, it has been reported that signaling factors, such as Rac1, are necessary for phagocytosis and the subsequent control of anti-inflammatory cytokine release, key to inflammatory resolution [30]. Further insights into epithelial cell phagocytosis may well be found in the study of inflammatory cytokine biology.

A common place for epithelial phagocytosis study can be found in the retinal epithelium of the eye [113]. Separated by the blood-retina barrier [114, 115], the retinal epithelium is able to maintain a certain level of immune privilege from circulating leukocytes [116]. Whilst there is evidence for resident and infiltrating myeloid cells in these tissues [117], it is primarily the retinal epithelium that maintains homeostasis through phagocytic functions [113]. Aside from immune recognition, phagocytosis by the retinal epithelium is important for the biological process of photoreception [118]. The distal portions of photoreceptors in the eye, known as "Photoreceptor Outer Segments" (POS) are in direct contact with the retinal epithelium [119] and rich in membranous discs packaged with proteins known as opsins [120], which are photosensitive. Exposure to light bleaches opsins to allow for signal transduction [121]. Extended exposure to these opsin-rich discs results in phototoxic damage and mature discs are shed from the distal tip to allow for the synthesis of new discs [113]. The retinal epithelium is perpetually "ensheathed" around the distal tips of photoreceptors [122], which upon shedding are phagocytosed into the retinal epithelium [119, 123]. The phagosome undergoes phagolysosomal maturation, including acidification and breakdown of the photoreceptor distal tips [113]. This entire process allows for the maintenance of long-term photoreceptors with short-lived distal tips by the retinal epithelial cells in an immune-privileged tissue. The retinal epithelium represents a prime example of a nonmyeloid cell performing specialized phagocytosis as a primary function in the homeostatic maintenance of its niche.

Internalization of pathogens by mucosal epithelium is well documented [5, 22–27]. Epithelial cells utilize both zipper and trigger mechanisms to internalize invading pathogens and engage in phagocytosis [6]. After internalization of the pathogen, the maturation of the phagosome in epithelia is akin to that of professional phagocytes [59], including markers of maturation, phagosome acidification, and lysosomal fusion [124]. The primary difference lies in the speed and efficiency when compared to professional phagocytes [125]. Despite this lack of efficiency, the contribution of phagocytosis of epithelial cells is still remarkably significant when considering cell numbers and so the impact of epithelial cell phagocytosis in pathogen clearance should not be ignored, having distinctive implications in both homeostasis and disease.

4. Endothelial cell phagocytosis

Like epithelial cells, endothelial cells also form a physical barrier, specifically in the walls of fluid systems, such as the circulatory and lymphatic systems [126]. These barriers comprise squamous endothelial cells, which form a single cell layer lining the entire system [126]. Their primary functions are to maintain the barrier and act as a filtration system for fluid-containing cells or substances into, and out of, the circulatory system [127, 128]. Significant cross talk occurs between endothelial cells and professional phagocytes as the endothelium allows leukocytes to cross through the barrier into tissues during times of infection and stress [129]. The concept of endothelial cells acting as phagocytes is not new, with some reports dating back as early as the 1920s [130]. Such a process is important for the endothelium to maintain circulatory homeostasis with effective phagocytic clearance mechanisms [129]. Phagocytosis is clearly an important function for endothelial cells to possess and execute efficiently, failure to do so can lead to serious complications such as stroke [131, 132]. Due to its importance, phagocytic clearance by endothelial cells has been termed "Angiophagy" [131, 132].

In situations of physical damage to endothelial tissue, endothelial cells can often be the first to encounter potentially pathogenic insults, particularly pathogens that enter circulation. Like epithelial cells, endothelial cells strongly express PRRs, including TLRs, NLRs, and RIG receptors [133–137]. During times of inflammation, endothelial cell PRR expression is increased [138], an important process for innate recognition of potentially invasive pathogens. It is also imperative for endothelial cells to recognize endogenous material, such as aged red blood cells, to both prevent and clear micro emboli blockages [139]. Endothelial cells express Lectin-like oxLDL receptor 1 (LOX-1), a transmembrane protein that is capable of recognizing these aged red blood cells that express phosphatidylserine [36]. Endothelial cells can also clear other cellular material, such as apoptotic cell bodies of circulating leukocytes, including that of circulating professional phagocytes, such as neutrophils [140], and do so *via* recognition of lactadherin [141]. Endothelial cells capable of recognizing and engulfing circulating cellular material is not just a function of cellular turnover homeostasis, but this is important in reducing coagulative activity.

Angiophagy, as a phagocytic process, can be considered distinct from other mechanisms such as efferocytosis, as a specialized method of clearing vascular occlusions, which may or may not have "eat-me" recognition molecules. In several organ systems, angiophagy of large particulates, such as blood clots and fibrin, has been observed by endothelial cells in microvascular capillary structures, releasing the phagocytosed particles into the basolateral parenchyma [132, 142]. While the overall result remains consistent, angiophagy efficiency can vary between different organs [142]. The biomechanical processes of angiophagy are not well understood. Studies have demonstrated that projections of the endothelial cell wall known as "lamellipodia" extend into the occluded lumen after extensive cellular remodeling [142]. Engulfment of the occluding body occurs within a few hours, relatively quickly when compared to the entire angiophagy process, which can take several days. Post engulfment, the occluding body is trafficked to the underlying tissue where it can be further processed, often by myeloid cells [142]. A more comprehensive characterization, beyond engulfment in angiophagy, is lacking although mechanisms of phagocytosis are certainly present. Further reports have demonstrated that microparticles are internalized and retained intracellularly without any impact on barrier integrity [143].

A common endpoint of phagocytosis in some professional phagocytes is antigen presentation. After a functional inactivation of the pathogen, components of the pathogen are "presented" on the cellular surface of the phagocyte and used to activate specific lymphocytes, to initiate adaptive immune responses. This specialized function of antigen presentation is typically associated with dendritic cells but is also observed in other myeloid cells. Interestingly, antigen presentation has been observed in endothelial cells [144, 145], and even express MHCII, typically restricted to professional antigen-presenting cells, as a result of inflammatory stimulation [146]. As endothelial cells are not professional antigen-presenting cells and lack migrating capabilities important for effective antigen presentation, it is somewhat unclear as to why endothelial cells have developed antigen-presentation capabilities. It has been postulated to be important for T-cell-specific trafficking to sites of infection and stress [144]. Either way, strong phagocytosis machinery is required to process and present antigens on the cell surface.

Phagocytosis for endothelial cells is an important homeostatic process that allows luminal vasculature to remain clear of blockages and underlying tissues to remain clear of potentially pathogenic infection. The process of angiophagy to allow the extravasation of occlusions, and restoring luminal perfusion is arguably unique to endothelial cells as a process that even myeloid cells do not possess. Further work on the capabilities of endothelial cell phagocytosis could well lead to a better understanding and even treatment options for serious acute macro and microvascular disease.

5. Mesenchymal stem cell phagocytosis

Mesenchymal stem cells (MSCs) are multipotent cells capable of regeneration and differentiation into multiple cell types [147]. They reside in a wide number of tissues and give rise to cells and tissues necessary for growth, development, and tissue repair. MSCs are frequently referred to as adult stem cells, along with hematopoietic stem cells (HSCs), which of course give rise to professional phagocytes. Adult stem cells, such as MSCs, are multipotent and distinguished from embryonic stem cells (ESCs) or laboratory-generated induced pluripotent stem cells (iPSCs), which are pluripotent with a differentiation capacity to generate cells of all three germ layers. MSCs are stromal cells, and distinct from their HSC counterparts, it is therefore perhaps surprising that an advanced cellular function such as phagocytosis has been observed. Several reports, however, have demonstrated that MSCs are indeed capable of phagocytosis. This was first reported in 2000 by Wood *et. al*, who demonstrated the ability of mesenchymal cells to clear apoptotic cells through efferocytosis in the absence of macrophages in PU.1 knock-out mice [11] and later established in 2010 when Tso *et. al* confirmed efferocytosis-like clearance of apoptotic cells by MSCs [10]. Since then, other reports have corroborated this finding in a variety of situations, confirming MSCs capabilities of efferocytosis and clearance of apoptotic cells [12, 148]. What is also surprising is the inflammatory response when apoptotic bodies are recognized by mesenchymal cells, including NF-κB signaling pathway activation [12], and MSCs can express a number of distinctive markers more closely associated with immune cells [149]. Furthermore, MSCs are capable of secreting antimicrobial peptides [150, 151] to aid in pathogen killing and clearance.

MSCs do possess a certain level of PRRs, including TLRs [152] and NOD-like receptors [153]; however, reports are lacking that definitively demonstrate exogenous pathogen phagocytosis although have suggested its plausibility [154]. Similar to endothelial cells, MSCs are capable of MHC-II type antigen presentation [155], considered to be unique to professional phagocytes, and these antigen-presenting MSCs are capable of presenting and activating T cells [156, 157]. This would suggest that phagocytosis of pathogens, to present antigens *via* MHC-II is possible; however, this has yet to be confirmed. The primary function is therefore that of a supporting role for professional phagocytes as opposed to being primary phagocytes themselves.

6. Smooth muscle cell phagocytosis

Smooth muscle is found in multiple organ systems and can provide a variety of roles, often important for the physical functions of the organ or tissue in which they reside. Unlike skeletal muscle, smooth muscle involuntarily can maintain its tone over extended periods of time [158]. The functional cellular units of smooth muscle are described as nonstriated, in that they lack the sarcomeres that their skeletal striated counterparts possess. Smooth muscle cells are rich in actin and myosin which allows for efficient contraction [159]. It would be easy to describe smooth muscle cells (SMCs) as monofunctional and homogenous; however, it would appear that they have stromal-like properties and are capable of further differentiation into multiple "macrophage-like" phenotypes capable of phagocytosis [160]. The concept of phagocytosis by SMCs was first suggested observed in 1971 by Campbell and colleagues [161], and later confirmed by Garfield *et. al* in 1975, who demonstrated uptake of yeast and latex beads by guinea pig smooth muscle [14]. Like other nonprofessional phagocytes, SMCs express the phosphatidylserine receptor and functionally recognize phosphatidylserine-rich apoptotic bodies, resulting in efferocytosis [13, 16]. Like the other nonprofessional phagocytes discussed in this chapter, SMC phagocytosis has been studied and implicated in diseases, where pathological phagocytosis is considered to play a major role, such as atherosclerosis [162, 163]. In fact, SMC phagocytosis has been a focus of investigation in atherosclerosis.

Atherosclerosis is the buildup of plaques in the subendothelial tissues of arterial macrovascular walls [164]. These plaques can obstruct blood flow through the arterial lumen, which can result in a series of vascular-related diseases. Atherosclerotic plaques comprise of "foam cells," which have phagocytosed low-density lipoproteins, which they are seemingly unable to efficiently process and resolve. Foam cells as active phagocytes are myeloid in origin, more specifically they are macrophages derived from monocytes [165] recruited into the subendothelial tissues as a result of vascular damage. However, foam cells of atherosclerotic plaques can also be derived from SMCs [49, 166], with some reports even suggesting the majority of foam cells in atherosclerotic legions to be of SMC origin [167]. Such SMCs resemble an undifferentiated precursor capable of a phenotypic switch under varying conditions [168]. The specific conditions that trigger SMCs to switch to a macrophage-like foam cell are not well known, although it appears to be KLF-4 dependent [169]. SMCs have a high abundance of LRP1, a key scavenger receptor for lipoproteins [170]. LRP1 activation will result in an influx of lipoproteins into the cell, generating a "foam cell" phenotype [171]. It is the inefficiency of SMC-derived foam cells as phagocytes that appears to be a significant factor in atherosclerosis. Despite the recognition that phagocytosis, or lack thereof, by SMCs is clearly playing a significant role in the pathophysiology of atherosclerosis, little is known about the internalization mechanism compared to the process of autophagy [172]. Studies to date have mainly focused their efforts to recreate SMC-derived foam cells and compare them to foam cells of macrophage origin in attempts to highlight key differences, instead of addressing the specific mechanisms relating to phagocytosis in SMC-derived foam cells.

7. Conclusions

Historically most investigations with regard to phagocytosis have focused on the role of myeloid cells as professional phagocytes. In this review, we have discussed nonmyeloid cell types, where roles in phagocytosis have been established. It is becoming increasingly evident that many tissue types are capable, to some extent, of phagocytosis [173]. Indeed, there are even situations of specialized phagocytic function, such as that observed in the retinal epithelia and angiophagy in vascular endothelial cells. Despite nonprofessional phagocytes being less effective when it comes to pathogen recognition, internalization, phagosome maturation, and pathogen killing, they still provide a significant contribution to phagocytosis, and, in more immune-privileged tissues, phagocytosis by nonprofessional phagocytes is imperative to maintain physiological functions.

Acknowledgements

ALR is supported by Cystic Fibrosis Foundation awards FIRTH21XX0 and FIRTH17XX0 and the Tyler Health and Education Fund.

Conflict of interest

The authors declare no conflict of interest.

Author details

Ben A. Calvert and Amy L. Ryan*
Department of Anatomy and Cell Biology, Carver College of Medicine, University of Iowa, Iowa City, IA, USA

*Address all correspondence to: amy-l-ryan@uiowa.edu

References

[1] Stegelmeier AA et al. Myeloid cells during viral infections and inflammation. Viruses. 2019;**11**(2):168-193

[2] Silva MT, Correia-Neves M. Neutrophils and macrophages: The main partners of phagocyte cell systems. Frontiers in Immunology. 2012;**3**:174

[3] Kantari C, Pederzoli-Ribeil M, Witko-Sarsat V. The role of neutrophils and monocytes in innate immunity. Contributions to Microbiology. 2008;**15**:118-146

[4] Dale DC, Boxer L, Liles WC. The phagocytes: Neutrophils and monocytes. Blood. 2008;**112**(4):935-945

[5] Sharma L et al. Mechanisms of epithelial immunity evasion by respiratory bacterial pathogens. Frontiers in Immunology. 2020;**11**:91

[6] Günther J, Seyfert HM. The first line of defence: Insights into mechanisms and relevance of phagocytosis in epithelial cells. Seminars in Immunopathology. 2018;**40**(6):555-565

[7] Sihombing M et al. Unexpected role of nonimmune Cells: Amateur phagocytes. DNA and Cell Biology. 2021;**40**(2):157-171

[8] Visan I. Amateur phagocytes. Nature Immunology. 2019;**20**(3):245-245

[9] Kirsch T et al. Engulfment of apoptotic cells by microvascular endothelial cells induces proinflammatory responses. Blood. 2007;**109**(7):2854-2862

[10] Tso GH et al. Phagocytosis of apoptotic cells modulates mesenchymal stem cells osteogenic differentiation to enhance IL-17 and RANKL expression on CD4+ T cells. Stem Cells. 2010;**28**(5):939-954

[11] Wood W et al. Mesenchymal cells engulf and clear apoptotic footplate cells in macrophageless PU.1 null mouse embryos. Development. 2000;**127**(24):5245-5252

[12] Zhang Z et al. Clearance of apoptotic cells by mesenchymal stem cells contributes to immunosuppression via PGE2. eBioMedicine. 2019;**45**:341-350

[13] Bennett MR et al. Binding and phagocytosis of apoptotic vascular smooth muscle cells is mediated in part by exposure of phosphatidylserine. Circulation Research. 1995;**77**(6):1136-1142

[14] Garfield RE, Chacko S, Blose S. Phagocytosis by muscle cells. Laboratory Investigation. 1975;**33**(4):418-427

[15] Gordon-Weeks P, Gabella G. Degeneration of varicose axons and their phagocytosis by smooth muscle cells. Journal of Neurocytology. 1977;**6**(6):711-721

[16] Kolb S et al. The phosphatidylserine receptor mediates phagocytosis by vascular smooth muscle cells. The Journal of Pathology. 2007;**212**(3):249-259

[17] Fais S. Cannibalism: A way to feed on metastatic tumors. Cancer Letters. 2007;**258**(2):155-164

[18] Rabinovitch M. Mononuclear Phagocytes. Oxford: Blackwell Scientific Publishers; 1970. pp. 299-315

[19] Rabinovitch M. Professional and non-professional phagocytes: An

introduction. Trends in Cell Biology. 1995;**5**(3):85-87

[20] Mudd S, McCutcheon M, Lucké B. Phagocytosis. Physiological Reviews. 1934;**14**(2):210-275

[21] Schwegler M et al. Clearance of primary necrotic cells by non-professional phagocytes. Biology of the Cell. 2015;**107**(10):372-387

[22] Plotkowski MC et al. Pseudomonas aeruginosa internalization by human epithelial respiratory cells depends on cell differentiation, polarity, and junctional complex integrity. American Journal of Respiratory Cell and Molecular Biology. 1999;**20**(5):880-890

[23] Fumagalli O et al. N-glycosylated proteins are involved in efficient internalization of Klebsiella pneumoniae by cultured human epithelial cells. Infection and Immunity. 1997;**65**(11):4445-4451

[24] Watson RO, Galán JE. Campylobacter jejuni survives within epithelial cells by avoiding delivery to lysosomes. PLoS Pathogens. 2008;**4**(1):e14

[25] Capasso D et al. Elimination of Pseudomonas aeruginosa through Efferocytosis upon binding to apoptotic Cells. PLoS Pathogens. 2016;**12**(12):e1006068

[26] Cortés G et al. Role of lung epithelial cells in defense against Klebsiella pneumoniae pneumonia. Infection and Immunity. 2002;**70**(3):1075-1080

[27] Couzinet S et al. Phagocytic uptake of Encephalitozoon cuniculi by nonprofessional phagocytes. Infection and Immunity. 2000;**68**(12):6939-6945

[28] Herrera EM et al. Mediation of Trypanosoma cruzi invasion by heparan sulfate receptors on host cells and penetrin counter-receptors on the trypanosomes. Molecular and Biochemical Parasitology. 1994;**65**(1):73-83

[29] Monks J et al. Epithelial cells as phagocytes: Apoptotic epithelial cells are engulfed by mammary alveolar epithelial cells and repress inflammatory mediator release. Cell Death and Differentiation. 2005;**12**(2):107-114

[30] Juncadella IJ et al. Apoptotic cell clearance by bronchial epithelial cells critically influences airway inflammation. Nature. 2013;**493**(7433):547-551

[31] Cao WM et al. Phosphatidylserine receptor cooperates with high-density lipoprotein receptor in recognition of apoptotic cells by thymic nurse cells. Journal of Molecular Endocrinology. 2004;**32**(2):497-505

[32] Wakefield JS, Hicks RM. Erythrophagocytosis by the epithelial cells of the bladder. Journal of Cell Science. 1974;**15**(3):555-573

[33] Rong G-H et al. Human intrahepatic biliary epithelial cells engulf blebs from their apoptotic peers. Clinical and Experimental Immunology. 2013;**172**(1):95-103

[34] Sexton DW, Blaylock MG, Walsh GM. Human alveolar epithelial cells engulf apoptotic eosinophils by means of integrin- and phosphatidylserine receptor-dependent mechanisms: A process upregulated by dexamethasone. The Journal of Allergy and Clinical Immunology. 2001;**108**(6):962-969

[35] Ichimura T et al. Kidney injury molecule-1 is a phosphatidylserine receptor that confers a phagocytic

phenotype on epithelial cells. The Journal of Clinical Investigation. 2008;**118**(5):1657-1668

[36] Oka K et al. Lectin-like oxidized low-density lipoprotein receptor 1 mediates phagocytosis of aged/apoptotic cells in endothelial cells. Proceedings of the National Academy of Sciences of the United States of America. 1998;**95**(16):9535-9540

[37] Guo F et al. ABCF1 extrinsically regulates retinal pigment epithelial cell phagocytosis. Molecular Biology of the Cell. 2015;**26**(12):2311-2320

[38] Penberthy KK, Juncadella IJ, Ravichandran KS. Apoptosis and engulfment by bronchial epithelial cells. Implications for allergic airway inflammation. Annals of American Thoracic Society. 2014;**5**(Suppl. 5): S259-S262

[39] Petrovski G et al. Clearance of dying ARPE-19 cells by professional and nonprofessional phagocytes in vitro- implications for age-related macular degeneration (AMD). Acta Ophthalmologica. 2011;**89**(1):e30-e34

[40] Mesa KR et al. Niche-induced cell death and epithelial phagocytosis regulate hair follicle stem cell pool. Nature. 2015;**522**(7554):94-97

[41] Lee CS et al. Boosting apoptotic cell clearance by colonic epithelial Cells attenuates inflammation In vivo. Immunity. 2016;**44**(4):807-820

[42] Burstyn-Cohen T et al. Genetic dissection of TAM receptor-ligand interaction in retinal pigment epithelial cell phagocytosis. Neuron. 2012;**76**(6):1123-1132

[43] Rengarajan M, Hayer A, Theriot JA. Endothelial cells use a formin-dependent phagocytosis-like process to internalize the bacterium listeria monocytogenes. PLoS Pathogens. 2016;**12**(5):e1005603

[44] Dini L et al. Phagocytosis of apoptotic bodies by liver endothelial cells. Journal of Cell Science. 1995;**108**(Pt 3):967-973

[45] Ramirez-Ortiz ZG et al. The scavenger receptor SCARF1 mediates the clearance of apoptotic cells and prevents autoimmunity. Nature Immunology. 2013;**14**(9):917-926

[46] Ji S et al. Phagocytosis by endothelial cells inhibits procoagulant activity of platelets of essential thrombocythemia in vitro. Journal of Thrombosis and Haemostasis. 2020;**18**(1):222-233

[47] Zhou T et al. Microvascular endothelial cells engulf myelin debris and promote macrophage recruitment and fibrosis after neural injury. Nature Neuroscience. 2019;**22**(3):421-435

[48] Goldman R. Lectin-mediated attachment and ingestion of yeast cells and erythrocytes by hamster fibroblasts. Experimental Cell Research. 1977;**104**(2):325-334

[49] Cooke PH, Smith SC. Smooth muscle cells: The source of foam cells in atherosclerotic white Carneau pigeons. Experimental and Molecular Pathology. 1968;**8**(2):171-189

[50] Rong JX et al. Transdifferentiation of mouse aortic smooth muscle cells to a macrophage-like state after cholesterol loading. Proceedings of the National Academy of Sciences of the United States of America. 2003;**100**(23):13531-13536

[51] Canbay A et al. Apoptotic body engulfment by a human stellate cell line is Profibrogenic. Laboratory Investigation. 2003;**83**(5):655-663

[52] Soji T et al. Evidence that hepatocytes can phagocytize exogenous substances. The Anatomical Record. 1992;**233**(4):543-546

[53] Shiratsuchi A et al. Role of class B scavenger receptor type I in phagocytosis of apoptotic rat spermatogenic cells by Sertoli cells. The Journal of Biological Chemistry. 1999;**274**(9):5901-5908

[54] Hughes J et al. Human glomerular mesangial cell phagocytosis of apoptotic neutrophils: Mediation by a novel CD36-independent vitronectin receptor/thrombospondin recognition mechanism that is uncoupled from chemokine secretion. The Journal of Immunology. 1997;**158**(9):4389-4397

[55] Lu Z et al. Phagocytic activity of neuronal progenitors regulates adult neurogenesis. Nature Cell Biology. 2011;**13**(9):1076-1083

[56] Jiao K et al. The identification of CD163 expressing phagocytic chondrocytes in joint cartilage and its novel scavenger role in cartilage degradation. PLoS One. 2013;**8**(1):e53312

[57] Uribe-Querol E, Rosales C. Phagocytosis: Our current understanding of a universal biological process. Frontiers in Immunology. 2020;**11**:1066

[58] Arias CF, Silva-Ayala D, López S. Rotavirus entry: A deep journey into the cell with several exits. Journal of Virology. 2015;**89**(2):890-893

[59] Pauwels AM et al. Patterns, receptors, and signals: Regulation of phagosome maturation. Trends in Immunology. 2017;**38**(6):407-422

[60] Vieira OV et al. Distinct roles of class I and class III phosphatidylinositol 3-kinases in phagosome formation and maturation. The Journal of Cell Biology. 2001;**155**(1):19-25

[61] Wilson JM et al. EEA1, a tethering protein of the early sorting endosome, shows a polarized distribution in hippocampal neurons, epithelial cells, and fibroblasts. Molecular Biology of the Cell. 2000;**11**(8):2657-2671

[62] Bucci C et al. The small GTPase rab5 functions as a regulatory factor in the early endocytic pathway. Cell. 1992;**70**(5):715-728

[63] Gorvel JP et al. rab5 controls early endosome fusion in vitro. Cell. 1991;**64**(5):915-925

[64] Balaji K et al. The RAB5-GEF function of RIN1 regulates multiple steps during Listeria monocytogenes infection. Traffic. 2014;**15**(11):1206-1218

[65] Saitoh S et al. Rab5-regulated endocytosis plays a crucial role in apical extrusion of transformed cells. Proceedings of the National Academy of Sciences of the United States of America. 2017;**114**(12):E2327-e2336

[66] Schnatwinkel C et al. The Rab5 effector Rabankyrin-5 regulates and coordinates different endocytic mechanisms. PLoS Biology. 2004;**2**(9):E261

[67] Tan JY et al. Rab5a-mediated autophagy regulates the phenotype and behavior of vascular smooth muscle cells. Molecular Medicine Reports. 2016;**14**(5):4445-4453

[68] Maxfield FR, McGraw TE. Endocytic recycling. Nature Reviews. Molecular Cell Biology. 2004;**5**(2):121-132

[69] Vieira OV et al. Modulation of Rab5 and Rab7 recruitment to phagosomes by phosphatidylinositol 3-kinase.

Molecular and Cellular Biology. 2003;**23**(7):2501-2514

[70] Cantalupo G et al. Rab-interacting lysosomal protein (RILP): The Rab7 effector required for transport to lysosomes. The EMBO Journal. 2001;**20**(4):683-693

[71] Huynh KK et al. LAMP proteins are required for fusion of lysosomes with phagosomes. The EMBO Journal. 2007;**26**(2):313-324

[72] Jordens I et al. The Rab7 effector protein RILP controls lysosomal transport by inducing the recruitment of dynein-dynactin motors. Current Biology. 2001;**11**(21):1680-1685

[73] Serizier SB, McCall K. Scrambled eggs: Apoptotic cell clearance by non-professional phagocytes in the Drosophila ovary. Frontiers in Immunology. 2017;**2017**:8

[74] Henson PM. Cell Removal: Efferocytosis. Annual Review of Cell and Developmental Biology. 2017;**33**:127-144

[75] Naeini MB et al. The role of phosphatidylserine recognition receptors in multiple biological functions. Cellular & Molecular Biology Letters. 2020;**25**(1):23

[76] Nagata S et al. Exposure of phosphatidylserine on the cell surface. Cell Death & Differentiation. 2016;**23**(6):952-961

[77] Jansen F et al. Endothelial microparticle uptake in target cells is annexin I/phosphatidylserine receptor dependent and prevents apoptosis. Arteriosclerosis, Thrombosis, and Vascular Biology. 2012;**32**(8):1925-1935

[78] Arai S et al. Apoptosis inhibitor of macrophage protein enhances intraluminal debris clearance and ameliorates acute kidney injury in mice. Nature Medicine. 2016;**22**(2):183-193

[79] Nakaya M et al. Cardiac myofibroblast engulfment of dead cells facilitates recovery after myocardial infarction. The Journal of Clinical Investigation. 2017;**127**(1):383-401

[80] Swanson JA, Baer SC. Phagocytosis by zippers and triggers. Trends in Cell Biology. 1995;**5**(3):89-93

[81] Tollis S et al. The zipper mechanism in phagocytosis: Energetic requirements and variability in phagocytic cup shape. BMC Systems Biology. 2010;**4**:149

[82] Bianco C, Griffin FM Jr, Silverstein SC. Studies of the macrophage complement receptor. Alteration of receptor function upon macrophage activation. The Journal of Experimental Medicine. 1975;**141**(6):1278-1290

[83] Griffin FM Jr, Griffin JA, Silverstein SC. Studies on the mechanism of phagocytosis. II. The interaction of macrophages with anti-immunoglobulin IgG-coated bone marrow-derived lymphocytes. The Journal of Experimental Medicine. 1976;**144**(3):788-809

[84] Cieza RJ et al. The IbeA invasin of adherent-invasive Escherichia coli mediates interaction with intestinal epithelia and macrophages. Infection and Immunity. 2015;**83**(5):1904-1918

[85] Coburn B, Sekirov I, Finlay BB. Type III secretion systems and disease. Clinical Microbiology Reviews. 2007;**20**(4):535-549

[86] Wallden K, Rivera-Calzada A, Waksman G. Type IV secretion systems: Versatility and diversity

in function. Cellular Microbiology. 2010;**12**(9):1203-1212

[87] Dickinson BL et al. Bidirectional FcRn-dependent IgG transport in a polarized human intestinal epithelial cell line. The Journal of Clinical Investigation. 1999;**104**(7):903-911

[88] Koenderman L. Inside-Out Control of Fc-Receptors. Frontiers in Immunology. 2019;**10**:544

[89] Leach JL et al. Isolation from human placenta of the IgG transporter, FcRn, and localization to the syncytiotrophoblast: Implications for maternal-fetal antibody transport. Journal of Immunology. 1996;**157**(8):3317-3322

[90] Roopenian DC, Akilesh S. FcRn: The neonatal fc receptor comes of age. Nature Reviews. Immunology. 2007;**7**(9):715-725

[91] Schlachetzki F, Zhu C, Pardridge WM. Expression of the neonatal fc receptor (FcRn) at the blood-brain barrier. Journal of Neurochemistry. 2002;**81**(1):203-206

[92] Spiekermann GM et al. Receptor-mediated immunoglobulin G transport across mucosal barriers in adult life: Functional expression of FcRn in the mammalian lung. The Journal of Experimental Medicine. 2002;**196**(3):303-310

[93] Vidarsson G et al. FcRn: An IgG receptor on phagocytes with a novel role in phagocytosis. Blood. 2006;**108**(10):3573-3579

[94] Pyzik M et al. The neonatal fc receptor (FcRn): A misnomer? Frontiers in Immunology. 2019;**10**:1540

[95] Larsen SB, Cowley CJ, Fuchs E. Epithelial cells: Liaisons of immunity. Current Opinion in Immunology. 2020;**62**:45-53

[96] Groeger S, Meyle J. Oral mucosal epithelial cells. Frontiers in Immunology. 2019;**10**:208

[97] Proud D, Leigh R. Epithelial cells and airway diseases. Immunological Reviews. 2011;**242**(1):186-204

[98] Buckley A, Turner JR. Cell biology of tight junction barrier regulation and mucosal disease. Cold Springer Harbor Perspective Biology. 2018;**10**(1):a029314

[99] Nanavati BN, Yap AS, Teo JL. Symmetry breaking and epithelial cell extrusion. Cells. 2020;**9**(6):cells9061416

[100] Pardo-Camacho C et al. Epithelial immunity: Priming defensive responses in the intestinal mucosa. American Journal of Physiology. Gastrointestinal and Liver Physiology. 2018;**314**(2):G247-g255

[101] Weitnauer M, Mijošek V, Dalpke AH. Control of local immunity by airway epithelial cells. Mucosal Immunology. 2016;**9**(2):287-298

[102] Takeuchi O, Akira S. Pattern recognition receptors and inflammation. Cell. 2010;**140**(6):805-820

[103] Wells JM et al. Epithelial crosstalk at the microbiota-mucosal interface. Proceedings of the National Academy of Sciences of the United States of America. 2011;**108**:4607-4614

[104] Hennessy C, D.P. McKernan anti-viral pattern recognition receptors as therapeutic targets. Cells. 2021;**10**:cells10092258

[105] Hornef MW et al. Intracellular recognition of lipopolysaccharide by toll-like receptor 4 in intestinal epithelial

cells. The Journal of Experimental Medicine. 2003;**198**(8):1225-1235

[106] Hill AA, Diehl GE. Identifying the patterns of pattern recognition receptors. Immunity. 2018;**49**(3):389-391

[107] Yu S, Gao N. Compartmentalizing intestinal epithelial cell toll-like receptors for immune surveillance. Cellular and Molecular Life Sciences. 2015;**72**(17):3343-3353

[108] McClure R, Massari P. TLR-dependent human mucosal epithelial cell responses to microbial pathogens. Frontiers in Immunology. 2014;**5**:386

[109] Lavelle EC et al. The role of TLRs, NLRs, and RLRs in mucosal innate immunity and homeostasis. Mucosal Immunology. 2010;**3**(1):17-28

[110] Moretti J, Blander JM. Insights into phagocytosis-coupled activation of pattern recognition receptors and inflammasomes. Current Opinion in Immunology. 2014;**26**:100-110

[111] Kingeter LM, Lin X. C-type lectin receptor-induced NF-κB activation in innate immune and inflammatory responses. Cellular & Molecular Immunology. 2012;**9**(2):105-112

[112] Goodridge HS, Simmons RM, Underhill DM. Dectin-1 stimulation by Candida albicans yeast or zymosan triggers NFAT activation in macrophages and dendritic cells. Journal of Immunology. 2007;**178**(5):3107-3115

[113] Kwon W, Freeman SA. Phagocytosis by the retinal pigment epithelium: Recognition, resolution, recycling. Frontiers in Immunology. 2020;**11**:604205

[114] Cunha-Vaz J, Bernardes R, Lobo C. Blood-retinal barrier. European Journal of Ophthalmology. 2011;**21**(Suppl. 6): S3-S9

[115] Lehmann GL et al. Plasma membrane protein polarity and trafficking in RPE cells: Past, present and future. Experimental Eye Research. 2014;**126**:5-15

[116] Taylor AW, Hsu S, Ng TF. The role of retinal pigment epithelial Cells in regulation of macrophages/microglial Cells in retinal Immunobiology. Frontiers in Immunology. 2021;**12**:91-100

[117] Ronning KE, Karlen SJ, Burns ME. Structural and functional distinctions of co-resident microglia and monocyte-derived macrophages after retinal degeneration. Journal of Neuroinflammation. 2022;**19**(1):299

[118] Lakkaraju A et al. The cell biology of the retinal pigment epithelium. Progress in Retinal and Eye Research. 2020:100846

[119] Young RW, Bok D. Participation of the retinal pigment epithelium in the rod outer segment renewal process. The Journal of Cell Biology. 1969;**42**(2):392-403

[120] Terakita A. The opsins. Genome Biology. 2005;**6**(3):213

[121] Masland RH. The neuronal Organization of the retina. Neuron. 2012;**76**(2):266-280

[122] Matsumoto B, Defoe DM, Besharse JC. Membrane turnover in rod photoreceptors: Ensheathment and phagocytosis of outer segment distal tips by pseudopodia of the retinal pigment epithelium. Proceedings of the Royal Society of London - Series B: Biological Sciences. 1987;**230**(1260):339-354

[123] LaVail MM. Rod outer segment disk shedding in rat retina:

Relationship to cyclic lighting. Science. 1976;**194**(4269):1071-1074

[124] Blanchette CD et al. Decoupling internalization, acidification and phagosomal-endosomal/lysosomal fusion during phagocytosis of InlA coated beads in epithelial cells. PLoS One. 2009;**4**(6):e6056

[125] Saftig P. Physiology of the lysosome. In: Mehta A, Beck M, Sunder-Plassmann G, editors. Fabry Disease: Perspectives from 5 Years of FOS. Chapter 3. Oxford: Oxford PharmaGenesis; 2006

[126] Potente M, Mäkinen T. Vascular heterogeneity and specialization in development and disease. Nature Reviews. Molecular Cell Biology. 2017;**18**(8):477-494

[127] Satchell SC, Braet F. Glomerular endothelial cell fenestrations: An integral component of the glomerular filtration barrier. American Journal of Physiology. Renal Physiology. 2009;**296**(5):F947-F956

[128] Luissint A-C et al. Tight junctions at the blood brain barrier: Physiological architecture and disease-associated dysregulation. Fluids and Barriers of the CNS. 2012;**9**(1):23

[129] Stolarz AJ et al. Opinion: Endothelial Cells - macrophage-like gatekeepers? Frontiers in Immunology. 2022;**13**:902945

[130] Doan CA, Sabin FR. Normal and pathological fragmentation of red blood cells; the phagocytosis of these fragments by desquamated endothelial cells of the blood stream; the correlation of the peroxidase reaction with phagocytosis in mononuclear cells. The Journal of Experimental Medicine. 1926;**43**(6):839-850

[131] Grutzendler J. Angiophagy: Mechanism of microvascular recanalization independent of the fibrinolytic system. Stroke. 2013;**44** (6 Suppl. 1):S84-S86

[132] Lam CK et al. Embolus extravasation is an alternative mechanism for cerebral microvascular recanalization. Nature. 2010;**465**(7297):478-482

[133] Opitz B et al. Role of toll-like receptors, NOD-like receptors and RIG-I-like receptors in endothelial cells and systemic infections. Thrombosis and Haemostasis. 2009;**102**(6):1103-1109

[134] Mitchell JA et al. Role of pattern-recognition receptors in cardiovascular health and disease. Biochemical Society Transactions. 2007;**35**(Pt 6):1449-1452

[135] Salvador B et al. Modulation of endothelial function by toll like receptors. Pharmacological Research. 2016;**108**:46-56

[136] Nagyőszi P et al. Regulation of NOD-like receptors and inflammasome activation in cerebral endothelial cells. Journal of Neurochemistry. 2015;**135**(3):551-564

[137] Xu S, Jin T, Weng J. Endothelial Cells as a key cell type for innate immunity: A focused review on RIG-I Signaling pathway. Frontiers in Immunology. 2022;**13**:951614

[138] El Kebir D et al. Bacterial DNA activates endothelial cells and promotes neutrophil adherence through TLR9 signaling. Journal of Immunology. 2009;**182**(7):4386-4394

[139] Fens MH et al. Erythrophagocytosis by angiogenic endothelial cells is enhanced by loss of erythrocyte deformability. Experimental Hematology. 2010;**38**(4):282-291

[140] Gao C et al. Endothelial cell phagocytosis of senescent neutrophils decreases procoagulant activity. Thrombosis and Haemostasis. 2013;**109**(6):1079-1090

[141] Ma R et al. Phosphatidylserine-mediated platelet clearance by endothelium decreases platelet aggregates and procoagulant activity in sepsis. Scientific Reports. 2017;**7**(1):4978

[142] Grutzendler J et al. Angiophagy prevents early embolus washout but recanalizes microvessels through embolus extravasation. Science Translational Medicine. 2014;**6**(226):226ra31

[143] van der Wijk A-E et al. Microembolus clearance through angiophagy is an auxiliary mechanism preserving tissue perfusion in the rat brain. Acta Neuropathologica Communications. 2020;**8**(1):195

[144] Marelli-Berg FM, Jarmin SJ. Antigen presentation by the endothelium: A green light for antigen-specific T cell trafficking? Immunology Letters. 2004;**93**(2-3):109-113

[145] Rothermel AL et al. Endothelial cells present antigens in vivo. BMC Immunology. 2004;**5**:5

[146] Leeuwenberg JF et al. Effects of tumor necrosis factor on the interferon-gamma-induced major histocompatibility complex class II antigen expression by human endothelial cells. European Journal of Immunology. 1988;**18**(9):1469-1472

[147] Tonk CH et al. Mesenchymal stem cells. In: Brand-Saberi B, editor. Essential Current Concepts in Stem Cell Biology. Cham: Springer International Publishing; 2020. pp. 21-39

[148] Jiang D et al. Suppression of neutrophil-mediated tissue damage-a novel skill of mesenchymal stem Cells. Stem Cells. 2016;**34**(9):2393-2406

[149] Yang ZX et al. CD106 identifies a subpopulation of mesenchymal stem cells with unique immunomodulatory properties. PLoS One. 2013;**8**(3):e59354

[150] Krasnodembskaya A et al. Antibacterial effect of human mesenchymal stem cells is mediated in part from secretion of the antimicrobial peptide LL-37. Stem Cells. 2010;**28**(12):2229-2238

[151] Gupta N et al. Mesenchymal stem cells enhance survival and bacterial clearance in murine Escherichia coli pneumonia. Thorax. 2012;**67**(6):533-539

[152] Hwa Cho H, Bae YC, Jung JS. Role of toll-like receptors on human adipose-derived stromal cells. Stem Cells. 2006;**24**(12):2744-2752

[153] Kim HS et al. Implication of NOD1 and NOD2 for the differentiation of multipotent mesenchymal stem cells derived from human umbilical cord blood. PLoS One. 2010;**5**(10):e15369

[154] Lee JW et al. Therapeutic effects of human mesenchymal stem cells in ex vivo human lungs injured with live bacteria. American Journal of Respiratory and Critical Care Medicine. 2013;**187**(7):751-760

[155] Stagg J et al. Interferon-gamma-stimulated marrow stromal cells: A new type of nonhematopoietic antigen-presenting cell. Blood. 2006;**107**(6):2570-2577

[156] Chan JL et al. Antigen-presenting property of mesenchymal stem cells occurs during a narrow window at low levels of interferon-gamma. Blood. 2006;**107**(12):4817-4824

[157] Romieu-Mourez R et al. Regulation of MHC class II expression and antigen processing in murine and human mesenchymal stromal cells by IFN-gamma, TGF-beta, and cell density. Journal of Immunology. 2007;**179**(3):1549-1558

[158] Hafen BB, Shook M, Burns B. Anatomy, Smooth Muscle. Treasure Island: StatPearls; 2022

[159] Hafen BB, Burns B. Physiology, Smooth Muscle. Treasure Island: StatPearls; 2022

[160] Sorokin V et al. Role of vascular smooth muscle cell plasticity and interactions in Vessel Wall inflammation. Frontiers in Immunology. 2020;**11**:599415

[161] Campbell GR et al. Degeneration and regeneration of smooth muscle transplants in the anterior eye chamber. An ultrastructural study. Zeitschrift für Zellforschung und Mikroskopische Anatomie. 1971;**117**(2):155-175

[162] Bennett MR, Sinha S, Owens GK. Vascular smooth muscle Cells in atherosclerosis. Circulation Research. 2016;**118**(4):692-702

[163] Clarke MC et al. Apoptosis of vascular smooth muscle cells induces features of plaque vulnerability in atherosclerosis. Nature Medicine. 2006;**12**(9):1075-1080

[164] Libby P et al. Atherosclerosis. Nature Reviews Disease Primers. 2019;**5**(1):56

[165] Gui Y, Zheng H, Cao RY. Foam Cells in atherosclerosis: Novel insights into its origins, consequences, and molecular mechanisms. Frontier in Cardiovascular Medicine. 2022;**9**:845942

[166] Cookson FB. The origin of foam cells in atherosclerosis. British Journal of Experimental Pathology. 1971;**52**(1):62-69

[167] Allahverdian S et al. Contribution of intimal smooth muscle cells to cholesterol accumulation and macrophage-like cells in human atherosclerosis. Circulation. 2014;**129**(15):1551-1559

[168] Gomez D, Owens GK. Smooth muscle cell phenotypic switching in atherosclerosis. Cardiovascular Research. 2012;**95**(2):156-164

[169] Shankman LS et al. KLF4-dependent phenotypic modulation of smooth muscle cells has a key role in atherosclerotic plaque pathogenesis. Nature Medicine. 2015;**21**(6):628-637

[170] Herz J, Strickland DK. LRP: A multifunctional scavenger and signaling receptor. The Journal of Clinical Investigation. 2001;**108**(6):779-784

[171] Chen J et al. The dual role of low-density lipoprotein receptor-related protein 1 in atherosclerosis. Frontier in Cardiovascular Medicine. 2021;**8**:682389

[172] Grootaert MOJ et al. Vascular smooth muscle cell death, autophagy and senescence in atherosclerosis. Cardiovascular Research. 2018;**114**(4):622-634

[173] Seeberg JC et al. Non-professional phagocytosis: A general feature of normal tissue cells. Scientific Reports. 2019;**9**(1):11875

Chapter 8

Physiological Role of Alveolar Macrophage in Acute Lower Respiratory Tract Infection: Phagocytosis and Aging

Ken Shirato, Keisuke Kasuga, Shogo Sato and Haruyuki Ishii

Abstract

Acute lower respiratory tract infections (LRTIs) are the deadliest communicable diseases. Inhaled pathogens that reach the alveoli are eliminated by lung-resident alveolar macrophages. Bacteria and fungi are detected and phagocytosed by specific pattern recognition receptors (PRRs) that are highly expressed in alveolar macrophages. In addition, early pro-inflammatory responses assist alveolar macrophages in the efficient phagocytosis of these pathogens. Viruses are also directly or indirectly endocytosed by pinocytosis or opsonization, respectively, whereas alveolar macrophages contribute to the prevention of pneumonia by removing endogenous dead cells through an alternate type of phagocytosis, efferocytosis. Macrophage phagocytosis and efferocytosis require not only sufficient expression of the relevant PRRs but also the coordinated interplay of intracellular factors that regulate engulfment. Given the current situation in which emerging infectious diseases spread worldwide, this chapter summarizes the physiological roles of alveolar macrophages in acute LRTIs, focusing on phagocytosis, pro-inflammatory responses, efferocytosis, and their regulatory machinery. This chapter also reviews recent insights into age-associated dysfunction of alveolar macrophages and discusses their relevance to vulnerability to acute LRTIs in the elderly population.

Keywords: alveolar macrophage, acute lower respiratory tract infection, pneumonia, phagocytosis, pro-inflammatory response, efferocytosis, pattern recognition receptor, intracellular signaling, aging

1. Introduction

Lung-resident alveolar macrophages play a pivotal role in maintaining lung homeostasis by eliminating airborne pathogenic microorganisms. The process by which cells ingest particles >0.5 μm in diameter, such as bacteria (0.5 to 2 μm) and fungi (3 to 10 μm), is defined as phagocytosis, which is composed of recognition, engulfment, and subsequent steps of the digestion process [1, 2]. Pathogen recognition occurs by directly detecting microbe-specific molecular signatures, known as pathogen-associated molecular patterns (PAMPs), using the corresponding pattern recognition receptors (PRRs), which activate downstream intracellular signaling that regulates cytoskeletal rearrangement and cell motility, leading to engulfment of pathogens [2–4]. As a result, efficient pathogen clearance necessitates sufficient expression of scavenger receptors as well as the continued concerted action of downstream signaling molecules. In addition to triggering phagocytosis, PAMPs induce the production of pro-inflammatory cytokines and chemokines via interactions with another family of PRRs, toll-like receptors (TLRs), resulting in the recruitment and activation of circulating phagocytes in the foci of infection and assisting the enhancement of macrophage phagocytosis [5–7].

However, unbridled inflammation is detrimental to tissue homeostasis, leading to organ failure if not properly treated. A typical example is the coronavirus disease 2019 (COVID-19), wherein critically ill patients are characterized by manifesting cytokine storm syndrome, resulting in respiratory failure and multiple organ failure [8, 9]. During viral infection, alveolar macrophages have been suggested to contribute to the alleviation of pneumonia by removing apoptotic epithelial cells and neutrophils from fighting viruses rather than by endocytosing viruses via pinocytosis and/or opsonization [10, 11]. Indeed, critically ill patients with COVID-19 are depleted of alveolar macrophages, which is accompanied by a remarkable increase in the proportion of pro-inflammatory monocyte-derived macrophages in bronchoalveolar lavage fluid [12]. Since the alternative type of phagocytosis, termed efferocytosis, is indispensable for preventing excessive inflammation during host defense against viral infection, failure of this protective action leads to the exacerbation of pneumonia from mild to life-threatening.

Severe acute respiratory syndrome coronavirus 2 (SARS-CoV-2), the virus that causes COVID-19, has received much attention from researchers since its outbreak owing to its highly virulent and transmissible nature; notably, COVID-19 is not the only threat to people. Acute lower respiratory tract infections (LRTIs), caused predominantly by *Streptococcus pneumoniae* and influenza viruses, remain the deadliest epidemics [13–15] because the older population is particularly liable to develop pneumonia and thereby respiratory failure [16, 17]. The vulnerability of the elderly to acute LRTIs has been suggested to be associated with immune senescence. In line with this trend, age-associated declines in immune cell functions and their mechanisms have been discussed [18–20]. Moreover, age-related alterations in the tissue microenvironment deeply influence immune cell senescence [21–23], and recent progress has enabled the analysis of the reality of alveolar microenvironment degeneration with aging and its adverse effects on alveolar macrophages.

In this chapter, we summarized the physiological roles of alveolar macrophages in acute LRTIs, focusing on phagocytosis, pro-inflammatory responses, efferocytosis, and their regulatory mechanisms. This chapter then reviewed recent insights into age-associated dysfunction of alveolar macrophages and discussed their relevance to the vulnerability of the elderly population to acute LRTIs.

2. Global epidemiology of acute LRTIs

2.1 Top causes of death

The World Health Organization (WHO) estimated that 55.4 million people died worldwide in 2019, with the top 10 leading causes accounting for 55% of deaths [13]. Further, seven of these causes are non-communicable diseases (NCDs), with the first, second, and third leading causes being ischemic heart disease, stroke, and chronic obstructive pulmonary disease. The total number of deaths caused by all NCDs accounts for 74% of the total deaths in the world. However, among communicable diseases, acute LRTIs kill 2.6 million people worldwide, making them the fourth leading cause of death.

2.2 Morbidity and mortality of acute LRTIs in children

According to the analysis results of the Global Burden of Disease Study (GBD) in 2016, acute LRTIs caused 336 million episodes and 2.4 million deaths in 2016 [14]. The rates of episodes and deaths attributable to acute LRTIs in children under the age of 5 were 2.4 and 3.2 times higher, respectively, compared with those in people of all ages; in particular, the mortality rates in children were the highest in developing countries in sub-Saharan Africa and South Asia. However, worldwide deaths from acute LRTIs in children decreased by 36.4% between 2007 and 2017 [16]. The substantial improvement in mortality in children is suggested to be primarily due to the implementation of vaccines against *S. pneumoniae* and *Haemophilus influenzae*, antibiotic therapy, and continuous improvements in education, nutrition, water, sanitation, and hygiene [24].

2.3 Morbidity and mortality of acute LRTIs in the elderly

Notably, the rates of episodes and deaths attributable to acute LRTIs in the elderly over the age of 70 were also 3.4 and 8.3 times higher, respectively, compared with those in people of all ages, but the mortality rates in older adults were globally higher than those in people of all ages [14]. Worldwide deaths from acute LRTIs in the elderly increased by 33.6% between 2007 and 2017 compared with those in children [16]. The deterioration of mortality in the elderly is likely associated with the extended longevity of the frail older population, chronic diseases, comorbidities, multiple medication use, and functional disability in high-income countries; further, it is associated with the adverse effects of air pollution, smoking, and alcohol consumption in low-income countries [24].

2.4 Most common causative agent of pneumonia

Acute LRTIs are responsible for inflammation of either the mucous membranes that line the bronchi or the lung tissue in one or both lungs, accompanied by infiltration and inflammation of the alveoli, leading to bronchitis or pneumonia, respectively [25]. Of the two conditions, pneumonia is the major cause of death, as it causes respiratory failure by filling the alveoli with fluid and pus resulting from inflammation [26]. Notably, pneumonia is caused by various pathogens, including bacteria, fungi, and viruses. *S. pneumoniae*, a Gram-positive bacterium, is the most common bacterial cause of pneumonia. In fact, across generations, *S. pneumoniae* accounted for approximately half of the pathogens that caused deaths in 2016, contributing to a higher number of deaths compared with all other major etiologies combined (respiratory syncytial virus, *H. influenzae* type b, and influenza) [14].

2.5 Seasonal influenza

Seasonal influenza epidemics occur every winter, annually resulting in 3–5 million cases of severe illness and 290,000–650,000 deaths from respiratory illness [15].

According to the analysis results of the GBD 2017, acute LRTIs attributable to influenza were estimated to have caused 55.5 million episodes, 9.5 million hospitalizations, and 145,000 deaths in 2017, and the highest mortality rates were observed, especially among adults over the age of 70 [17]. Of the influenza A and B viruses that cause seasonal epidemics, influenza A viruses, in particular, have a high mutagenic capacity to generate new strains that can escape from acquired immunity, which causes a pandemic every few decades. Further, the influenza A(N1H1)pdm09 strain emerged in April 2009 and caused a pandemic, globally resulting in 200,000 respiratory and 80,000 cardiovascular deaths that year [27].

2.6 COVID-19

The ongoing pandemic is COVID-19, which is caused by SARS-CoV-2. Since the first case of COVID-19 was reported in Wuhan, China, in December 2019, the infection has rapidly spread worldwide and continues to be a global epidemic, regardless of the season. According to the WHO, as of January 2023, the confirmed cases of infected patients had reached approximately 750 million worldwide, and deaths had risen to >6.8 million [28]. As with other acute LRTIs, older adults are at a higher risk of severe illness or death from COVID-19, even after the Delta-virulent strain was replaced by the Omicron-attenuated strain [29–33].

3. Physiological roles of alveolar macrophage phagocytosis in acute LRTIs

3.1 Development and maintenance of alveolar macrophages

Lung-resident alveolar macrophages play a leading role in the clearance of airborne microorganisms that enter the alveoli during inspiration. Murine alveolar macrophages originate from fetal monocytes [34]. The development of alveolar macrophages from fetal monocytes is regulated by granulocyte-macrophage colony-stimulating factor (GM-CSF) and the downstream transcription factor peroxisome proliferator-activated receptor γ (PPARγ) [35]. After birth, however, alveolar macrophages are essentially not replenished by bone marrow-derived monocytes but are self-maintained by the paracrine action of GM-CSF secreted by epithelial cells [35]. Moreover, further maturation of alveolar macrophages requires transforming growth factor (TGF)-β1, which is secreted in an autocrine manner and upregulates PPARγ expression [36]. A similar developmental pathway is presumed to occur in humans since immunostaining of lung sections from stillborn infants revealed that interstitial macrophages were abundant in the interstitium, whereas mature alveolar macrophages were completely absent in the alveoli [37]. The acquisition of specific functions by alveolar macrophages, including advanced phagocytic capacity, is partly due to the unique maturation processes in the alveolar microenvironment, where GM-CSF acts as a key regulator.

3.2 Phagocytic receptors expressed on alveolar macrophages

3.2.1 Scavenger receptors and their functions

Among the PRRs, two members of the scavenger receptor superfamily proteins, macrophage scavenger receptor 1 (MSR1) and macrophage receptor with collagenous structure (MARCO), recognize both Gram-positive and Gram-negative bacteria by detecting their pyrogenic cell wall components, lipoteichoic acid (LTA) and lipopolysaccharide (LPS), respectively [38–40]. Alveolar macrophages constitutively express MSR1 and MARCO, which are essential to eliminate airborne pathogenic bacteria. Knockout mice lacking MSR1 or MARCO displayed an impaired ability to remove live bacteria, exacerbated pneumonia, and reduced survival after intranasal inoculation with *S. pneumoniae* [41, 42]. The expression and function of MSR1 and MARCO are conserved in human alveolar macrophages [43]. Further, mice lacking another scavenger receptor, CD36, exhibited similar phenotypes during pulmonary infection caused by the Gram-positive bacterium *Staphylococcus aureus* [44]. In addition, alveolar macrophages are characterized by higher expression of scavenger receptors with one or more C-type lectin-like domains, such as β-1,3/1,6-D-glucan receptor dectin-1 [45, 46] and the mannose receptor CD206 [37, 47], which pivotally contribute to the removal of fungi and bacteria from the alveoli by detecting their respective target carbohydrates that cover the cell wall surface.

3.2.2 Opsonin receptors and their functions

Murine alveolar macrophages highly express Fcγ receptors FcγRI/II/III and further enhance their phagocytic activity when Gram-negative bacteria, *Pseudomonas aeruginosa*, are opsonized with IgG, whereas they hardly express complement receptors CR1/2/3, and their ability is not affected by complement opsonization [48]. Further, the other subset of complement receptor CRIg is expressed in murine and human alveolar macrophages [49], but its ability to directly recognize Gram-positive bacteria by detecting LTA suggests that it can act as a PRR in the lungs [50]. Notably, alveolar macrophages isolated from GM-CSF-knockout mice were deficient in Fcγ receptors and had impaired phagocytic activity against both IgG-opsonized and non-opsonized latex beads and their phenotypes were restored by epithelial cell-specific expression of GM-CSF [51]. A recent study reported that human alveolar macrophages express FcγRI/II/III at higher levels than other systemic counterparts, such as macrophages in the bone marrow, spleen, and liver [52]. Moreover, peripheral blood monocyte-derived macrophages that differentiated in GM-CSF-containing culture exhibited properties that were partially similar to those of alveolar macrophages, expressing a larger amount of FcγRI/II compared with that of their counterparts [52].

3.3 Regulation of engulfment in alveolar macrophages

3.3.1 Roles of small-GTP binding proteins in engulfment

Pathogen recognition by scavenger and opsonin receptors initiates cytoskeleton remodeling, leading to pathogen engulfment. The regulatory signaling pathways rely on each receptor ligated to the particles, but all forms of engulfment require the recruitment of filamentous (F)-actin beneath tethered particles and subsequent rearrangement of F-actin. F-actin is primarily controlled by three small-GTP binding proteins, including Ras homolog (Rho) family member A (RhoA), Ras-related C3 botulinus toxin substrate 1 (Rac1), and cell division control protein 42 homolog (Cdc42), both of which are members of Rho family [2, 4]. The binding of particles to receptors causes RhoA, Rac1, and Cdc42 to be converted from the GDP-bound inactive form to active form and then recruited from the cytosol to the cell membrane under tethered particles, where they regulate F-actin rearrangement and subsequent cell motility by triggering the formation of stress fibers, lamellipodia, and filopodia, respectively [2].

3.3.2 Receptor-dependent roles of small-GTP binding proteins

The roles of these small-GTP binding proteins have been systematically studied after the ligation of Fcγ receptors. FcγRIIA-transfected COS fibroblasts treated with IgG-opsonized particles facilitated recruitment of all the small-GTP binding proteins to the nascent F-actin phagocytic cup, whereas blocking Rac1 and Cdc42 suppressed engulfment by preventing the formation of membrane ruffles and filopodia, respectively; however, blocking RhoA had no effects on the engulfment [53]. In contrast, when CR3-transfected COS fibroblasts were treated with complement-opsonized particles, only RhoA colocalized with F-actin, and blocking RhoA compromised CR3-mediated phagocytosis [53]. Dectin-1 has downstream signaling cascades that are highly similar to those of Fcγ receptors [54]. Although the downstream pathways of MSR1 and CD36 have not yet been reported, a recent study indicated that the Gram-negative bacterium *Escherichia coli* interacts with MARCO, which activates Rac1 to initiate F-actin polymerization, filopodia formation, and subsequent engulfment in murine alveolar macrophages [55].

4. Physiological roles of alveolar macrophage pro-inflammatory responses in acute LRTIs

4.1 PAMPs closely associated with activation of alveolar macrophages

In addition to phagocytosis, alveolar macrophages induce pro-inflammatory responses by detecting PAMPs using a wide variety of PRRs, including TLRs, to facilitate the immediate mobilization and activation of phagocytes such as neutrophils and monocytes. For instance, during pulmonary infection with *S. pneumoniae*, the cell wall components of Gram-positive bacteria, lipoproteins [56], LTA [57], peptidoglycan [58], and the structural ancillary pilus protein, RrgA oligomer [59], are detected by TLR2, while the pneumococcal virulence factor pneumolysin is detected by TLR4 [60, 61]. Endopeptidase O, a new pneumococcal virulence protein, induces pro-inflammatory responses in macrophages by activating both TLR2 and TLR4 signaling [62]. For Gram-negative bacteria such as *H. influenzae* type b, the cell wall components, LPS and porin proteins, are detected by TLR4 [63] and TLR2 [64], respectively. Further, TLR9 detects bacterial DNA [65]. Thus, bacterial infection stimulates multiple TLRs simultaneously, rather than singly, resulting in complex signal activation.

4.2 Downstream signaling of TLRs and their outcomes

Detailed figures illustrating downstream signaling by TLRs are available in a highly specialized review article [5]. When TLR4 is activated by its agonists, it engages two distinct adaptor proteins in the signaling process: myeloid differentiation factor 88 (MyD88) and toll/interleukin (IL)-1 receptor domain-containing adapter-inducing interferon (IFN)-β (TRIF). The MyD88-dependent pathway recruits IL-1 receptor-associated kinases 1 and 4, which phosphorylate tumor necrosis factor (TNF) receptor-associated factor 6 (TRAF6), leading to the activation of nuclear factor-κB (NF-κB), p44/42 mitogen-activated protein kinase (MAPK), p38 MAPK, and c-Jun N-terminal kinase (JNK). However, the TRIF-dependent pathway facilitates the formation of a complex consisting of TRAF3, TRAF family member-associated NF-κB activator (TANK), TANK-binding kinase 1, and inhibitor of NF-κB kinase subunit ε, which phosphorylates IFN regulatory factor 3, resulting in the activation of dimers to translocate from the cytoplasm into the nucleus. The MyD88-dependent pathway elicits the production of pro-inflammatory cytokines (TNF-α, IL-6, and IL-1β), chemokines (IL-8 and monocyte chemoattractant protein 1), and anti-microbial proteins (inducible nitric oxide synthase), whereas the TRIF-dependent pathway triggers the production of type I IFNs (IFN-α/β). Unlike TLR4, TLR2 and TLR9 only initiate the MyD88-dependent pathway.

4.3 Roles of TLRs in pneumococcal infection

Studies using TLR2-, TLR4-, or TLR9-knockout or mutant mice suggested the protective role of TLR2, TLR4, and TLR9 against pneumococcal infection. However, TLRs are ubiquitously expressed in cells other than immune cells. Therefore, the phenotypes observed in these studies are attributable to the lack of TLR signaling not only in alveolar macrophages but also in alveolar structural cells.

4.3.1 Roles of TLR2 in pneumococcal infection

The comparison of TLR2-knockout mice with wild-type mice indicated only a partial reduction in pro-inflammatory cytokine production after intranasal *S. pneumoniae* inoculation, with no significant difference in survival rate or bacterial clearance, suggesting that TLR2 signaling plays a minor role in eliciting local inflammation and bactericidal activity against *S. pneumoniae* [66]. Further, no differences were observed between TLR2-knockout and wild-type mice in bacterial growth, lung inflammation, or pro-inflammatory cytokine and chemokine production in post-influenza pneumococcal pneumonia [67]. Similar results were obtained in splenectomized mice [68].

4.3.2 Roles of TLR4 in pneumococcal infection

On inoculation with a non-lethal dose of *S. pneumoniae*, TLR4 mutant mice exhibited decreased survival rates, accompanied by increased bacterial growth, monocyte and lymphocyte infiltration, and interstitial inflammation in the lungs [69]. Notably, a recent study demonstrated that although mice lacking TLR4 also displayed lower viability and augmented colonization in the lung after intranasal *S. pneumoniae* inoculation compared with that of wild-type mice, this exacerbation of infection was accompanied by an attenuated pro-inflammatory profile, reduced live alveolar macrophages, diminished infiltration of neutrophils and monocytes, and inhibition of monocyte differentiation into macrophages [70]. In addition, MyD88 deletion was not able to completely reproduce these phenotypes, implying that pro-inflammatory responses via both MyD88- and TRIF-dependent TLR4 signaling are necessary for the mobilization and activation of phagocytes [70]. Therefore, TLR4 signaling could have led to the sufficient elimination of bacteria and subsequent protection of alveolar macrophages from pneumococcal cytotoxicity.

4.3.3 Roles of TLR9 in pneumococcal infection

Both TLR9-knockout and wild-type mice developed pulmonary inflammation during *S. pneumoniae* infection, but TLR9-knockout mice exhibited worse survival and more bacterial invasion from the bronchoalveolar fluids into the lung tissue and blood stream, with abrogated upregulation of phagocytic activity in alveolar macrophages [71]. This early finding indicates that the activation of TLR9 signaling is indispensable for maximizing phagocytosis in alveolar macrophages during pneumococcal infection. The priming effects of TLR agonists have also been investigated. A prior inhalational challenge with the TLR9 agonist ODN2395 in combination with the TLR2 agonist Pam2CSK4 protected mice from death due to *S. pneumoniae* infection, although administration of agonists of any individual TLR had no protective effect [72]. However, ODN2395/Pam2CSK4 stimulation enhanced intracellular bacterial death in isolated tracheal epithelial cells, but not in alveolar macrophages. Taken together, maintaining basal levels of TLR9 expression and signaling in alveolar macrophages is likely to be critical for defensing the host from pneumococcal infection.

5. Physiological roles of alveolar macrophage efferocytosis in acute LRTIs

5.1 Roles of alveolar macrophages in viral infection

Alveolar macrophages can directly or indirectly endocytose viruses via pinocytosis or opsonization, respectively. In the case of SARS-CoV-2, alveolar macrophages also recognize viral components such as envelop protein [73], spike protein [74–77], and single-stranded RNA [78, 79] using TLR2, TLR4, and TLR3/7, respectively, which trigger pro-inflammatory responses. However, the phagocytic and pro-inflammatory responses of alveolar macrophages against viruses appear to be dispensable for protecting the host from viral infection. Indeed, the absence of mature alveolar macrophages in GM-CSF-deficient mice resulted in severe respiratory failure and increased mortality after pulmonary infection with a non-lethal dose of influenza A virus, and these conditions were improved by neonatal transplantation of alveolar macrophage progenitor cells from wild-type mice [11]; however, alveolar macrophage-depleted mice exhibited severe manifestations, with viral clearance not being largely impaired and the functions of antibody-producing B lymphocytes and cytotoxic CD8-positive T-lymphocytes being normally activated [11]. Similarly, critically ill patients with COVID-19 have been characterized by a depletion of alveolar macrophages and a remarkably increased proportion of recruited pro-inflammatory monocyte-derived macrophages in bronchoalveolar lavage fluid [12]. These suggest that alveolar macrophages contribute to host survival by suppressing excessive pulmonary inflammation, which is caused by removing endogenous apoptotic cells rather than by phagocytosing the exogenous virus itself during infection.

5.2 Regulation and roles of efferocytosis in alveolar macrophages

Notably, clearance of apoptotic cells, termed efferocytosis, is an essential process for maintaining tissue homeostasis under both healthy and diseased conditions. Efferocytosis differs morphologically and mechanistically from the classical form of phagocytosis against pathogens and requires the expression of receptors that recognize "eat me" signatures such as phosphatidylserine (Ptd-L-Ser) exposed on the membrane surface of apoptotic cells [80]. Macrophages perform efferocytosis primarily using tyrosine receptor kinases as Ptd-L-Ser receptors, including Tyro 3, Axl, and proto-oncogene c-mer tyrosine kinase (MerTK) (collectively abbreviated as TAM) [81]. In a recent study, transcriptome and flow-cytometric analyses revealed that murine alveolar macrophages highly express Axl and MerTK, but little or no expression was found in lung-mobilized monocytes after the LPS challenge [82]. Moreover, human alveolar macrophages predominantly express Axl, and peripheral monocytes do not express either Axl or MerTK [83]. Although Axl-knockout mice did not manifest inflammatory disorders under healthy conditions, they exhibited exaggerated severity during pulmonary infection with influenza A virus, accompanied by increased accumulation of apoptotic cells, elevated infiltration of neutrophils and T-lymphocytes, and increased secretion of pro-inflammatory cytokines and chemokines, without compromising virus clearance [10]. In addition, during acute lung injury after LPS challenge in mice, alveolar macrophages engulfed Pst-L-Ser-exposed microparticles but not lung-mobilized monocytes, and deletion of MerTK abrogated efferocytosis activity in both in vivo and in vitro experiments [82]. Therefore, alveolar macrophages prevent excessive pulmonary inflammation via efferocytosis using Axl and MerTK in lung injuries caused by viruses and bacteria; notably, lung-mobilized pro-inflammatory monocytes do not contribute to efferocytosis, at least at the early stage of infection.

5.3 Anti-inflammatory properties of efferocytosis in alveolar macrophages

Notably, TAM receptor-mediated recognition of Ptd-L-Ser requires soluble cross-linking molecules in the serum (growth arrest-specific gene 6 or protein S) [84]. Similar to pathogen recognition by phagocytic receptors, ligation of TAM receptors results in the activation of Rac1, leading to membrane ruffling to engulf apoptotic bodies [85, 86]. Phagocytic receptors are linked to pro-inflammatory responses [4, 87], whereas TAM receptors activate anti-inflammatory responses in macrophages. For example, TAM receptor ligation activates type I IFN receptor signaling to upregulate the expression of suppressors of cytokine signaling 1 and 3. This induces negative feedback to suppress type I IFN receptor signaling and both MyD88- and TRIF-dependent TLR signaling [88]. Moreover, the detailed molecular mechanisms underlying the promotion of anti-inflammatory IL-10 and TGF-β production during efferocytosis in macrophages have also been elucidated. The coenzyme NAD^+, generated by mitochondrial β-oxidation of apoptotic cell-derived fatty acids, activates sirtuin-1 and downstream transcription factor PBX homeobox 1, producing IL-10 in macrophages [89]. Higher expression of cholesterol 25-hydroxylase, characteristically found in alveolar macrophages, contributes to the biosynthesis of 25-hydroxycholesterol, which stimulates the nuclear receptor liver X receptor to increase transcriptional activity during efferocytosis, leading to the escalation of TGF-β production [90]. Thus, alveolar macrophages have advanced efferocytosis activity, enabling them to promptly and effectively eliminate the apoptotic bodies that prominently appear during viral infection. Furthermore, this property is indispensable for preventing excessive pulmonary inflammation owing to the massive production of viruses and damage-associated molecular patterns (DAMPs) from apoptotic bodies that lose cell membrane integrity.

6. Age-associated dysfunction of alveolar macrophages

As discussed in Section 2, recent epidemiological data indicate that older adults are vulnerable to acute LRTIs that are attributable to either bacteria or viruses, and the globally increasing life expectancy further reinforces this fact. Phagocytosis by alveolar macrophages is responsible for the frontline defense against inhaled bacteria and fungi (Section 3), and the pro-inflammatory responses assist the defense by promoting phagocytosis (Section 4). During viral infection, efferocytosis of alveolar macrophages is indispensable to prevent uncontrolled pneumonia caused by DAMPs that leak from damaged and dead cells (Section 5). Since alveolar macrophages are characterized by advanced phagocytosis and efferocytosis, the decline in their activity is likely associated with the age-dependent exacerbation of acute LRTIs (**Figure 1**). In this section, we discussed the past and recent progress in the findings regarding age-related dysfunction of alveolar macrophages.

6.1 Age-associated decline in alveolar macrophage phagocytosis

A previous study demonstrated that macrophages accounted for approximately 95% of the bronchoalveolar lavage fluid cells in both young and aged mice [91]. The absolute numbers of alveolar macrophages were also similar, but they indicated an age-related decrease when adjusted for lung weight, as discussed later (subsection 6.5). The percentage of alveolar macrophages capable of phagocytosing latex beads was approximately 80% and 60% in young and aged mice, respectively, and the difference was statistically significant. Like bacteria, phagocytosis against non-opsonized latex beads is mediated by MSR1 and CD36 [92]. Thus, these results suggest that aging is associated with reduced expression of scavenger receptors and/or an impaired ability to transduce engulfment signals, leading to an age-dependent decline in alveolar macrophage phagocytosis (**Figure 1A**). This finding is supported by recent evidence from in vivo studies. The phagocytic capacity of each alveolar macrophage for intranasally instilled latex beads was lower in aged mice than in young mice [93]. In this study, aged mice also exhibited decreased cell surface expression levels of MSR1, but not of CD36 and CD206, in alveolar macrophages (**Figure 1A**).

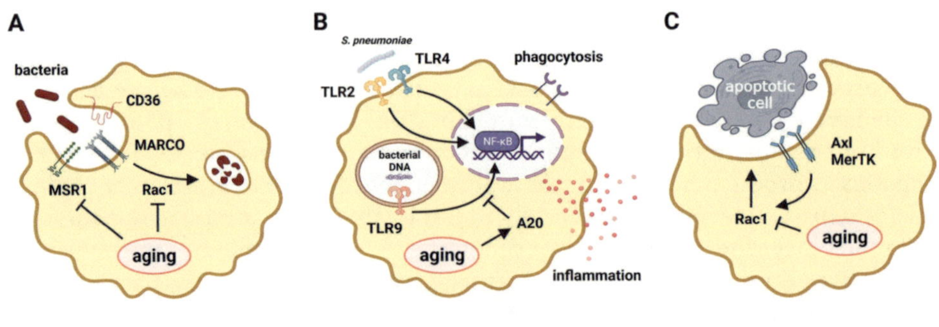

Figure 1.
Intracellular events involved in age-associated dysfunction of phagocytosis (A), pro-inflammatory responses (B), and efferocytosis (C) in alveolar macrophages. (A) Age-associated decline in phagocytosis is mediated by reduced expression levels of MSR1 and Rac1. (B) Age-associated decline in pro-inflammatory responses is due to elevated expression levels of A20, which inactivates TRAF6, an upstream signaling protein of NF-κB, to suppress Streptococcus pneumoniae-stimulated signaling activation of TLRs. (C) Age-associated decline in efferocytosis is possible to be dependent on reduced expression levels of Rac1, which transmits engulfment signal associated with the TAM receptors Axl and MerTK.

Moreover, alveolar macrophages in aged mice exhibited reduced phagocytosis after intratracheal injection of *E. coli*, which could be attributed to the reduced constitutive expression levels of Rac1 and resultant attenuated F-actin polymerization and filopodia formation (**Figure 1A**) [55]. No studies on human alveolar macrophages have been reported; however, unlike animal studies wherein the laboratory environment is maintained, identifying only the pure effects of aging in humans without other confounding factors is challenging. This is because smoking habits [94–96], chronic alcohol abuse [95, 97], and exposure to air pollutants [95] have been found to adversely influence alveolar macrophage phagocytosis.

6.2 Age-associated decline in alveolar macrophage pro-inflammatory responses

Studies indicate that increased susceptibility to pneumococcal infection in elderly people is associated with a compromised initial response to TLR signaling in alveolar macrophages (**Figure 1B**). For instance, alveolar macrophages from aged mice exhibit suppressed responsiveness to in vitro LPS stimulation [98]. Notably, aged mice exhibited reduced survival, impaired bacterial clearance, and attenuated prompt pro-inflammatory cytokine production after intratracheal challenge with *S. pneumoniae*, which was accompanied by attenuated *S. pneumoniae*- or its cell wall-stimulated phosphorylation of NF-κB p65 subunit, p38 MAPK, and JNK, in alveolar macrophages (**Figure 1B**) [99]. Further result was presented as a possible mechanism. In aged mice, the expression of A20 is specifically elevated in alveolar macrophages, which reduces *S. pneumoniae* exposure-induced IL-6 production (**Figure 1B**) [100]. A20 is known to inactivate TRAF6 in the cytosol, resulting in defects in its common downstream NF-κB, p38 MAPK, and JNK signaling cascades [101]. Thus, during pneumococcal infection, TLR9 signaling-mediated upregulation of alveolar macrophage phagocytosis can also be impaired in aged mice or humans (subsection 4.3.3) (**Figure 1B**). Notably, in an in vitro *Mycobacterium tuberculosis* infection model, compared with alveolar macrophages from young mice, those from aged mice constitutively expressed similar levels of TLR2, TLR4, and TLR9. They were able to produce equivalent levels of IL-12 and TNF-α in response to infection, while the contribution of TLR2 signaling to pro-inflammatory cytokine production was distinctly reduced in aged mice [102]. This suggests that phenotypes associated with age-dependent deterioration of TLR signaling differ according to the type of bacteria and possibly the composition of their virulence factors.

6.3 Age-associated decline in alveolar macrophage efferocytosis

Aged mice indicated significant deterioration in survival rate and clinical score after intranasal instillation with influenza A virus, which also caused increased inflammation, accumulation of apoptotic cells in the alveoli, and impaired ability to bind to and engulf apoptotic neutrophils in alveolar macrophages [93]. In this study, alveolar macrophages from aged mice retained normal Axl expression levels but had markedly reduced levels of MSR1, as discussed above (Section 6.1). Further, MSR1 suppresses excessive inflammation by mediating the internalization of DAMPs by macrophages in a mouse model of ischemic stroke brain injury [103]. In addition, MSR1 participates in Tyro 3 signaling in macrophages to mediate efferocytosis in a mouse model of acute aortic dissection [104]. However, since alveolar macrophages express Axl or MerTK, but not Tyro 3 (Section 5.2), whether the age-associated decline in efferocytosis is caused by defects in the MSR1-Tyro 3 signaling axis is unclear. Engulfment of apoptotic cells via TAM receptors requires Rac1 activation (Section 5.3), and Rac1 expression is depleted in alveolar macrophages from aged mice (Section 6.1), implying that reduced Rac1 expression is involved in the age-associated decline in efferocytosis (**Figure 1C**). In summary, the decreased processing capacity for DAMPs due to suppressed MSR1 expression and decreased efferocytosis activity due to suppressed Rac1 expression in alveolar macrophages can be involved in the exacerbation of viral infection.

6.4 Age-associated change in alveolar macrophage subpopulation

Lung macrophages (a crude fraction containing both alveolar and interstitial macrophages) from aged mice has a high baseline level of dysfunctional expression of IFN-γ target genes, and IFN-γ fails to boost ex vivo *M. tuberculosis* infection-induced phagosome-lysosome fusion and IL-12 production in aged mouse cells [105]. The so-called inflammaging phenotype in alveolar macrophages and lining fluid extends further to a wide variety of pro-inflammatory cytokine and chemokine levels, which was caused by an increased subpopulation of CD11b-positive alveolar macrophages originating from peripheral monocytes [106]. Such inflammaging systemically occurs in humans as well [107]. Although inflammaging of alveolar macrophages has been suggested to increase susceptibility to *M. tuberculosis* in the elderly [105, 106, 108, 109], the relationship between inflammaging and vulnerability to acute LRTIs remains to be elucidated [110]. Further, recruitment of circulating monocytes to the alveoli has been demonstrated in several longitudinal studies using mice in which bone marrow-derived monocytes were labeled with specific reporters [111, 112] and was systematically discussed in a review article [113]. In contrast, another recent genetic lineage-tracing analysis using CD45.1/CD45.2 chimeric mice yielded contradictory observations that the proportion of CD45.1-positive monocyte-derived macrophages and CD45.2-positive tissue-resident macrophages in the alveoli were preserved throughout life [114]. However, when infected with a sublethal dose of the influenza A virus, monocyte-derived macrophages were recruited into the alveoli, and the macrophages persisted for at least 60 days. These results underpin previous findings that alveolar macrophages are not replenished by bone marrow-derived monocytes [35]. Further experimental results and an integrated understanding are required to clarify the age-associated changes in alveolar macrophage subpopulations and their role in susceptibility to acute LRTIs.

6.5 Age-associated change in alveolar macrophage abundance

A previous study reported a significantly reduced proportion of alveolar macrophages in bronchoalveolar lavage fluid cells in the elderly [115]. Likewise, aged mice indicated decreased numbers of alveolar macrophages per unit lung weight in two strains (BALB/c and C57BL/6 J), which was accompanied by the downregulation of gene expression that regulates the cell cycle [93]. These findings suggest that the quantitative decline in alveolar macrophages with age partially contributes to the high vulnerability to acute LRTIs in the elderly. In another recent study, the gene expression profile was reproduced in murine as well as human alveolar macrophages; however, this property could be mediated by the inhibition of GM-CSF signaling in alveolar macrophages due to age-dependent alterations in the alveolar microenvironment (especially, increased hyaluronan levels in the alveolar epithelial lining fluid), but not due to cell-autonomous mechanisms such as alterations in intracellular signaling protein levels or circulating monocyte migration [114]. Indeed, the transplantation of alveolar macrophages from aged mice into the alveoli of young mice reverted age-related changes in the transcriptome to a state resembling young alveolar macrophages [114]. Although the importance of age-associated changes in the tissue microenvironment has long been proposed [21], recent advances in research methods and techniques have made it possible to elucidate the role of age-related alterations in the alveolar microenvironment. Therefore, the mechanism by which aging reduces phagocytosis, pro-inflammatory responses, and efferocytosis can be primarily explained by the inhibition of the differentiation or maturation of alveolar macrophages through microenvironmental degeneration.

7. Conclusion

Alveolar macrophages acquire heterogeneity with other lineages by receiving unique signals in the alveolar microenvironment. The advanced phagocytosis and efferocytosis activities of alveolar macrophages enable efficient clearance of continuously inhaled pathogens and endogenous dead cells, respectively, which contributes to the prevention of uncontrolled pneumonia. Previous studies have addressed the reasons for the vulnerability of the elderly to acute LRTIs, mainly shedding light on the senescence process of alveolar macrophages from a cell-autonomous aspect. However, in addition to the knowledge gained from such studies, recent progress in experimental methods and techniques is beginning to provide insightful evidence that age-associated alterations in the alveolar microenvironment mediate reversible dysfunction of alveolar macrophages. In other words, to improve age-related dysfunction of alveolar macrophages, an approach that targets the cells is inefficient, whereas exploring methods to recover age-related alterations in the alveolar microenvironment is appropriate. As the average life expectancy is estimated to further increase in the future, exploring health promotion activities (i.e., habitual exercise, healthy diet, and regular sleep cycle) or supplements that influence the alveolar microenvironment and whether such factors can reduce the risk of acute LRTIs in the elderly is essential. We hope that this chapter will help students, trainees, and researchers in their education and research in health and life sciences.

Acknowledgements

K.S. was supported by a Grant-in-Aid for Scientific Research (C) (21 K11472) from the Ministry of Education, Culture, Sports, Science and Technology, Japan. S.S. was funded by the Brain & Behavior Research Foundation (NARSAD Young Investigator Grant, 28681) and start-up funds from Texas A&M University. We would like to express our deepest gratitude to Dr. Takako Kizaki (Visiting Professor, Kyorin University Faculty of Medicine, Mitaka, Japan) and Dr. Kazuhiko Imaizumi (Professor Emeritus, Faculty of Human Sciences, Waseda University, Tokorozawa, Japan) for their consistent guidance on macrophage biology and physiological science, respectively. The figure was created using BioRender.com.

Conflict of interest

The authors declare no conflict of interest.

Author details

Ken Shirato[1*], Keisuke Kasuga[2], Shogo Sato[3] and Haruyuki Ishii[2]

1 Department of Molecular Predictive Medicine and Sport Science, Kyorin University Faculty of Medicine, Mitaka, Japan

2 Department of Respiratory Medicine, Kyorin University Faculty of Medicine, Mitaka, Japan

3 Center for Biological Clocks Research, Department of Biology, Texas A&M University, College Station, TX, USA

*Address all correspondence to: shirato@ks.kyorin-u.ac.jp

References

[1] Gordon S. Phagocytosis: An Immunobiologic process. Immunity. 2016;**44**(3):463-475

[2] Mao Y, Finnemann SC. Regulation of phagocytosis by Rho GTPases. Small GTPases. 2015;**6**(2):89-99

[3] Lee HJ, Woo Y, Hahn TW, Jung YM, Jung YJ. Formation and maturation of the phagosome: A key mechanism in innate immunity against intracellular bacterial infection. Microorganisms. 2020;**8**(9):1298

[4] Moretti J, Blander JM. Insights into phagocytosis-coupled activation of pattern recognition receptors and inflammasomes. Current Opinion in Immunology. 2014;**26**:100-110

[5] Kawasaki T, Kawai T. Toll-like receptor signaling pathways. Frontiers in Immunology. 2014;**5**:461

[6] Orecchioni M, Matsunami H, Ley K. Olfactory receptors in macrophages and inflammation. Frontiers in Immunology. 2022;**13**:1029244

[7] Doyle SE, O'Connell RM, Miranda GA, Vaidya SA, Chow EK, Liu PT, et al. Toll-like receptors induce a phagocytic gene program through p38. The Journal of Experimental Medicine. 2004;**199**(1):81-90

[8] Merad M, Martin JC. Author correction: Pathological inflammation in patients with COVID-19: A key role for monocytes and macrophages. Nature Reviews. Immunology. 2020;**20**(7):448

[9] Mehta P, McAuley DF, Brown M, Sanchez E, Tattersall RS, Manson JJ. COVID-19: Consider cytokine storm syndromes and immunosuppression. Lancet. 2020;**395**(10229):1033-1034

[10] Fujimori T, Grabiec AM, Kaur M, Bell TJ, Fujino N, Cook PC, et al. The Axl receptor tyrosine kinase is a discriminator of macrophage function in the inflamed lung. Mucosal Immunology. 2015;**8**(5):1021-1030

[11] Schneider C, Nobs SP, Heer AK, Kurrer M, Klinke G, van Rooijen N, et al. Alveolar macrophages are essential for protection from respiratory failure and associated morbidity following influenza virus infection. PLoS Pathogens. 2014;**10**(4):e1004053

[12] Liao M, Liu Y, Yuan J, Wen Y, Xu G, Zhao J, et al. Single-cell landscape of bronchoalveolar immune cells in patients with COVID-19. Nature Medicine. 2020;**26**(6):842-844

[13] World Health Organization. The top 10 causes of death. 2020. Available from: https://www.who.int/news-room/fact-sheets/detail/the-top-10-causes-of-death

[14] GBD 2016 Lower Respiratory Infections Collaborators. Estimates of the global, regional, and national morbidity, mortality, and aetiologies of lower respiratory infections in 195 countries, 1990-2016: A systematic analysis for the Global Burden of Disease Study 2016. Lancet Infectious Diseases. 2018;**18**(11):1191-1210

[15] World Health Organization. Influenza (Seasonal) 2023. Available from: https://www.who.int/news-room/fact-sheets/detail/influenza-(seasonal)

[16] GBD 2017 Causes of Death Collaborators. Global, regional, and national age-sex-specific mortality for 282 causes of death in 195 countries and territories, 1980-2017:

A systematic analysis for the Global Burden of Disease Study 2017. Lancet. 2018;**392**(10159):1736-1788

[17] GBD 2017 Influenza Collaborators. Mortality, morbidity, and hospitalisations due to influenza lower respiratory tract infections, 2017: An analysis for the Global Burden of Disease Study 2017. Lancet Respiratory Medicine. 2019;**7**(1):69-89

[18] Crooke SN, Ovsyannikova IG, Poland GA, Kennedy RB. Immunosenescence and human vaccine immune responses. Immunity & Ageing. 2019;**16**:25

[19] Aiello A, Farzaneh F, Candore G, Caruso C, Davinelli S, Gambino CM, et al. Immunosenescence and its hallmarks: How to oppose aging strategically? A review of potential options for therapeutic intervention. Frontiers in Immunology. 2019;**10**:2247

[20] Pawelec G, Akbar A, Caruso C, Solana R, Grubeck-Loebenstein B, Wikby A. Human immunosenescence: Is it infectious? Immunological Reviews. 2005;**205**:257-268

[21] Stout RD, Suttles J. Immunosenescence and macrophage functional plasticity: Dysregulation of macrophage function by age-associated microenvironmental changes. Immunological Reviews. 2005;**205**:60-71

[22] Tan Q, Liang N, Zhang X, Li J. Dynamic aging: Channeled through microenvironment. Frontiers in Physiology. 2021;**12**:702276

[23] Zhao Y, Yang Y, Li Q, Li J. Understanding the unique microenvironment in the aging liver. Frontiers in Medicine (Lausanne). 2022;**9**:842024

[24] Torres A, Cilloniz C, Niederman MS, Menéndez R, Chalmers JD, Wunderink RG, et al. Pneumonia. Nature Review Disease Primers. 2021;**7**(1):25

[25] Nowicki J, Murray MT. Bronchitis and pneumonia. Textbook of Natural Medicine. 2020;**2020**:1196-201.e1

[26] World Health Organization. Pneumonia in children 2022. Available from: https://www.who.int/news-room/fact-sheets/detail/pneumonia

[27] Dawood FS, Iuliano AD, Reed C, Meltzer MI, Shay DK, Cheng PY, et al. Estimated global mortality associated with the first 12 months of 2009 pandemic influenza A H1N1 virus circulation: A modelling study. The Lancet Infectious Diseases. 2012;**12**(9):687-695

[28] World Health Organization. WHO Coronavirus (COVID-19) Dashboard 2023. Available from: https://covid19.who.int/?adgroupsurvey={adgroupsurvey}&gclid=EAIaIQobChMItqXFnLXu_AIVz34rCh1w9wUWEAAYASABEgJgX_D_BwE

[29] Ho FK, Petermann-Rocha F, Gray SR, Jani BD, Katikireddi SV, Niedzwiedz CL, et al. Is older age associated with COVID-19 mortality in the absence of other risk factors? General population cohort study of 470,034 participants. PLoS One. 2020;**15**(11):e0241824

[30] Lu G, Zhang Y, Zhang H, Ai J, He L, Yuan X, et al. Geriatric risk and protective factors for serious COVID-19 outcomes among older adults in Shanghai Omicron wave. Emerg Microbes Infectious. 2022;**11**(1):2045-2054

[31] O'Driscoll M, Ribeiro Dos Santos G, Wang L, Cummings DAT, Azman AS, Paireau J, et al. Age-specific mortality

and immunity patterns of SARS-CoV-2. Nature. 2021;**590**(7844):140-145

[32] Ward IL, Bermingham C, Ayoubkhani D, Gethings OJ, Pouwels KB, Yates T, et al. Risk of covid-19 related deaths for SARS-CoV-2 omicron (B.1.1.529) compared with delta (B.1.617.2): Retrospective cohort study. BMJ. 2022;**378**:e070695

[33] Yanez ND, Weiss NS, Romand JA, Treggiari MM. COVID-19 mortality risk for older men and women. BMC Public Health. 2020;**20**(1):1742

[34] Guilliams M, De Kleer I, Henri S, Post S, Vanhoutte L, De Prijck S, et al. Alveolar macrophages develop from fetal monocytes that differentiate into long-lived cells in the first week of life via GM-CSF. The Journal of Experimental Medicine. 2013;**210**(10):1977-1992

[35] Schneider C, Nobs SP, Kurrer M, Rehrauer H, Thiele C, Kopf M. Induction of the nuclear receptor PPAR-γ by the cytokine GM-CSF is critical for the differentiation of fetal monocytes into alveolar macrophages. Nature Immunology. 2014;**15**(11):1026-1037

[36] Yu X, Buttgereit A, Lelios I, Utz SG, Cansever D, Becher B, et al. The cytokine TGF-β promotes the development and homeostasis of alveolar macrophages. Immunity. 2017;**47**(5):903-12.e4

[37] Bharat A, Bhorade SM, Morales-Nebreda L, McQuattie-Pimentel AC, Soberanes S, Ridge K, et al. Flow cytometry reveals similarities between lung macrophages in humans and mice. American Journal of Respiratory Cell and Molecular Biology. 2016;**54**(1):147-149

[38] Dunne DW, Resnick D, Greenberg J, Krieger M, Joiner KA. The type I macrophage scavenger receptor binds to gram-positive bacteria and recognizes lipoteichoic acid. Proceedings of the National Academy of Sciences of the United States of America. 1994;**91**(5):1863-1867

[39] Hampton RY, Golenbock DT, Penman M, Krieger M, Raetz CR. Recognition and plasma clearance of endotoxin by scavenger receptors. Nature. 1991;**352**(6333):342-344

[40] SankalaM,BrännströmA,SchulthessT, Bergmann U, Morgunova E, Engel J, et al. Characterization of recombinant soluble macrophage scavenger receptor MARCO. The Journal of Biological Chemistry. 2002;**277**(36):33378-33385

[41] Arredouani MS, Yang Z, Imrich A, Ning Y, Qin G, Kobzik L. The macrophage scavenger receptor SR-AI/II and lung defense against pneumococci and particles. American Journal of Respiratory Cell and Molecular Biology. 2006;**35**(4):474-478

[42] Arredouani M, Yang Z, Ning Y, Qin G, Soininen R, Tryggvason K, et al. The scavenger receptor MARCO is required for lung defense against pneumococcal pneumonia and inhaled particles. The Journal of Experimental Medicine. 2004;**200**(2):267-272

[43] Arredouani MS, Palecanda A, Koziel H, Huang YC, Imrich A, Sulahian TH, et al. MARCO is the major binding receptor for unopsonized particles and bacteria on human alveolar macrophages. Journal of Immunology. 2005;**175**(9):6058-6064

[44] Sharif O, Matt U, Saluzzo S, Lakovits K, Haslinger I, Furtner T, et al. The scavenger receptor CD36 downmodulates the early inflammatory response while enhancing bacterial phagocytosis during pneumococcal pneumonia. Journal of Immunology. 2013;**190**(11):5640-5648

[45] Steele C, Marrero L, Swain S, Harmsen AG, Zheng M, Brown GD, et al. Alveolar macrophage-mediated killing of pneumocystis carinii f. sp. muris involves molecular recognition by the Dectin-1 beta-glucan receptor. The Journal of Experimental Medicine. 2003;**198**(11):1677-1688

[46] Steele C, Rapaka RR, Metz A, Pop SM, Williams DL, Gordon S, et al. The beta-glucan receptor dectin-1 recognizes specific morphologies of Aspergillus fumigatus. PLoS Pathogens. 2005;**1**(4):e42

[47] Mitsi E, Kamng'ona R, Rylance J, Solórzano C, Jesus Reiné J, Mwandumba HC, et al. Human alveolar macrophages predominately express combined classical M1 and M2 surface markers in steady state. Respiratory Research. 2018;**19**(1):66

[48] Berger M, Norvell TM, Tosi MF, Emancipator SN, Konstan MW, Schreiber JR. Tissue-specific Fc gamma and complement receptor expression by alveolar macrophages determines relative importance of IgG and complement in promoting phagocytosis of Pseudomonas aeruginosa. Pediatric Research. 1994;**35**(1):68-77

[49] Nagre N, Cong X, Terrazas C, Pepper I, Schreiber JM, Fu H, et al. Inhibition of macrophage complement receptor CRIg by TRIM72 polarizes innate immunity of the lung. American Journal of Respiratory Cell and Molecular Biology. 2018;**58**(6):756-766

[50] Zeng Z, Surewaard BG, Wong CH, Geoghegan JA, Jenne CN, Kubes P. CRIg functions as a macrophage pattern recognition receptor to directly bind and capture blood-borne gram-positive Bacteria. Cell Host & Microbe. 2016;**20**(1):99-106

[51] Berclaz PY, Shibata Y, Whitsett JA, Trapnell BC. GM-CSF, via PU.1, regulates alveolar macrophage Fcgamma R-mediated phagocytosis and the IL-18/IFN-gamma -mediated molecular connection between innate and adaptive immunity in the lung. Blood. 2002;**100**(12):4193-4200

[52] Bruggeman CW, Houtzager J, Dierdorp B, Kers J, Pals ST, Lutter R, et al. Tissue-specific expression of IgG receptors by human macrophages ex vivo. PLoS One. 2019;**14**(10):e0223264

[53] Caron E, Hall A. Identification of two distinct mechanisms of phagocytosis controlled by different Rho GTPases. Science. 1998;**282**(5394):1717-1721

[54] Goodridge HS, Reyes CN, Becker CA, Katsumoto TR, Ma J, Wolf AJ, et al. Activation of the innate immune receptor Dectin-1 upon formation of a 'phagocytic synapse'. Nature. 2011;**472**(7344):471-475

[55] Li Z, Jiao Y, Fan EK, Scott MJ, Li Y, Li S, et al. Aging-impaired filamentous actin polymerization Signaling reduces alveolar macrophage phagocytosis of Bacteria. Journal of Immunology. 2017;**199**(9):3176-3186

[56] Tomlinson G, Chimalapati S, Pollard T, Lapp T, Cohen J, Camberlein E, et al. TLR-mediated inflammatory responses to Streptococcus pneumoniae are highly dependent on surface expression of bacterial lipoproteins. Journal of Immunology. 2014;**193**(7):3736-3745

[57] Schröder NW, Morath S, Alexander C, Hamann L, Hartung T, Zähringer U, et al. Lipoteichoic acid (LTA) of Streptococcus pneumoniae and Staphylococcus aureus activates immune cells via toll-like receptor (TLR)-2, lipopolysaccharide-binding protein (LBP), and CD14, whereas

TLR-4 and MD-2 are not involved. The Journal of Biological Chemistry. 2003;**278**(18):15587-15594

[58] Yoshimura A, Lien E, Ingalls RR, Tuomanen E, Dziarski R, Golenbock D. Cutting edge: Recognition of gram-positive bacterial cell wall components by the innate immune system occurs via toll-like receptor 2. Journal of Immunology. 1999;**163**(1):1-5

[59] Basset A, Zhang F, Benes C, Sayeed S, Herd M, Thompson C, et al. Toll-like receptor (TLR) 2 mediates inflammatory responses to oligomerized RrgA pneumococcal pilus type 1 protein. The Journal of Biological Chemistry. 2013;**288**(4):2665-2675

[60] Dessing MC, Hirst RA, de Vos AF, van der Poll T. Role of Toll-like receptors 2 and 4 in pulmonary inflammation and injury induced by pneumolysin in mice. PLoS One. 2009;**4**(11):e7993

[61] Malley R, Henneke P, Morse SC, Cieslewicz MJ, Lipsitch M, Thompson CM, et al. Recognition of pneumolysin by toll-like receptor 4 confers resistance to pneumococcal infection. Proceedings of the National Academy of Sciences of the United States of America. 2003;**100**(4):1966-1971

[62] Zhang H, Kang L, Yao H, He Y, Wang X, Xu W, et al. Streptococcus pneumoniae endopeptidase O (PepO) elicits a strong innate immune response in mice via TLR2 and TLR4 Signaling pathways. Frontiers in Cellular and Infection Microbiology. 2016;**6**:23

[63] Hoshino K, Takeuchi O, Kawai T, Sanjo H, Ogawa T, Takeda Y, et al. Cutting edge: Toll-like receptor 4 (TLR4)-deficient mice are hyporesponsive to lipopolysaccharide: Evidence for TLR4 as the Lps gene product. Journal of Immunology. 1999;**162**(7):3749-3752

[64] Galdiero M, Galdiero M, Finamore E, Rossano F, Gambuzza M, Catania MR, et al. Haemophilus influenzae porin induces toll-like receptor 2-mediated cytokine production in human monocytes and mouse macrophages. Infection and Immunity. 2004;**72**(2):1204-1209

[65] Hemmi H, Takeuchi O, Kawai T, Kaisho T, Sato S, Sanjo H, et al. A toll-like receptor recognizes bacterial DNA. Nature. 2000;**408**(6813):740-745

[66] Knapp S, Wieland CW, van Veer C, Takeuchi O, Akira S, Florquin S, et al. Toll-like receptor 2 plays a role in the early inflammatory response to murine pneumococcal pneumonia but does not contribute to antibacterial defense. Journal of Immunology. 2004;**172**(5):3132-3138

[67] Dessing MC, van der Sluijs KF, Florquin S, Akira S, van der Poll T. Toll-like receptor 2 does not contribute to host response during postinfluenza pneumococcal pneumonia. American Journal of Respiratory Cell and Molecular Biology. 2007;**36**(5):609-614

[68] Lammers AJ, de Porto AP, de Boer OJ, Florquin S, van der Poll T. The role of TLR2 in the host response to pneumococcal pneumonia in absence of the spleen. BMC Infectious Diseases. 2012;**12**:139

[69] Branger J, Knapp S, Weijer S, Leemans JC, Pater JM, Speelman P, et al. Role of Toll-like receptor 4 in gram-positive and gram-negative pneumonia in mice. Infection and Immunity. 2004;**72**(2):788-794

[70] Sánchez-Tarjuelo R, Cortegano I, Manosalva J, Rodríguez M, Ruíz C, Alía M, et al. The TLR4-MyD88 Signaling Axis regulates lung monocyte differentiation pathways in response to

Streptococcus pneumoniae. Frontiers in Immunology. 2020;**11**:2120

[71] Albiger B, Dahlberg S, Sandgren A, Wartha F, Beiter K, Katsuragi H, et al. Toll-like receptor 9 acts at an early stage in host defence against pneumococcal infection. Cellular Microbiology. 2007;**9**(3):633-644

[72] Duggan JM, You D, Cleaver JO, Larson DT, Garza RJ, Guzmán Pruneda FA, et al. Synergistic interactions of TLR2/6 and TLR9 induce a high level of resistance to lung infection in mice. Journal of Immunology. 2011;**186**(10):5916-5926

[73] Zheng M, Karki R, Williams EP, Yang D, Fitzpatrick E, Vogel P, et al. TLR2 senses the SARS-CoV-2 envelope protein to produce inflammatory cytokines. Nature Immunology. 2021;**22**(7):829-838

[74] Li X, Li W, Liu Z, Kang Y, Zhang X, Xu Z, et al. A comparative study of spike protein of SARS-CoV-2 and its variant omicron (B.1.1.529) on some immune characteristics. Scientific Reports. 2022;**12**(1):17058

[75] Shirato K, Kizaki T. SARS-CoV-2 spike protein S1 subunit induces pro-inflammatory responses via toll-like receptor 4 signaling in murine and human macrophages. Heliyon. 2021;**7**(2):e06187

[76] Shirato K, Takanari J, Kizaki T. Standardized extract of Asparagus officinalis stem attenuates SARS-CoV-2 spike protein-induced IL-6 and IL-1β production by suppressing p44/42 MAPK and Akt phosphorylation in murine primary macrophages. Molecules. 2021;**26**(20):6189

[77] Zhao Y, Kuang M, Li J, Zhu L, Jia Z, Guo X, et al. Publisher correction: SARS-CoV-2 spike protein interacts with and activates TLR4. Cell Research. 2021;**31**(7):825

[78] Bortolotti D, Gentili V, Rizzo S, Schiuma G, Beltrami S, Strazzabosco G, et al. TLR3 and TLR7 RNA sensor activation during SARS-CoV-2 infection. Microorganisms. 2021;**9**(9):1820

[79] Salvi V, Nguyen HO, Sozio F, Schioppa T, Gaudenzi C, Laffranchi M, et al. SARS-CoV-2-associated ssRNAs activate inflammation and immunity via TLR7/8. JCI Insight. 2021;**6**(18):e150542

[80] Doran AC, Yurdagul A Jr, Tabas I. Efferocytosis in health and disease. Nature Reviews. Immunology. 2020;**20**(4):254-267

[81] Seitz HM, Camenisch TD, Lemke G, Earp HS, Matsushima GK. Macrophages and dendritic cells use different Axl/Mertk/Tyro3 receptors in clearance of apoptotic cells. Journal of Immunology. 2007;**178**(9):5635-5642

[82] Mohning MP, Thomas SM, Barthel L, Mould KJ, McCubbrey AL, Frasch SC, et al. Phagocytosis of microparticles by alveolar macrophages during acute lung injury requires MerTK. American Journal of Physiology. Lung Cellular and Molecular Physiology. 2018;**314**(1):L69-l82

[83] Grabiec AM, Denny N, Doherty JA, Happonen KE, Hankinson J, Connolly E, et al. Diminished airway macrophage expression of the Axl receptor tyrosine kinase is associated with defective efferocytosis in asthma. The Journal of Allergy and Clinical Immunology. 2017;**140**(4):1144-6.e4

[84] Elliott MR, Koster KM, Murphy PS. Efferocytosis Signaling in the regulation of macrophage inflammatory

responses. Journal of Immunology. 2017;**198**(4):1387-1394

[85] Todt JC, Hu B, Curtis JL. The receptor tyrosine kinase MerTK activates phospholipase C gamma2 during recognition of apoptotic thymocytes by murine macrophages. Journal of Leukocyte Biology. 2004;**75**(4):705-713

[86] Wu Y, Singh S, Georgescu MM, Birge RB. A role for Mer tyrosine kinase in alphavbeta5 integrin-mediated phagocytosis of apoptotic cells. Journal of Cell Science. 2005;**118**(Pt 3):539-553

[87] Fu YL, Harrison RE. Microbial phagocytic receptors and their potential involvement in cytokine induction in macrophages. Frontiers in Immunology. 2021;**12**:662063

[88] Rothlin CV, Ghosh S, Zuniga EI, Oldstone MB, Lemke G. TAM receptors are pleiotropic inhibitors of the innate immune response. Cell. 2007;**131**(6):1124-1136

[89] Zhang S, Weinberg S, DeBerge M, Gainullina A, Schipma M, Kinchen JM, et al. Efferocytosis fuels requirements of fatty acid oxidation and the Electron transport chain to polarize macrophages for tissue repair. Cell Metabolism. 2019;**29**(2):443-56.e5

[90] Madenspacher JH, Morrell ED, Gowdy KM, McDonald JG, Thompson BM, Muse G, et al. Cholesterol 25-hydroxylase promotes efferocytosis and resolution of lung inflammation. JCI Insight. 2020;**5**(11):e137189

[91] Higashimoto Y, Fukuchi Y, Shimada Y, Ishida K, Ohata M, Furuse T, et al. The effects of aging on the function of alveolar macrophages in mice. Mechanisms of Ageing and Development. 1993;**69**(3):207-217

[92] Nagao G, Ishii K, Hirota K, Makino K, Terada H. Role of lipid rafts in phagocytic uptake of polystyrene latex microspheres by macrophages. Anticancer Research. 2010;**30**(8):3167-3176

[93] Wong CK, Smith CA, Sakamoto K, Kaminski N, Koff JL, Goldstein DR. Aging impairs alveolar macrophage phagocytosis and increases influenza-induced mortality in mice. Journal of Immunology. 2017;**199**(3):1060-1068

[94] Jasper AE, Sapey E, Thickett DR, Scott A. Understanding potential mechanisms of harm: The drivers of electronic cigarette-induced changes in alveolar macrophages, neutrophils, and lung epithelial cells. American Journal of Physiology. Lung Cellular and Molecular Physiology. 2021;**321**(2):L336-Ll48

[95] Karavitis J, Kovacs EJ. Macrophage phagocytosis: Effects of environmental pollutants, alcohol, cigarette smoke, and other external factors. Journal of Leukocyte Biology. 2011;**90**(6):1065-1078

[96] Lugg ST, Scott A, Parekh D, Naidu B, Thickett DR. Cigarette smoke exposure and alveolar macrophages: Mechanisms for lung disease. Thorax. 2022;**77**(1):94-101

[97] Yeligar SM, Mehta AJ, Harris FL, Brown LA, Hart CM. Peroxisome proliferator-activated receptor γ regulates chronic alcohol-induced alveolar macrophage dysfunction. American Journal of Respiratory Cell and Molecular Biology. 2016;**55**(1):35-46

[98] Ito Y, Betsuyaku T, Moriyama C, Nasuhara Y, Nishimura M. Aging affects lipopolysaccharide-induced upregulation of heme oxygenase-1 in the lungs and alveolar macrophages. Biogerontology. 2009;**10**(2):173-180

[99] Boyd AR, Shivshankar P, Jiang S, Berton MT, Orihuela CJ. Age-related defects in TLR2 signaling diminish the cytokine response by alveolar macrophages during murine pneumococcal pneumonia. Experimental Gerontology. 2012;**47**(7):507-518

[100] Hinojosa CA, Akula Suresh Babu R, Rahman MM, Fernandes G, Boyd AR, Orihuela CJ. Elevated A20 contributes to age-dependent macrophage dysfunction in the lungs. Experimental Gerontology. 2014;**54**:58-66

[101] Shembade N, Harhaj EW. Regulation of NF-κB signaling by the A20 deubiquitinase. Cellular & Molecular Immunology. 2012;**9**(2):123-130

[102] Rottinghaus EK, Vesosky B, Turner J. TLR-2 independent recognition of mycobacterium tuberculosis by CD11c+ pulmonary cells from old mice. Mechanisms of Ageing and Development. 2010;**131**(6):405-414

[103] Shichita T, Ito M, Morita R, Komai K, Noguchi Y, Ooboshi H, et al. MAFB prevents excess inflammation after ischemic stroke by accelerating clearance of damage signals through MSR1. Nature Medicine. 2017;**23**(6):723-732

[104] Zhang Z, Jiang Y, Zhou Z, Huang J, Chen S, Zhou W, et al. Scavenger receptor A1 attenuates aortic dissection via promoting efferocytosis in macrophages. Biochemical Pharmacology. 2019;**168**:392-403

[105] Canan CH, Gokhale NS, Carruthers B, Lafuse WP, Schlesinger LS, Torrelles JB, et al. Characterization of lung inflammation and its impact on macrophage function in aging. Journal of Leukocyte Biology. 2014;**96**(3):473-480

[106] Lafuse WP, Rajaram MVS, Wu Q, Moliva JI, Torrelles JB, Turner J, et al. Identification of an increased alveolar macrophage subpopulation in old mice that displays unique inflammatory characteristics and is permissive to mycobacterium tuberculosis infection. Journal of Immunology. 2019;**203**(8):2252-2264

[107] Hearps AC, Martin GE, Angelovich TA, Cheng WJ, Maisa A, Landay AL, et al. Aging is associated with chronic innate immune activation and dysregulation of monocyte phenotype and function. Aging Cell. 2012;**11**(5):867-875

[108] Moliva JI, Duncan MA, Olmo-Fontánez A, Akhter A, Arnett E, Scordo JM, et al. The lung mucosa environment in the elderly increases host susceptibility to mycobacterium tuberculosis infection. The Journal of Infectious Diseases. 2019;**220**(3):514-523

[109] Piergallini TJ, Turner J. Tuberculosis in the elderly: Why inflammation matters. Experimental Gerontology. 2018;**105**:32-39

[110] Torrelles JB, Restrepo BI, Bai Y, Ross C, Schlesinger LS, Turner J. The impact of aging on the lung alveolar environment, predetermining susceptibility to respiratory infections. Frontier in Aging. 2022;**3**:818700

[111] Gomez Perdiguero E, Klapproth K, Schulz C, Busch K, Azzoni E, Crozet L, et al. Tissue-resident macrophages originate from yolk-sac-derived erythro-myeloid progenitors. Nature. 2015;**518**(7540):547-551

[112] Liu Z, Gu Y, Chakarov S, Bleriot C, Kwok I, Chen X, et al. Fate mapping via Ms4a3-expression history traces monocyte-derived cells. Cell. 2019;**178**(6):1509-25.e19

[113] Bain CC, MacDonald AS. The impact of the lung environment on macrophage development, activation and function: Diversity in the face of adversity. Mucosal Immunology. 2022;**15**(2):223-234

[114] McQuattie-Pimentel AC, Ren Z, Joshi N, Watanabe S, Stoeger T, Chi M, et al. The lung microenvironment shapes a dysfunctional response of alveolar macrophages in aging. The Journal of Clinical Investigation. 2021;**131**(4):e140299

[115] Zissel G, Schlaak M, Müller-Quernheim J. Age-related decrease in accessory cell function of human alveolar macrophages. Journal of Investigative Medicine. 1999;**47**(1):51-56

Chapter 9

Immunometabolic Processes of Macrophages in Disease States

Filex Otieno

Abstract

Macrophages are immune cells functioning primarily as antigen-presenting cells. They are professional phagocytes and patrol tissues within the body contributing to immunological surveillance. The majority of circulating macrophages and to some extend tissue-resident macrophages differentiate from monocytes. A few of resident macrophages do however originate from embryo during fetal development and remain capable of self-renewal even in adulthood. Macrophages are highly plastic seeing that they play a dual function in inflammatory conditions: either pro-inflammatory or anti-inflammatory. Depending on state of the body, whether disease, healing or homeostatic state, macrophages can be polarized to either one of two phenotypes-M1 macrophages or M2 macrophages. The former phenotype is associated with pro-inflammatory processes, while the latter mediates anti-inflammatory process. Metabolic process and intermediate substrates influence macrophage activation, polarization and functioning within the body. Moreover, within macrophages themselves, the metabolic pathways activated also influences their polarization. As such inflammatory conditions from either infectious agents or metabolic diseases are a major drive for macrophage activation that determines disease severity and prognosis seemingly because macrophages also activate other immune cells. This interplay between immune system and metabolism is of interest especially in development newer treatment strategies for metabolic diseases and infectious agents.

Keywords: immune response, infections, metabolic diseases, metabolism, polarization

1. Introduction

Macrophages are innate immune cells derived either from blood-circulating monocytes or tissue-resident persistent embryonic stem cells [1]. Monocytes are hematopoietic stem cells formed in adult bone marrow and once mature are released into systemic circulation from where they go into different body tissues [2]. Once in the tissue, monocytes differentiate into and become macrophages [2]. Depending on the body tissue invaded, monocyte-derived macrophages function primarily to add onto the pool of total tissue macrophages during an immune response [3]. Contrary, during embryogenesis, macrophage stem cells and monocyte progenitor cells remain localized within body tissues permanently till adulthood. These cells are capable of self-renewal and in adults result in formation of resident macrophages i.e. the progenitor cells of embryonic origin directly differentiate into tissue-specific resident macrophage with signature molecules explicit for a given tissue [4]. Primarily, they serve homeostatic functions within tissues such as iron metabolism, removal of dead apoptotic cellular debris, synthesis of surfactant etc. [5]. They, however, are also involved in immune response against foreign particles in conjunction with monocyte-derived macrophages. In fact, during an immune response in a particular tissue, tissue-specific macrophages are the first type of macrophages to respond. As their population diminishes within the tissue, monocyte-derived macrophages migrate into the tissue to add to the pool and also fight the invading foreign particle.

In general, macrophages are phagocytic cells that function as antigen processing cells during a foreign invasion [6]. They use pattern recognition receptors (PRRs) to detect pathogen associated molecular patterns (PAMPs) in pathogens and damage associated molecular patterns (DAMPs) in damaged cells [7]. These patterns constitute molecules express on cellular surface that denote cellular damage or presence of a pathogenic microbe etc. Once detected, macrophages engulf the supposed recognized particle through a cell eating process termed phagocytosis [8]. The foreign materials are then digested in a sac-like organelle called the phagolysosomes into smaller particles [9]. These breakdown particles are then expressed on surface of macrophage membrane together with major histocompatibility molecules (MHC) for lymphocytes to recognized and trigger cytotoxic and humoral effects [10].

Although the functioning of macrophages seems straightforward, it is rather a complex process of active immune response. Presence of foreign particles within tissue surroundings alters the tissue microenvironment [11]. This microenvironment acts as a signaling pathway for activating of naïve macrophages [11]. Macrophages can either be polarized to be pro-inflammatory or anti-inflammatory in nature. Classically activated macrophages are pro-inflammatory in nature and function to eradicate foreign particle [12]. They are also known as M1 macrophages. Alternatively activated macrophages or M2 macrophages are anti-inflammatory in nature and are recruited during resolution of inflammation when invader has been eradicated to promote tissue healing and removal of debris [12].

Altogether, the entire process from activation, polarization, functioning and return to homeostatic steady-state, the macrophage cell is regulated by the microenvironment surrounding it. This consist of signaling molecules and metabolites, either intermediate or finished, that influence the working of the cell. While immune signaling molecules such as cytokines is discussed in detailed in the field of immunology, the latter has been recently recognized and its crucial role in chronic inflammation associated with specific chronic diseases; especially those inflammatory in nature. Noteworthy, it has led to emergence of the field of immunometabolism which focuses on how metabolism affects functioning of immune components. This chapter reviews current knowledge of how metabolic processes and metabolites influences functioning of macrophages.

2. Immunometabolic processes of macrophages

The term metabolism sums up chemical processes that occur within the body of a living organism to maintain life. The basic unit of life, which is a cell, utilizes cellular processes to break down large organic compounds into energy depending on their biogenetics. Metabolism can be viewed as either cellular or systemic. Cellular metabolism occurs within a cell while the latter depicts metabolism in which specific organs/tissues are regarded as producers of metabolites which are then utilized by consumer organs/tissues. For instance, the liver metabolizes much of carbohydrate and iron to form metabolites e.g. glucose that other organs such as the brain and bone tissue utilize for their own cellular processes. However, the general outlook of metabolism predominates around cellular metabolism and for this review; five metabolic pathways will be discussed in relation to influence on macrophage function. These are: glycolysis, pentose phosphate pathway (PPP), Tri-carboxylic acid cycle (TCA), amino acid (AA) and fatty acid (FA) metabolism.

In terms of macrophage activation, hypoxia and danger signals induce HIF1-α which that stimulates the glycolytic pathway [13]. This leads to rapid generation of ATP and macrophage polarization to M1 phenotype. Contrary, helminths stimulate interleukin 4 release which in addition to normoxia activates the TCA and electron transport chain pathways typical of M2 macrophages [14].

2.1 Glycolysis

Glycolysis defines the breakdown of glucose into pyruvate. The process occurs within the cytosol. Glucose is a monosaccharide which represents the unit molecule for carbohydrate compounds. Glycolysis can occur under either aerobic or anaerobic conditions. In aerobic conditions, pyruvate is converted to acetyl CoA which enters the TCA cycle or FA synthesis [15]. In anaerobic conditions, pyruvate is converted to lactate which is removed from cells and taken to the liver to be converted back to pyruvate for gluconeogenesis. Glycolysis is a 10-step process that results in a net amount of 2-ATP molecules being formed per unit of glucose [15]. Additionally, NAD^+ is reduced to NADH which is used as a cofactor in various anabolic conditions [16].

During an immune response, naïve macrophages are polarized to the M1 subset due to changes in the microenvironment. In particular, when macrophages are stimulated by lipopolysaccharide (LPS) and interferon γ (IFN-γ), expression of glucose transporter 1 (GLUT1) increases significantly unlike that of succinate dehydrogenase A (SDHA), which is a component of electron transport chain [17]. High levels of intracellular glucose activates the glycolytic process which has been seen to be significantly ongoing during infectious conditions and carcinogenesis [18]. Inhibition of hexokinase using 2-deoxy-D-glucose, the first glycolytic enzyme that phosphorylates glucose leads to a reduction in the amount of TNF-α and interleukin-12 (IL-12) produced [19]. Notably, the cytokines stated previous mediate pro-inflammatory reaction. In addition, hexokinase inhibition also reduces expression of CD80, CD86 and inducible nitric oxide syntheses (iNOS) which are co-stimulatory molecules in macrophages and marker of M1 differentiation respectively [20, 21]. Hexokinase 1 also functions as a regulator of NOD-LRR and pyrin domain-containing 3 (NLRP3) found in the outer membrane of mitochondria [22]. NLRP3 functions to regulate activity of caspase 1 which is involved in generation of active and mature IL-18 and -1β respectively. Increased glycolytic activity activates hexokinase 1 which in turn activates NLRP3 to induce cell death via pyroptosis in macrophages [22].

Noteworthy is the effect of isomeric forms of pyruvate kinase on macrophage polarization. Pyruvate kinase mediates last step of glycolysis by converting intermediate metabolite- phosphoenolpyruvate to pyruvate with concomitant generation of ATP. The enzyme exists as two isoforms either as pyruvate kinase M1 (PKM1) or M2 (PKM2) [23]. Macrophage stimulation by LPS induces expression of PKM2 which is associated with slowing the rate of pyruvate formation unlike PKM1 [24]. This allows glycolytic intermediate metabolites to accumulate and divert to other pathways. For instance, glucose-6-phosphate is diverted to the PPP pathway to generate ribose for nucleotide synthesis while 3-phosphoglycerate is shunted to serine synthesis process.

In addition, the PKM2 enzyme translocate into the nucleus where it interacts with HIF1-α and induce expression of HIF1-α genes [24]. These genes are responsible for expression of inflammatory proteins such as IL-1β and glycolytic enzymes [23]. At times however, the PKM2 enzyme is stabilized in the tetrameric form rather than dimeric. This inhibits its translocation into the nucleus [24]. The enzyme then becomes more concentrated in cytosol and predominantly participate in glycolysis reducing its immune-related function.

Ultimately, interference with glycolytic process in macrophages during an immune response reduces their pro-inflammatory activity. This is because, M1 macrophages depend largely on glycolysis for energy production and subsequent use of such energy for survival and synthesis of mediator molecules [25]. Furthermore, it would seem that in organisms with dysfunctional glycolytic process, a chronic inflammatory process is likely to ensue with fibrotic resolution and formation of granulomas; as the pathogen is not sufficiently eradicated.

2.2 Pentose phosphate pathway

The pentose phosphate pathway is a shunt from the glycolytic process occurring in the cytosol and leads to formation of pentoses and a major contributor of total NADPH produced in the human body. The pathway is branched into oxidative branch leading to generation of NADPH and non-oxidative branch leading to formation of pentoses [26]. Pentose sugars are ultimately utilized in the synthesis of nucleotides and amino acids. Pentose phosphate pathway starts with glucose-6-phosphate branching off from glycolytic process to form 6-phosphogluconolactone that is oxidized via intermediates to form ribulose-5-phosphate and NADPH molecules. Ribulose-5-phosphate in turn is converted to ribose- and xylulose-5-phosphate. These metabolites can be further metabolizes into intermediate molecules that enter the glycolytic pathway.

Macrophages and neutrophils are phagocytic in nature and during phagocytosis induce a respiratory burst that synthesizes reactive oxygen species (ROS) which oxidizes and interfere with integrity of biological structures of a pathogen. Macrophages utilize NADPH oxidase to synthesize ROS from NADPH [27]. Additionally, NADPH is used to generate glutathione which is an antioxidant that minimizes oxidative stress subjected to tissues [28]. Macrophage activation via LPS increases activity of the PPP shunt [29]. Noteworthy, the enzyme carbohydrate kinase-like protein (CARKL) which is a sedoheptulose kinase is critical in macrophage polarization. The enzyme phosphorylates sedoheptulose to sedoheptulose-7-phosphate which is an intermediate metabolite in the PPP pathway. This reaction is coupled to conversion of glyceraldehyde-3-phosphate into the non-oxidative branch of PPP. LPS activation of macrophages represses expression of CARKL genes leading to the intermediate product being used to synthesized pentose phosphates [30]. It remains unclear why such a regulatory activity occurs in M1 macrophages which for the larger part are not proliferative in nature and would not require much of the nucleotides. On the other hand, IL-4 activated macrophages (M2 polarization), show enhanced expression of the CARKL genes thus the enzyme's catalyzed reactions increase in M2 macrophages [29].

2.3 Tri-carboxylic cycle

The TCA cycle or commonly known as Krebs cycle is an energy efficient mode of energy generation in form of ATP. Comparatively, from a single glucose molecule, glycolysis yields two ATP molecules while Krebs cycle yields a total of 36 ATP molecules.

The process occurs within the mitochondrion and is commonly utilized by non-proliferative cells for energy generation. Krebs cycle has multiple input points notably via acetyl CoA and α-ketoglutarate (α-KG). Acetyl CoA together with oxaloacetate undergoes aldol condensation to form citrate while glutamate is converted to α-KG and altogether join the TCA. Ultimately, the cycle is meant to generate NADH and $FADH_2$ by sequentially reducing the carbon atoms from acetyl CoA. Formed NADH and $FADH_2$ enters ETC to generate ATP molecules.

M2 macrophages utilizes more or less the intact TCA cycle for energy production and further allows intermediates of UDP-GlcNAc to be generated which are utilized for glycosylation of M2-associated proteins e.g. mannose receptors [31]. Contrary, polarization of macrophages to the M1-phenotype is associated with break points in the intracellular TCA cycle [32]. First, conversion of citrate to isocitrate and secondly succinate to fumarate. This results in accumulation of citrate and succinate [32]. Citrate molecules are then directed to synthesis of fatty acid and itaconate and nitric oxide formation while the latter activates HIF1-α and production of IL-1β [33].

The first breakpoint occurs during the third reaction of Krebs cycle where isocitrate is converted to α-KG by the enzyme isocitrate dehydrogenase (IDH). M1 polarized macrophages transcriptional represses levels of IDH mRNA responsible for synthesis of IDH1 [34]. This leads to accumulation of isocitrate which isomerizes back to citrate via a two-step reaction process: isocitrate is first dehydrated to cis-aconitate which is then rehydrated to citrate. Ultimately, it is citrate and cis-aconitate that accumulates within mitochondrial matrix. As a result, cis-aconitate is diverted to synthesis of itaconate through decarboxylation reaction catalyzed by the immune-responsive gene 1 (IRG1). Itaconate is bactericidal in nature especially against *Salmonella typhimurium* and *Mycobacterium tuberculosis* [35]. Additionally, itaconate inhibits succinyl dehydrogenase (SDH) [36] which converts succinate to fumarate, the second break point in TCA cycle. Itaconate also alkylates the Kelch-like ECH-associated protein 1 which subsequently activates nuclear factor erythroid 2-related factor 2 (NRF2) that has anti-inflammatory activity [37].

Accumulation of citrate in M1 macrophages inhibits pyruvate dehydrogenase (PDH) and SDH ultimately decreasing formation of Acetyl CoA and $FADH_2$ respectively. This additionally promotes consumption of ATP [38]. Accumulated citrate is transported from mitochondria matrix to cytosol via citrate transporter. Expression of citrate transporter is increased in proinflammatory macrophages in a NF-KB-dependent fashion [29]. Exported mitochondrial citrate is catabolized into products utilized in synthesis of inflammatory mediators e.g. nitric oxide and prostaglandins (PGE_2) [29]. In M2 macrophages, since the TCA cycle is intact, much of α-KG is accumulated. α-KG has been shown to be immunosuppressive in nature by: preventing expression of pro-inflammatory IL-1β, inhibiting stabilization of HIF-1α and inactivating NF-Kβ signaling pathways [39]. Glutamate and glutamine provide precursors for formation of α-KG once deaminated via anaplerosis and will be discussed further under AA metabolism.

Conversion of α-KG to succinyl-CoA is a rate limiting step in the TCA cycle as it is one of the oxidoreductase reactions that result in formation of NADH. The reaction is catalyzed by the enzyme α-KG dehydrogenase (α-KGDH) which is highly sensitive to levels of ROS [40]. LPS activation and cytosolic accumulation of calcium within macrophages enhances activity of α-KGDH and limit production of anti-inflammatory IL-10 [29]. The intermediate product, succinyl-CoA is used to succinylate lysine residues within proteins such as SDH, PDH, Acyl-CoA and carbamoyl phosphate synthase 1 [32]. Notably, in LPS-activated macrophages, a lot of succinyl-CoA is produced which leads to succinylation of lysine 311 present on PKM2 [41–43]. As a result, the enzyme acquires a dimeric form which as earlier discussed facilitates entry of the enzyme into nucleus and consequent association with HIF-1α [41]. However, not all proteins succinylated activates pro-inflammatory activity as some have been shown to be immunosuppressive when succinylated. Formed succinyl-CoA is hydrolyzed by succinyl-CoA synthetase to succinate. Alternatively, succinate can also be produced via the gamma-aminobutyric acid shunt through which glutamine is deaminated to glutamate which is further catabolized to succinic semialdehyde and eventually succinate [17]. The latter product is of special importance in situations of inflammation and metabolic stress where it has been shown to regulate tumorigenesis, cellular inflammatory activity, signal transduction and epigenetics.

The second break occurs during conversion of succinate to fumarate by the enzyme SDH. Notably, the increased accumulation of succinate is not largely depended on SDH inhibition rather on glutamine anaplerosis as discussed above. Increased succinate is exported outside the mitochondria where it stabilizes HIF-1α and activate inflammatory genes leading to sustained production of IL-1β [32]. Within the mitochondrion, oxidation of succinate by SDH drives formation of ROS required during an immune response [44]. Although conversion of succinate to fumarate may be disrupted in M1 macrophages, LPS-activation has been shown to induce the aspartate-arginosuccinate shunt which feeds fumarate precursor molecules and leads to formation of fumarate [45]. Moreover, activation of the above stated shunt has been associated with upregulation of synthesis of NO and IL-6 [46] which are pro-inflammatory. At the same time, excess fumarate levels being formed inhibit pyroptosis increasing formation of gasdermin D [47]. Most likely, intermediates of aspartate-arginosuccinate shunt drives pro-inflammatory activities while the final product fumarate is anti-inflammatory in nature. Notably, might be another reason behind the second break that prevents conversion of succinate to fumarate in M1 macrophages.

Overall, metabolites of the TCA cycle on their own and in homeostatic concentrations seems to be immunosuppressive but activity of such metabolites on other pathways within and out of mitochondria most likely activate inflammatory pathways.

2.4 Lipid metabolism

Lipid metabolism functions to deliver lipid compounds to peripheral tissues and at the same time recycle lipids from peripheral tissues within the liver. It entails three pathways: exogenous, reverse cholesterol transport and endogenous pathways [48]. Dietary lipids are metabolized via exogenous pathway while endogenous pathways metabolize lipids synthesized in the liver. Reverse cholesterol transport pathway describes how cholesterol is removed from body tissues and transported to the liver for recycling since most peripheral tissue are not able to metabolize cholesterol.

Broadly, lipids entails triglycerides (TG), cholesterol and transporting molecules. Dietary lipids absorbed from intestinal lumen are package into chylomicrons and transported via lymphatic system where they become associated with apolipoproteins (ApoB, ApoC-II, -III, ApoE etc.) and enter systemic circulation to be delivered to various body tissues [49]. Apolipoproteins enable different body tissues to identify and uptake lipids; lipids bound to ApoC-II are recognized by adipose tissue which upon cellular entry are hydrolyzed to free fatty acids (FFA) and chylomicron remnants by lipoprotein lipase (LPL). Similarly, endogenously synthesized TGs and cholesterol get packaged into very low-density lipoprotein (VLDL) and ApoB respectively and then transported to body tissues. Adipocyte LDL hydrolyzes VLDL-bound TGs to FFAs and IDLs (VLDL remnants) [48]. The lipid transporting remnants are transported to the liver where hepatic lipases convert IDLs to low density lipoproteins (LDLs) which transport cholesterol across body tissues. In conditions such as chronic high fat intake where LDL is secreted in high amounts, excess LDL binds to free ApoA and resulting compound binds extracellular matrix within walls of vessels [50]. This has been implicated in the pathogenesis of atherosclerosis.

Macrophages are well fashioned to metabolize lipids especially liver, lung and adipose macrophages. They readily absorb and release lipoproteins and cholesterol respectively from dying cells. Lipoproteins, LDL and VLDL are absorbed either via phagocytosis, micropinocytosis or scavenger receptors such as CD36 and digested in the lysosomes by action of lysosomal acid lipase to form free FAs or cholesterol molecules [48]. Cytosolic esterification of free cholesterol to esters results in formation of lipid droplets that makes macrophages look like foam cells [51]. Additionally, free cytosolic cholesterol activates transcription factors such as peroxisome proliferator-activated receptor (PPAR), liver X receptor (LXR) and retinoid X receptor (RXR) [52]. The latter two receptors regulate lipogenesis in a more complex manner and in terms of macrophage function, their deficiency increases susceptibility to infections by *Listeria monocytogenes* [53] and *mycobacterium tuberculosis* [54] but at the same time confers protection from leishmania infections [55]. Nevertheless, binding of LXR by agonists inhibits expression of inflammatory genes that lead to synthesis of NO, PG and IL-6 [56].

Formed FFA on the other hand, enters mitochondria where it is oxidized to generate acetyl CoA and the reducing agents $FADH_2$ and NADH. This latter process is largely seen in M2 polarized macrophages where lipolysis is registered but also occurs in M1 macrophages [57]. Blocking of the fatty acid oxidation pathway, as seen by use of etomoxir which inhibits carnitine palmitoyl-transferase 1, leads to inhibition of M2 macrophages polarization [58]. Additionally, formation of reducing agents $FADH_2$ and NADH enables metabolism within macrophages to take an oxidative shift and by so doing activates PPAR-γ which activates expression of M2 signature genes. Activated PPAR-γ also enhances oxidation of glutamine within via anaplerosis which activates the TCA cycle [57]. In M1 macrophages on the other hand, fatty acid synthesis (FAS) is a more predominantly seen feature when macrophages are activated by TLR, LPS or IFN-γ [59]. Fatty acid synthesis ultimately leads to lipid formation which are necessary for macrophage cell membrane expansion during remodeling. Additionally, activation of FAS pathway induces the NLRP3 inflammasome with subsequent secretion of IL-1β [60].

2.5 Amino acid metabolism

Amino acids are essential building blocks for proteins that constitutively have an amino and carboxyl group attached to a central carbon. In mammals, 20 amino acids are utilized in protein synthesis out of which 9 are essential while the rest are non-essential. Noteworthy, there exist more than 20 amino acids but consensually, the 20 essential and non-essential amino acids are mostly described in biochemistry for cell function. The human body cannot synthesize essential amino acids and have to be supplied by dietary intake unlike non-essential amino acids [61]. They include valine, phenylalanine, lysine, methionine, tryptophan, isoleucine, leucine and histidine. Contrary, non-essential amino acids include arginine, tyrosine, alanine, serine, aspartate, glycine, asparagine, proline, glutamine and glutamate [61]. The role of amino acids and their metabolites during immune response is quite complex, varied and still an enigma. Of importance in macrophage functioning is tryptophan, arginine, serine, methionine and glutamine metabolism.

Tryptophan can either be metabolized via kynurenine or serotonin pathway [62]. Kynurenine pathway is key for de novo synthesis of NAD^+ which is essential during redox reactions in glycolytic, TCA, fatty acid and electron transport chain pathways [63]. Contrary, serotonin pathway leads to formation of serotonin, a neurotransmitter, via action of tryptophan hydroxylase and aromatic amino acid decarboxylase [62]. Tryptophan can also be metabolized to indole-pyruvate that is skewed into TCA via anaplerosis. Kynurenine pathway starts with conversion of tryptophan to N-formyl-kynurenine mediated by indoleamine-2,3-dioxigenases (IDO) especially IDO1. Presences of infectious agents, TNF-α and IFN-γ stimulates expression of IDO genes which upregulates enzyme expression and tipping of tryptophan metabolism to the kynurenine pathway [64]. This additionally denies pathogens growth substrates within body tissues. In macrophages, serotonin formed from tryptophan is used to synthesize melatonin by action of N-acetyltransferase and O-methyltransferase. The product, melatonin has regulatory functions in terms of cytokine production by macrophages [65].

Serine and methionine are important during one-carbon metabolism in which methylation reactions occurs [62]. Serine, obtained exogenously or endogenously from 3-phosphoglycerate, donates one carbon atom to the folate and methionine cycles whereby in the latter, methionine acts as an intermediate donor in form of S-adenosylmethionine (SAM) thus not consumed. Macrophages utilize SAM to methylate histone molecules and synthesized IL-1beta in M1 phenotypes [66]. Additionally, LPS-activated macrophages utilize serine as a precursor molecule for synthesis of glycine which is subsequently used for glutathione synthesis. This enables rapid provision of the antioxidant as the NRF2-driven pathways generates glutathione molecules slowly [67].

Arginine can be catabolized either via arginase pathway or the nitric oxide synthesis pathway [62]. TNF-α and IFN-γ upregulate expression of inducible NO synthase (iNOS) in M1 macrophages to catabolize arginine into NO [68]. The enzyme iNOS mediates conversion of arginine to citrulline with concomitant production of NO which is an inflammatory mediator [68]. Upregulation of arginase enzyme, especially arginase 1, has been noted in macrophages stimulated by IL-4, -5 and -13 which are signature activators for naïve macrophages to M2 phenotype [69]. The enzyme converts arginine to ornithine limiting available substrate for iNOS within the cell. Ornithine is an important source of polyamines such as spermine which inhibits mitochondrial respiration and synthesis of pro-inflammatory cytokines [10].

In macrophages, glutamine is an important amino acid especially in M2 macrophages where it serves as a fuel source via anaplerotic processes [62]. In response to stimulation by IL-4, macrophages upregulate glutaminolysis to produce α-KG which mediates epigenetic reprogramming. Additionally, glutamine together with glycine and cysteine are used to synthesize glutathione which is a potent intracellular antioxidant. Glutamine is also a substrate for arginine biosynthesis [67] which is important for generation of NO in M1 macrophages.

Branched chain amino acids (leucine, isoleucine and valine) are major sources of carbon, and generation of glutamine, acetyl- and succinyl-CoA [67]. Increased uptake of leucine by macrophages activates the mTORC1 pathway leading to increased production of TNF-α and IL-1β in M1 macrophages [67].

3. Metabolic modulation of functions of tissue-specific resident macrophages

Resident macrophages especially in adults are formed through self-renewal of progenitor cells i.e. progenitor stem cells formed during embryogenesis that were responsible for primitive hematopoiesis persist in adulthood in various tissues though in smaller proportions [4]. These stem cells under the influence of factors such as colony stimulating factor-1 and IL-34 mediate activation of proliferation of stem cells to tissue macrophages dictated by transcription factors e.g. PU.1. Stem cell derived macrophages have differing transcriptional and gene expression profiles when compared to monocyte-derived macrophages [70]. They however, all perform similar functions depending on resident tissue and to which polarization end they are activated. Below is a discussion of some of tissue specific macrophages extensively studied and how they are metabolically programmed to function.

3.1 Alveolar macrophages

Alveolar macrophages are derived from fetal liver monocytes which during birth colonized the lungs and maintained self-perpetuation to adulthood. Primarily, their main function is to clear pulmonary surfactant that constantly being secreted into the alveolar space to maintain lung compliance [71]. Additionally, they also carry out immune surveillance and phagocytosis of foreign particles that have been inhaled [71]. Surfactants are predominately made up of lipids and as such, alveolar macrophages are metabolically equipped to handle lipid metabolism. During development, alveolar macrophages, under the influence of TGF-β and GM-CSF, activate the transcription factor PPARγ which regulates metabolism of fatty acids [72]. PPARγ activate genes responsible for increased fatty acid oxidation, esterification and efflux of cholesterol from cells [72]. Inability of alveolar macrophages to metabolize lipids leads to an accumulation of lung surfactant; a disease termed alveolar proteinosis [73]. Metabolically, alveolar macrophages conduct oxidation-phosphorylation reaction, fatty acid metabolism and cholesterol homeostasis.

3.2 Interstitial macrophages

Interstitial macrophages take residence in the space between epithelium and capillaries. They are derived from circulating blood monocytes and though are present in smaller numbers, their concentration increases in cases of immune response. Interstitial macrophages majorly junction as immune sentinels and once activated by a foreign particle, they differentiate to M1 phenotype [25]. Thus metabolically, interstitial cells conduct predominantly glycolysis and induction of nitric oxide synthase resulting in inhibition of mitochondrial oxidation-phosphorylation reaction [25].

3.3 Liver macrophages

Two types of liver macrophages have been documented: Kupffer cells and liver capsular macrophages [25]. Kupffer cells, located in the sinusoidal lumen, are derived from precursors of fetal liver monocytes and are capable of renewal. They carry out three major functions: clearance of damaged erythrocytes, immunological tolerance, clearance of blood-borne antigens [74]. In the presence of an antigen, Kupffer cells shift cellular metabolism towards glycolysis. This leads to increased glucose uptake and subsequently secretion of interleukin 10 [75]. Liver capsular macrophages on the other hand apart from performing immune surveillance, they also participate in neutrophil recruitment during an inflammatory episode. Less predominantly, liver macrophages conduct iron metabolism which is a major function of splenic macrophages [25]. During differentiation of Kupffer cells, notch ligands from endothelial cells of liver sinusoids induces expression of Spi-C. the latter is involved in activating genes that are responsible for iron metabolism 74].

3.4 Microglia

Microglia are CNS macrophages derived from embryonic yolk sac. They function to surveil the brain for pathogens, regulate neurogenesis and synaptic activity and have a role in clearance of apoptotic cells. Notably, microglia are active conductors of oxidative phosphorylation in inactive states to meet their energy requirement [76]. However, upon activation, they shift to a glycolytic model similar to that of blood monocyte derived macrophages. The metabolic profile of microglia is highly dynamic in nature and largely being influenced by the environment [76]. In steady state homeostatic conditions, microglia utilize oxidative phosphorylation for energy production; however, in hypoglycemic conditions, they switch to glutamine metabolism to support energy production [25].

3.5 Osteoclasts

Osteoclasts are multinucleated terminally differentiated monocyte-derived macrophages that are majorly found in the bone marrow. Predominantly, their function is bone resorption which they conduct via dissolution of collagen and mineral it the bone matrix [25]. This process is highly energy deficient thus osteoclasts have mitochondria not only in great numbers but size and complexity [25]. Formation of new osteoclasts is dependent on the factors RANK and osteoprotegerin. Activation of these systems is highly dependent on oxidative phosphorylation and mitochondrial biogenesis thus hypoxic conditions limit osteoclastogenesis process. Additionally, the metabolic profile of osteoclasts consists of elevate fatty acid oxidation, glutaminolysis, decreased glycolysis and activity of pentose phosphate pathway [77]. The former two serve to fuel oxidative phosphorylation processes which is required to produce energy for the energy driven process of bone resorption. Lactate, the end product of glycolysis has been shown to inhibit the osteoclastogenesis process [77]. During bone absorption by osteoclast, the metabolically switch to glycolysis.

3.6 Peritoneal macrophages

Two types of macrophages populate the peritoneum: large peritoneal macrophage (LPM) and small peritoneal macrophage. The former is derived from yolk sac progenitors with self-renewal capability thus forming the resident macrophages [25]. They function to phagocytose dead cells and bacteria. Small peritoneal macrophages are derived from circulating blood monocytes and predominantly function as immune sentinels, regulate immune response. In normal health conditions large peritoneal macrophages are more than small peritoneal macrophages but status changes often during immune stimulation or an ongoing inflammatory condition. Metabolically, Large peritoneal macrophages upon inflammatory stimulation exhibit increased activity in the mitochondria and electron transport chain which is linked to production of mtROS [78]. This high oxidative metabolism is fueled by fatty acids and glutamine whereby stimulated LPMs incorporate mitochondria into the phagosome and ensuing glutaminolysis induces complex II of the electron transport chain [78]. Notably, genes involved in lipid metabolism such as PPAR$\gamma$are downregulated in LPMS. SPMs on the other hand have higher glycolytic activity with reduced fatty acid oxidation and oxidative phosphorylation [78]. Stimulation of SPMs activates NF-kB which is associated with production of inflammatory cytokines.

3.7 Splenic macrophages

Currently, four different types of macrophages have been known to colonize the spleen: marginal zone macrophages, marginal metalophilic macrophages, tangible body macrophages and red pulp macrophages [25]. All except red pulp macrophages are derived from circulating blood monocytes. Red pulp macrophages differentiated from yolk sac and fetal liver progenitors that took residence in the spleen during embryogenesis. Red pulp macrophages act immune sentinels and in healthy conditions they primarily phagocytose platelets and red blood cells for iron metabolism [25]. Tangible body macrophages on the other hand phagocytose B cells that have undergone apoptosis. Marginal zone and marginal metallophillic macrophages function to blood-borne pathogens and clear them from circulation.

4. Conclusions

Macrophages, derived from either bone marrow monocytes or embryonic stem cells have crucial functions during immune response and homeostasis. Stem cell derived tissue specific macrophages are metabolically and functionally specialized to enable them play their role within specific tissues. In terms of immune response, macrophages are highly dynamic largely due to influence of low weight molecules such as intermediate metabolites within the tissue matrix. In turn, metabolic process occurring within macrophages and by extend extracellularly tend to modify the functioning of activated macrophages. As described, classically activated macrophages perform much of glycolysis and fatty acid synthesis to rapidly produce energy and remodel cell membrane. They also have breakpoints in the TCA cycle which allows intermediate products to accumulate and activate proinflammatory pathways. Contrary, alternatively activated macrophages predominantly utilize oxidative phosphorylation reactions and fatty acid oxidation to fuel their cellular activities and have an intact TCA cycle. However, to be noted, is that both M1 and M2 macrophages have been shown to depict a mixed metabolic picture. Additionally, the complexity of how metabolic processes are woven within cells makes it difficult to pin point a single pathway as either specialized in M1 or M2 macrophages. As such, we cannot conclusively state that above metabolic processes are delineated to specific macrophage polarization; rather it suggests that some metabolic pathways predominate either during inflammatory or anti-inflammatory events.

Conflict of interest

The author declares no conflict of interest.

Author details

Filex Otieno
School of Pharmacy, Kabarak University, Nakuru, Kenya

*Address all correspondence to: filexotieno27@gmail.com

References

[1] Epelman S, Lavine K, Randolph G. Origin and functions of tissue macrophages. Immunity. 2014;**41**(1):21-35. DOI: 10.1016/j.immuni.2014.06.013

[2] Yang J, Zhang L, Yu C, Yang X, Wang H. Monocyte and macrophage differentiation: Circulation inflammatory monocyte as biomarker for inflammatory diseases. Biomarker Research. 2014;**2**(1):1-9. DOI: 10.1186/2050-7771-2-1

[3] Italiani P, Boraschi D. From monocytes to M1/M2 macrophages: Phenotypical vs. functional differentiation. Frontiers in Immunology. 2014;**5**(514):1-22. DOI: 10.3389/fimmu.2014.00514

[4] Röszer T. Understanding the biology of self-renewing macrophages. Cell. 2018;**7**(8):103. DOI: 10.3390/cells7080103

[5] Caputa G, Castoldi A, Pearce EJ. Metabolic adaptations of tissue-resident immune cells. Nature Immunology. 2019;**20**(7):793-801. DOI: 10.1038/s41590-019-0407-0

[6] Pollard JW. Trophic macrophages in development and disease. Nature Reviews Immunology. 2009;**9**(4):259-270. DOI: 10.1038/nri2528

[7] Plüddemann A, Mukhopadhyay S, Gordon S. Innate immunity to intracellular pathogens: Macrophage receptors and responses to microbial entry. Immunological Reviews. 2011;**240**(1):11-24. DOI: 10.1111/j.1600-065x.2010.00989.x

[8] Rosales C, Uribe-Querol E. Phagocytosis: A fundamental process in immunity. BioMed Research International. 2017;**2017**:1-18. DOI: 10.1155/2017/9042851

[9] Lee H, Woo Y, Hahn T, Jung YM, Jung Y. Formation and maturation of the phagosome: A key mechanism in innate immunity against intracellular bacterial infection. Microorganisms. 2020;**8**(9):1298. DOI: 10.3390/microorganisms8091298

[10] Hesterberg R, Cleveland J, Epling-Burnette P. Role of polyamines in immune cell functions. Medical Science. 2018;**6**(1):22. DOI: 10.3390/medsci6010022

[11] Ivashkiv LB. Epigenetic regulation of macrophage polarization and function. Trends in Immunology. 2013;**34**(5):216-223. DOI: 10.1016/j.it.2012.11.001

[12] Yunna C, Mengru H, Lei W, Weidong C. Macrophage M1/M2 polarization. European Journal of Pharmacology. 2020;**877**:173090. DOI: 10.1016/j.ejphar.2020.173090

[13] Corrado C, Fontana S. Hypoxia and HIF signaling: One axis with divergent effects. International Journal of Molecular Sciences. 2020;**21**(16):5611. DOI: 10.3390/ijms21165611

[14] Gauthier T, Chen W. Modulation of macrophage Immunometabolism: A new approach to fight infections. Frontiers in Immunology. 2022;**13**(780839):1-21. DOI: 10.3389/fimmu.2022.780839

[15] Harris RA, Harper ED. Glycolytic pathway. In: Encyclopedia of Life Sciences. 3rd ed. Chichester: John Wiley & Sons, Ltd; 2015. pp. 1-8

[16] Brito-Arias M. Glycolysis. Enzymes Involved in Glycolysis, Fatty Acid and Amino Acid Biosynthesis: Active Site Mechanism and Inhibition. Sharjah, United Arab Emirates: Bentham Science Publishers; 2020. ISBN: 978-981-14-6088-3

[17] Viola A, Munari F, Sánchez-Rodríguez R, Scolaro T, Castegna A. The metabolic signature of macrophage responses. Frontiers in Immunology. 2019;**10**(1462):1-16. DOI: 10.3389/fimmu.2019.01462

[18] Rodríguez-Prados J, Través PG, Cuenca J, Rico D, Aragonés J, Martín-Sanz P, et al. Substrate fate in activated macrophages: A comparison between innate, classic, and alternative activation. The Journal of Immunology. 2010;**185**(1):605-614. DOI: 10.4049/jimmunol.0901698

[19] Michl J, Ohlbaum DJ, Silverstein SC. 2-Deoxyglucose selectively inhibits Fc and complement receptor-mediated phagocytosis in mouse peritoneal macrophages. I. Description of the inhibitory effect. Journal of Experimental Medicine. 1976;**144**(6):1465-1483. DOI: 10.1084/jem.144.6.1465

[20] Koo S, Garg NJ. Metabolic programming of macrophage functions and pathogens control. Redox Biology. 2019;**24**:101198. DOI: 10.1016/j.redox.2019.101198

[21] Yu Q, Wang Y, Dong L, He Y, Liu R, Yang Q, et al. Regulations of glycolytic activities on macrophages functions in tumor and infectious inflammation. Frontiers in cellular and infection. Microbiology. 2020;**10**(287):1-14. DOI: 10.3389/fcimb.2020.00287

[22] Wolf AJ, Reyes CN, Liang W, Becker C, Shimada K, Wheeler ML, et al. Hexokinase is an innate immune receptor for the detection of bacterial peptidoglycan. Cell. 2016;**166**(3):624-636. DOI: 10.1016/j.cell.2016.05.076

[23] Min B, Park S, Kang H, Kim DW, Ham HJ, Ha C, et al. Pyruvate dehydrogenase kinase is a metabolic checkpoint for polarization of macrophages to the M1 phenotype. Frontiers in Immunology. 2019;**10**(944):1-14. DOI: 10.3389/fimmu.2019.00944

[24] Palsson-McDermott E, Curtis A, Goel G, Lauterbach M, Sheedy F, Gleeson L, et al. Pyruvate kinase M2 regulates hif-1α activity and IL-1β induction and is a critical determinant of the Warburg effect in LPS-activated macrophages. Cell Metabolism. 2015;**21**(1):65-80. DOI: 10.1016/j.cmet.2014.12.005

[25] Wculek SK, Dunphy G, Heras-Murillo I, Mastrangelo A, Sancho D. Metabolism of tissue macrophages in homeostasis and pathology. Cellular & Molecular Immunology. 2021;**19**(3):384-408. DOI: 10.1038/s41423-021-00791-9

[26] Stincone A, Prigione A, Cramer T, Wamelink MM, Campbell K, Cheung E, et al. The return of metabolism: Biochemistry and physiology of the pentose phosphate pathway. Biological Reviews. 2014;**90**(3):927-963. DOI: 10.1111/brv.12140

[27] Panday A, Sahoo MK, Osorio D, Batra S. NADPH oxidases: An overview from structure to innate immunity-associated pathologies. Cellular & Molecular Immunology. 2014;**12**(1):5-23. DOI: 10.1038/cmi.2014.89

[28] Aranda-Rivera AK, Cruz-Gregorio A, Arancibia-Hernández YL, Hernández-Cruz EY, Pedraza-Chaverri J. RONS and oxidative stress: An overview of basic concepts. Oxygen. 2022;**2**(4):437-478. DOI: 10.3390/oxygen2040030

[29] O'Neill LA, Kishton RJ, Rathmell J. A guide to immunometabolism for immunologists. Nature Reviews Immunology. 2016;**16**(9):553-565. DOI: 10.1038/nri.2016.70

[30] Haschemi A, Kosma P, Gille L, Evans C, Burant C, Starkl P, et al. The

Sedoheptulose kinase CARKL directs macrophage polarization through control of glucose metabolism. Cell Metabolism. 2012;**15**(6):813-826. DOI: 10.1016/j.cmet.2012.04.023

[31] Jha A, Huang S, Sergushichev A, LampropoulouV, IvanovaY, LoginichevaE, et al. Network integration of parallel metabolic and transcriptional data reveals metabolic modules that regulate macrophage polarization. Immunity. 2015;**42**(3):419-430. DOI: 10.1016/j.immuni.2015.02.005

[32] Ryan DG, O'Neill LA. Krebs cycle reborninmacrophageImmunometabolism. Annual Review of Immunology. 2020;**38**(1):289-313. DOI: 10.1146/annurev-immunol-081619-104850

[33] Infantino V, Iacobazzi V, Menga A, Avantaggiati ML, Palmieri F. A key role of the mitochondrial citrate carrier (SLC25A1) in tnfα- and ifnγ-triggered inflammation. Biochimica et Biophysica Acta (BBA) - Gene Regulatory Mechanisms. 2014;**1839**(11):1217-1225. DOI: 10.1016/j.bbagrm.2014.07.013

[34] Tannahill GM, Curtis AM, Adamik J, Palsson-McDermott EM, McGettrick AF. Succinate is an inflammatory signal that induces IL-1β through HIF-1α. Nature. 2013;**496**:238-242. DOI: 10.1038/nature11986

[35] Michelucci A, Cordes T, Ghelfi J, Pailot A, Reiling N, Goldmann O, et al. Immune-responsive gene 1 protein links metabolism to immunity by catalyzing itaconic acid production. Proceedings of the National Academy of Sciences. 2013;**110**(19):7820-7825. DOI: 10.1073/pnas.1218599110

[36] Lampropoulou V, Sergushichev A, Bambouskova M, Nair S, Vincent E, Loginicheva E, et al. Itaconate links inhibition of succinate dehydrogenase with macrophage metabolic remodeling and regulation of inflammation. Cell Metabolism. 2016;**24**(1):158-166. DOI: 10.1016/j.cmet.2016.06.004

[37] Cheng C, Ku H, Shen T. The potential of using itaconate as treatment for inflammation-related heart diseases. Tzu Chi Medical Journal. 2022;**34**(2):113. DOI: 10.4103/tcmj.tcmj_83_21

[38] Williams NC, O'Neill LA. A role for the Krebs cycle intermediate citrate in metabolic reprogramming in innate immunity and inflammation. Frontiers in Immunology. 2018;**9**(141):1-11. DOI: 10.3389/fimmu.2018.00141

[39] Liu S, Yang J, Wu Z. The regulatory role of α-ketoglutarate metabolism in macrophages. Mediators of Inflammation. 2021;**2021**(11):1-7. DOI: 10.1155/2021/5577577

[40] Tretter L, Adam-Vizi V. Alpha-ketoglutarate dehydrogenase: A target and generator of oxidative stress. Philosophical Transactions of the Royal Society B: Biological Sciences. 2005;**360**(1464):2335-2345. DOI: 10.1098/rstb.2005.1764

[41] Harber KJ, De Goede KE, Verberk SG, Meinster E, De Vries HE, Van Weeghel M, et al. Succinate is an inflammation-induced immunoregulatory metabolite in macrophages. Metabolites. 2020;**10**(9):372. DOI: 10.3390/metabo10090372

[42] Wang F, Wang K, Xu W, Zhao S, Ye D, Wang Y, et al. SIRT5 Desuccinylates and activates pyruvate kinase M2 to block macrophage IL-1β production and to prevent DSS-induced colitis in mice. Cell Reports. 2017;**19**(11):2331-2344. DOI: 10.1016/j.celrep.2017.05.065

[43] Park J, Chen Y, Tishkoff D, Peng C, Tan M, Dai L, et al. SIRT5-mediated

lysine Desuccinylation impacts diverse metabolic pathways. Molecular Cell. 2013;**50**(6):919-930. DOI: 10.1016/j.molcel.2013.06.001

[44] Mills E, O'Neill LA. Succinate: A metabolic signal in inflammation. Trends in Cell Biology. 2014;**24**(5):313-320. DOI: 10.1016/j.tcb.2013.11.008

[45] Fall F, Lamy E, Brollo M, Naline E, Lenuzza N, Thévenot E, et al. Metabolic reprograming of LPS-stimulated human lung macrophages involves tryptophan metabolism and the aspartate-arginosuccinate shunt. PLoS One. 2020;**15**(4):e0230813. DOI: 10.1371/journal.pone.0230813

[46] Nassef MZ, Hanke JE, Hiller K. Mitochondrial metabolism in macrophages. American Journal of Physiology-Cell Physiology. 2021;**321**(6):C1070-C1081. DOI: 10.1152/ajpcell.00126.2021

[47] Humphries F, Shmuel-Galia L, Ketelut-Carneiro N, Li S, Wang B, Nemmara VV, et al. Succination inactivates gasdermin D and blocks pyroptosis. Science. 2020;**369**(6511):1633-1637. DOI: 10.1126/science.abb9818

[48] Remmerie A, Scott CL. Macrophages and lipid metabolism. Cellular Immunology. 2018;**330**:27-42. DOI: 10.1016/j.cellimm.2018.01.020

[49] Gaudet D, Drouin-Chartier J, Couture P. Lipid metabolism and emerging targets for lipid-lowering therapy. Canadian Journal of Cardiology. 2017;**33**(7):872-882. DOI: 10.1016/j.cjca.2016.12.019

[50] Nordestgaard BG, Chapman MJ, Ray K, Borén J, Andreotti F, Watts GF, et al. Lipoprotein(a) as a cardiovascular risk factor: Current status. European Heart Journal. 2010;**31**(23):2844-2853. DOI: 10.1093/eurheartj/ehq386

[51] Moore KJ, Sheedy FJ, Fisher EA. Macrophages in atherosclerosis: A dynamic balance. Nature Reviews Immunology. 2013;**13**(10):709-721. DOI: 10.1038/nri3520

[52] Wang B, Tontonoz P. Liver X receptors in lipid signalling and membrane homeostasis. Nature Reviews Endocrinology. 2018;**14**(8):452-463. DOI: 10.1038/s41574-018-0037-x

[53] Matalonga J, Glaria E, Bresque M, Escande C, Carbó JM, Kiefer K, et al. The nuclear receptor LXR limits bacterial infection of host macrophages through a mechanism that impacts cellular NAD metabolism. Cell Reports. 2017;**18**(5):1241-1255. DOI: 10.1016/j.celrep.2017.01.007

[54] Korf H, Vander Beken S, Romano M, Steffensen KR, Stijlemans B, Gustafsson J, et al. Liver X receptors contribute to the protective immune response against mycobacterium tuberculosis in mice. Journal of Clinical Investigation. 2009;**119**(6):1626-1637. DOI: 10.1172/jci35288

[55] Bruhn KW, Marathe C, Maretti-Mira AC, Nguyen H, Haskell J, Tran TA, et al. LXR deficiency confers increased protection against visceral leishmania infection in mice. PLoS Neglected Tropical Diseases. 2010;**4**(11):e886. DOI: 10.1371/journal.pntd.0000886

[56] Ito A, Hong C, Rong X, Zhu X, Tarling EJ, Hedde PN, et al. LXRs link metabolism to inflammation through abca1-dependent regulation of membrane composition and TLR signaling. eLife. 2015;**4**(e08009):1-23. DOI: 10.7554/elife.08009

[57] Batista-Gonzalez A, Vidal R, Criollo A, Carreño LJ. New insights on the role of lipid metabolism in the metabolic reprogramming of

macrophages. Frontiers in Immunology. 2020;**10**(2993):1-7. DOI: 10.3389/fimmu.2019.02993

[58] Divakaruni AS, Hsieh WY, Minarrieta L, Duong TN, Kim KK, Desousa BR, et al. Etomoxir inhibits macrophage polarization by disrupting CoA homeostasis. Cell Metabolism. 2018;**28**(3):490-503.e7. DOI: 10.1016/j.cmet.2018.06.001

[59] Posokhova EN, Khoshchenko OM, Chasovskikh MI, Pivovarova EN, Dushkin MI. Lipid synthesis in macrophages during inflammation in vivo: Effect of agonists of peroxisome proliferator activated receptors α and γ and of retinoid X receptors. Biochemistry (Moscow). 2008;**73**(3):296-304. DOI: 10.1134/s0006297908030097

[60] Anand PK. Lipids, inflammasomes, metabolism, and disease. Immunological Reviews. 2020;**297**(1):108-122. DOI: 10.1111/imr.12891

[61] Kelly B, Pearce EL. Amino assets: How amino acids support immunity. Cell Metabolism. 2020;**32**(2):154-175. DOI: 10.1016/j.cmet.2020.06.010

[62] Miyajima M. Amino acids: Key sources for immunometabolites and immunotransmitters. International Immunology. 2020;**32**(7):435-446. DOI: 10.1093/intimm/dxaa019

[63] Badawy AA. Kynurenine pathway of tryptophan metabolism: Regulatory and functional aspects. International Journal of Tryptophan Research. 2017;**10**(1178646917691938):2-20. DOI: 10.1177/1178646917691938

[64] Cervenka I, Agudelo LZ, Ruas JL. Kynurenines: Tryptophan's metabolites in exercise, inflammation, and mental health. Science. 2017;**357**(6349):eaaf9794. DOI: 10.1126/science.aaf9794

[65] Xia Y, Chen S, Zeng S, Zhao Y, Zhu C, Deng B, et al. Melatonin in macrophage biology: Current understanding and future perspectives. Journal of Pineal Research. 2019;**66**(2):1-21. DOI: 10.1111/jpi.12547

[66] Yu W, Wang Z, Zhang K, Chi Z, Xu T, Jiang D, et al. One-carbon metabolism supports S-adenosylmethionine and histone methylation to drive inflammatory macrophages. Molecular Cell. 2019;**75**(6):1147-1160.e5. DOI: 10.1016/j.molcel.2019.06.039

[67] Halaby MJ, McGaha TL. Amino acid transport and metabolism in myeloid function. Frontiers in Immunology. 2021;**12**(695238):1-9. DOI: 10.3389/fimmu.2021.695238

[68] Rath M, Müller I, Kropf P, Closs EI, Munder M. Metabolism via arginase or nitric oxide synthase: Two competing arginine pathways in macrophages. Frontiers in Immunology. 2014;**5**(532):1-10. DOI: 10.3389/fimmu.2014.00532

[69] Yang Z, Ming X. Functions of arginase isoforms in macrophage inflammatory responses: Impact on cardiovascular diseases and metabolic disorders. Frontiers in Immunology. 2014;**5**(533):1-10. DOI: 10.3389/fimmu.2014.00533

[70] Yadav S, Priya A, Borade DR, Agrawal-Rajput R. Macrophage subsets and their role: Co-relation with colony-stimulating factor-1 receptor and clinical relevance. Immunologic Research. 2022:1-23. Advance online publication. DOI: 10.1007/s12026-022-09330-8. Available from: https://link.springer.com/content/pdf/10.1007/s12026-022-09330-8.pdf?pdf=button%20sticky

[71] Mass E. Delineating the origins, developmental programs and homeostatic functions of tissue-resident macrophages. International Immunology.

2018;**30**(11):493-501. DOI: 10.1093/intimm/dxy044

[72] Schneider C, Nobs SP, Kurrer M, Rehrauer H, Thiele C, Kopf M. Induction of the nuclear receptor PPAR-γ by the cytokine GM-CSF is critical for the differentiation of fetal monocytes into alveolar macrophages. Nature Immunology. 2014;**15**(11):1026-1037. DOI: 10.1038/ni.3005

[73] Kumar A, Abdelmalak B, Inoue Y, Culver DA. Pulmonary alveolar proteinosis in adults: Pathophysiology and clinical approach. The Lancet Respiratory Medicine. 2018;**6**(7):554-565. DOI: 10.1016/s2213-2600(18)30043-2

[74] Nguyen-Lefebvre AT, Horuzsko A. Kupffer cell metabolism and function. Journal of Enzymology and Metabolism. 2015;**1**(1):101

[75] Meszaros K, Bojta J, Bautista AP, Lang CH, Spitzer JJ. Glucose utilization by Kupffer cells, endothelial cells, and granulocytes in endotoxemic rat liver. American Journal of Physiology-Gastrointestinal and Liver Physiology. 1991;**260**(1):G7-G12. DOI: 10.1152/ajpgi.1991.260.1.g7

[76] Lauro C, Limatola C. Metabolic reprograming of microglia in the regulation of the innate inflammatory response. Frontiers in Immunology. 2020;**11**(493):1-8. DOI: 10.3389/fimmu.2020.00493

[77] Arnett TR, Orriss IR. Metabolic properties of the osteoclast. Bone. 2018;**115**:25-30. DOI: 10.1016/j.bone.2017.12.021

[78] Pavlou S, Wang L, Xu H, Chen M. Higher phagocytic activity of thioglycollate-elicited peritoneal macrophages is related to metabolic status of the cells. Journal of Inflammation. 2017;**14**(4):1-6. DOI: 10.1186/s12950-017-0151-x

Chapter 10

Close Encounters: Pathogenic Protists-Host Cell Interactions

María Cristina Vanrell and Patricia Silvia Romano

Abstract

In this chapter, we summarize the highlights of the early events in the interaction of parasitic protists and the host cell. Pathogenic protists are a group of eukaryotic organisms, responsible for causing different human diseases, such as malaria, Chagas disease, leishmaniasis, and toxoplasmosis. These pathogens display complex life cycles and go through different cellular transformations to adapt to the different hosts in which they live. Part of these life cycles takes place in mammals, inside the host cell. Host cell entry ends with the formation of phagosomes or parasitophorous vacuoles, which differ from each parasite and each type of host cell. While canonical phagocytosis involves the fusion of phagosomes with compartments of the endocytic pathway to produce normal maturation through the phagocytic route, pathogenic microorganisms have developed Different evasion mechanisms to resist the intracellular defense systems. These strategies, including phagosome maturation arrest, resistance to the harsh lysosomal environment, or exit to the host cell cytoplasm, will be also presented in this work.

Keywords: phagocytosis, parasitophorous vacuoles, phagosomes, pathogenic protists, parasites

1. Introduction

With the exception of *Trypanosoma brucei*, the etiological agent of African trypanosomiasis (sleeping sickness), pathogenic protists of Kinetoplastida and Apicomplexa lineages are intracellular pathogens causing broadly disseminated diseases: malaria (caused by species of the genus *Plasmodium spp.*), Chagas disease (caused by *Trypanosoma cruzi*), leishmaniasis (caused by species of *Leishmania spp.*), and toxoplasmosis (caused by *Toxoplasma gondii*). These illnesses kill millions of people worldwide; have a significant economic impact, and cause public health issues everywhere.

In the following paragraphs, we present the diseases caused by these pathogens as well as the life cycles they go through in order to adapt to the hosts in which they live.

1.1 Malaria *(Plasmodium spp)*

Different species of *Plasmodium spp.* can infect humans causing malaria disease; the most common, *Plasmodium falciparum*, is responsible for the majority of deaths.

In contrast, *Plasmodium vivax* is responsible for the majority of cases. The symptoms of malaria range from asymptomatic parasitemia to severe disease, including cerebral malaria and death. Pregnant women and children under the age of five are particularly vulnerable to the disease. A combination of infected red blood cell sequestration in the microvasculature, endothelial activation, procoagulant action, and, most importantly, pro-inflammatory responses are thought to be the cause of the pathology. This disease is a huge public health burden, with an estimated 241 million cases reported in 2020 in 85 malaria-endemic countries (including the territory of French Guiana), resulting in 405,000 deaths [1–3].

Female Anopheles mosquitoes transmit the parasites, which have a complex life cycle that alternates between sexual and asexual phases. The infection begins with the bite of the mosquito, which injects parasites into the host in the form of sporozoites, which then travel to the liver. After replicating in liver cells, they mature into merozoites and are released into the bloodstream to invade host erythrocytes. Although the high parasite burden (up to 30,000 merozoites) stresses the host cell, infected hepatocytes do not undergo stress-mediated apoptosis, implying that the parasite interferes with this process in the host cell, In the erythrocyte, the parasites develop into immature gametocytes or ring-stage trophozoites, which are followed by mature trophozoites, schizonts, and merozoites. The immune system attacks these parasites; sporozoites in the liver find hepatic macrophages known as Kupffer cells, while parasites in the blood can find circulating monocytes and neutrophils [4].

1.2 Chagas disease *(Trypanosoma cruzi)*

Trypanosoma cruzi is the causative agent of Chagas disease, also known as American trypanosomiasis. This is a public health problem in Latin America where it affects approximately 7 million people worldwide, and 100 million people are at risk of contracting it. Furthermore, it has become increasingly common in the United States of America, Canada, and many European and Western Pacific countries in recent decades [5, 6].

The life cycle of the protozoan parasite *Trypanosoma cruzi* involves both vertebrate and invertebrate hosts. Vectorial transmission to vertebrate hosts occurs via the bite of insect triatomine vectors (from the Reduviidae subfamily known as "kissing bugs"), which shed metacyclic trypomastigotes in their feces after feeding allowing the entry of trypomastigotes through skin wounds and mucosal membranes. Other infection routes are the oral ingestion of food contaminated with triatomine feces, such as fruit juices, blood transfusion or organ transplant, laboratory accidents, and congenital transmission from the mother to child during pregnancy. The last form became the most important nowadays and explains the presence of new cases in non-endemic countries as mentioned above.

Trypomastigotes can infect a wide range of nucleated cells, including macrophages, cardiac muscle cells, and nervous system glial cells, exploiting phagocytic or non-phagocytic mechanisms depending on the class of cell involved. After a brief residence in a parasitophorous vacuole, parasites go through the cytoplasm and differentiate into amastigotes. After several divisions (binary fission), amastigotes transform back into trypomastigotes, which are released from the host cell and can infect neighboring cells or reach the bloodstream and infect different organs, particularly the heart.

Trigonoscuta cruzi infection in humans is characterized by a brief acute phase with nonspecific symptoms and a long chronic phase in which most individuals do not exhibit pathology. In contrast, some infected people (around 10 to 30% of cases) develop specific pathology cardiomyopathy and mega syndromes of the digestive system, which cause significant morbidity and may lead to mortality [5–7]. The development of Chagas pathology is complex and multifactorial, involving parasite immune evasion strategies, genetically programmed deficiencies in host immunological homeostasis, and autoreactive events marked by the presence of autoantibodies. *T. cruzi* genetic material has been identified in tissues destroyed during chronic infection, showing that the parasite plays an active role in pathogenesis [8, 9]. In fact, despite a vigorous immune response, the host fails to clear the parasites from the tissues, allowing the infection to remain indefinitely.

1.3 Leishmaniasis *(Leishmania spp)*

To cause leishmaniasis, *Leishmania* parasites infect and develop into phagocytic cells [10]. Clinical symptoms of the disease range from skin or mucocutaneous disorders to visceral infections, which are caused by different parasite strains and the delicate balance of parasite proliferation, the patient's immune response, and the consequent degenerative alterations. Consequently, *L. major*, *L. tropica*, and *L. mexicana* produce mainly the cutaneous forms, *L. braziliensis* causes the mucocutaneous illness, and *L. donovani* causes the most severe visceral disease (called kala-azar which means black fever in Hindi language). Infections caused by *Leishmania spp.* are a major public health concern across the world. This illness is seen in 88 different nations. More than 350 million individuals worldwide are at risk of leishmaniasis [11, 12], with 12 million already infected.

The life cycle of *Leishmania* is rather straightforward, with two basic stages: motile flagellate promastigotes residing in the stomach of the sandfly vector and immotile amastigotes within the phagolysosomal vesicles of vertebrate host macrophages.

A variety of sandfly species from two primary genera, *Phlebotomus* and *Lutzomyia*, transmit the illness to the host. Female infected sandflies spread the illness by injecting the promastigote form into the skin during a blood meal. After being inoculated into the upper dermis, metacyclic promastigotes are phagocytosed by skin-resident macrophages and dendritic cells and largely localized to phagolysosomes [10]. The internal development of Leishmania metacyclic promastigotes into amastigotes devoid of exterior flagella takes 12 to 24 hours. Amastigotes reproduce and survive intracellularly inside the phagolysosomal compartment, acting as a reservoir for transmission [13]. Moreover, polymorphonuclear neutrophils are attracted to the site of infection to clear promastigotes [14]. Explaining the significant inflammatory response produced after roughly 3 weeks [15]. As a sandfly feeds on the blood of an infected vertebrate host, it consumes amastigotes-containing monocytes and macrophages. Amastigotes are discharged into the sandfly's midgut, where they evolve into flagellated promastigotes through a process known as metacyclogenesis. Metacyclic promastigotes enter the throat and oral cavity, where they will be transmitted during the next blood meal.

1.4 Toxoplasmosis *(Toxoplasma gondii)*

Toxoplasma gondii is an obligate intracellular parasite of the order *Coccidia* with felines as the unique definitive hosts. It is a zoonotic illness that regularly affects a range of wild and domestic animals, with humans serving as unwitting hosts.

The protozoan parasite *T. gondii* infects 25 to 30% of the world's human population, with significant prevalences in South America and tropical African countries.

As of 2020, the World Health Organization reported around 240 million illnesses and 600,000 deaths [16] (World malaria report 2021). Infected fetuses (congenital toxoplasmosis) and immunocompromised people are the most vulnerable to this illness. More than 80% of cases of primary acquired infection in immunocompetent people in Europe or North America are asymptomatic. In other instances, patients may develop fever or cervical lymphadenopathy, which may be accompanied by myalgia, asthenia, or other nonspecific clinical symptoms. Toxoplasmosis is extremely dangerous in immunocompromised patients, and toxoplasmic encephalitis, the most common manifestation of the disease in these patients can cause a variety of symptoms ranging from headache, lethargy, lack of coordination, or ataxia to hemiparesis, loss of memory, dementia, or focal major motor seizures, usually associated with fever. The lungs, eyes, and heart are also often damaged, leading to myocarditis, while *Toxoplasma* has been isolated from other organs such as the liver, pancreas, bone marrow, bladder, lymph nodes, kidney, spleen, and skin. Toxoplasmic retinochoroiditis is a less prevalent complication.

Congenital infection is typically the outcome of a primary infection acquired by the mother during pregnancy. The incidence of vertical transmission and the severity of fetal harm is determined by the stage of pregnancy at which the mother becomes infected. It is more dangerous when the infection develops in the early trimester of pregnancy, resulting in significant abnormalities or termination. The parasite's replication causes necrosis and severe inflammation, resulting in serious abnormalities in the brain and eye organs. Mental retardation, convulsions, microcephaly, hydrocephalus, hearing, and psychomotor impairment are all serious consequences. Microphthalmia, cataracts, increased intraocular pressure, strabismus, optic neuritis, and retinal necrosis can also be detected, as can uveitis and retinochoroiditis, which can lead to blindness. Retinochoroiditis is a typical characteristic that can be present regardless of the period of maternal infection [17].

Intermediate hosts become infected by the consumption of sporulated oocytes present in contaminated meat. In the intestinal epithelial cells, *T. gondii* develops in rapidly growing tachyzoites which travel throughout the body. In the infected cells, parasites proliferate in parasitophorous vacuoles. In response to immunological pressure, the parasites encyst as bradyzoites, a slow-growing form. Tissue cysts are most commonly found in long-lived cells like muscular, endothelium, or neural cells.

When members of the cat family consume bradyzoites, they undergo sexual development within intestinal epithelial cells, ending in the discharge of oocysts that undergo meiosis in the environment to generate eight haploid sporozoites. The consumption of oocysts by a wide range of hosts results in acute infection. Humans become infected by consuming oocysts that can contaminate food or drink, or by eating undercooked meat with tissue cysts [7].

To survive in the host cell, *T. gondii* typically resides in a vacuole, which inhibits lysosomal degradation and promotes parasite reproduction.

2. Phagocytosis

The first person to describe the absorption of particles by cells was Élie Metchnikoff (1845–1916), who also highlighted the significance of this process for the host's reaction to damage and infection. Phagocytosis is a sophisticated mechanism for ingesting and eliminating infections that also plays a crucial role in the elimination of apoptotic cells, which is essential for maintaining tissue homeostasis.

Target particle identification, signaling to start the internalization machinery, phagosome formation, and phagolysosome maturation are the four key stages of phagocytosis [18].

The key aspects of the early events of phagocytosis of protist parasites under study will be discussed in the following section.

2.1 Recognition and phagocytosis of *Plasmodium spp*

Microorganisms express molecules known as pathogen-associated molecular patterns (PAMPs), which are only expressed by pathogens and not by host cells. Glycosylphosphatidylinositol (GPI) anchors, nucleic acids, and Hemozoin are all Plasmodium PAMPs [2]. Pattern recognition receptors (PRRs) such as CD36, toll-like receptors (TLRs), and complement receptor 3 identify these PAMPs and trigger the parasite uptake.

Phagocytes, particularly monocytes, and macrophages, may also perform opsonic phagocytosis of *Plasmodium spp*. Certain opsonins, notably antibodies, have been found in functional investigations to increase successful phagocytosis. Protective immunity in malaria has been linked to the IgG1 and IgG3 subclasses. MSP (the merozoite surface proteins) 2 and 3, MSP-Duffy binding-like proteins 1 and 2, and glutamate-rich proteins have been discovered as targets of these opsonizing antibodies in merozoites [19].

Immune system cells have immunoglobulin (Ig) binding receptors, FcgR I receptors, FcgRII and FcgRIIII, and complement receptors CR1 and CR3. These factors, when combined, can aid in the phagocytic absorption of antigens opsonized with components such as IgG or C3b [1].

The complement receptor CR1 recognizes and phagocytoses ring-parasitized red blood cells opsonized by IgG and complement. Parasites cause changes in the membrane proteins of hosts' erythrocytes, exposing antigenic regions identified by autoantibodies. For example, band 3 protein is clustered and oxidized, and it is also underglycosylated [20]. Protein 1 (PfEMP1), which is expressed on the membrane of *Plasmodium falciparum*-infected erythrocytes, is also a significant target of opsonizing antibodies, with antibodies recognizing distinct domains of this protein [20].

When activated, neutrophils can produce reactive oxygen species (ROS), which are highly poisonous chemicals that can kill parasites by inflicting oxidative damage.

2.2 Enfermedad de Chagas-Phagocytosis of *Trypanosoma cruzi*

Tissue-resident macrophages are the first host cells invaded by *T. cruzi* during in vivo infection. Trypomastigotes and epimastigotes are both readily absorbed by macrophages and detected within phagolysosomes. Only the trypomastigotes may escape the phagolysosome and grow in the cytosol, while the epimastigotes are killed. The plasma membrane of macrophages has been demonstrated to envelop the parasite by producing a tubular structure, also known as a coiled phagosome. Although this mechanism appears to be comparable to phagocytosis, data shows that, unlike non-infectious epimastigotes, trypomastigotes actively strive to route their own infection to macrophages. The escape of trypomastigotes to the cytosol is important because nitric oxide (NO) produced in the parasitophorous vacuole is the most potent agent in activated macrophages [5].

The parasite's primary target organ is the heart. Tissue damage in the heart is associated with severe parasitism of the myocardium during acute illness. To regulate parasite proliferation, monocytes migrate and extravasate from the circulation to the heart, where they develop into macrophages [6].

The surface receptor for sialodhesin can be expressed by macrophages (Sn). This receptor detects sialic acid, which is abundant on the parasite's surface and appears to play a significant role in the adhesion process during *T. cruzi* phagocytosis. TLR2 and TLR9 on the surface of macrophages have also been implicated in the identification of *T. cruzi* antigens: GPI (glycosylphosphatidylinositol) anchors, a dominating glycolipid dispersed on the surface of the *T. cruzi* membrane, and parasite DNA, respectively. Classical activation causes profound metabolic changes in macrophages, such as increased inducible nitric oxide synthase (iNOS or NOS2) activity and respiratory burst, as well as secretory responses, such as the production of proinflammatory cytokines and chemokines that lead to phagocytosis, intracellular pathogen destruction, antigen presentation, and costimulation. During experimental mouse infection, NO released by activated macrophages was thought to be a significant chemical for host defense against the parasite. The infection has also been demonstrated to enhance splenic but not peritoneal macrophage production of hydrogen peroxide (H_2O_2), indicating that in vivo production of antimicrobial compounds appears to be connected to certain kinds of macrophages and/or the parasite's capacity to activate these cells [6, 7].

T. cruzi amastigotes engage in phagocytic processes to invade both professional and non-professional phagocytic cells, depending significantly on the actin cytoskeleton of the host cell [21]. The GTPases of the Rho family of the host cell and their effector proteins were involved in the actin-dependent invasion [22].

2.3 *Leishmania spp*

Leishmania promastigotes access macrophages after opsonization mainly through complement receptor 1 (CR1) or 3 (CR3), Other receptors have also been implicated such as the Toll-like receptor (TLR) family, the receptors for the Fc domain of immunoglobulins (FcR), mannose-fucose receptor (MR), and fibronectin receptors. In this regard, an important molecule is complement component 3 (C3), which mainly binds to gp63 and LPG (glycolipid lipophosphoglycan) *in vitro* after complement activation [23]. This is a RhoA-dependent phagocytosis process. RhoA is a small GTPase protein of the Rho family of GTPases that is primarily involved in the regulation of the cytoskeleton, specifically the formation of actin stress fibers and actomyosin contractility. Phagocytosis has been proposed to be the main mode of invasion of promastigotes since infection by macrophages is reduced in the absence of actin polymerization of the host cell [24]. Phagocytosis of promastigotes by macrophages appears to begin within 2 minutes of contact with the parasites *in vitro* [25]. It should be noted that, during the first few minutes of contact, 90% of promastigotes connect to macrophages with low affinity through their flagellar tip [25], implying a role for this structure in the formation of phagosome Caveolae-dependent phagocytosis is also activated by *Leishmania.* The entry of pathogenic metacyclic promastigotes into murine macrophages has been linked to caveolae, and this route is critical to prevent early lysosome fusion.

During the differentiation process, promastigotes arrest phagosome maturation and exhibit delayed or decreased recruitment of late endosomal lysosome markers such as rab7 and LAMP1. Arrested phagosomes are further distinguished by the presence of host actin coating, related polymerization factors, such as Arp 2, 3, Nck, and WASP, and the recruitment of a variety of host GTPases involved in actin polymerization. Further phagosome remodeling is related to the breakdown of the lipid raft and reduced formation of the NADPH oxidase complex.

Amastigotes, like promastigotes, are taken up by a conventional phagocytic process that may be opsonic or non-opsonic. Uncoated parasites are taken up by Rho and Cdc42, but IgG-coated parasites are phagocytosed by a Rac1-dependent mechanism. The FcR and CR receptors are mostly involved in amastigotes invading macrophages. Vacuoles containing amastigotes are fusogenic and acquire markers associated with phagosome development into phagolysosomes. The vacuole contains hydrolytic enzymes and is positive for H+ ATPase. It also includes markers such as Rab7, LAMP1, and LAMP2. Amastigotes are resistant to hydrolysis and multiplying the acidic environment (pH 4.5–5.5) of the phagolysosome. The ability of *Leishmania* to control phagosome maturation depends on a surface-abundant glycolipid called lipophosphoglucan (LGP), which is a member of the phosphoglycan family. In addition, the parasite membrane contains a proton translocating ATPase, which presumably helps maintain pH homeostasis inside the parasite and contributes to lysosomal acidification. The proton gradient thus established drives the active transport of nutrients necessary for the growth of the parasite [26].

It has also been described that *Leishmania mexicana* induces an autophagy-like pathway in infected cells, redirecting cytosolic proteins for destruction and making them accessible to parasites within the phagolysosome for nutrition [27, 28].

2.4 *Toxoplasma gondii*

Unlike *Leishmania*, *Toxoplasma gondii* infects by both phagocytic and non-phagocytic cells. The infection and subsequent demise of these cells following the parasite's rapid proliferation is a crucial event in the pathogenic course of this organism. The parasite may enter a cell as a macrophage using the well-known phagocytosis process without causing its own death within the cell.

Trophozoites may actively escape cells after phagocytosis, by reversion of the process of invasion. At the moment, it is considered that entrance into the host cell includes a complicated process that combines phagocytosis with aggressive invasion.

Macrophages can swallow the parasite, opsonized or not. *T. gondii* inhibits phagosome-lysosome fusion after phagocytosis [29, 30]. Toxoplasma phagocytosis occurs primarily via opsonins such as C3b and C3a, which are recognized by their corresponding receptors on macrophages [31].

3. The evasion mechanisms

3.1 *Plamodium* can control the phagocytosis process through a variety of methods

Plasmodium spp. can prevent phagocytosis by changing its interaction with host phagocytic receptors and controlling downstream signaling cascades.

Plasmodium yoelii parasites, for example, preferentially infect erythrocytes expressing large amounts of CD47, allowing them to evade phagocytosis by the red-pulp macrophages in the spleen. CD47 is a marker that inhibits phagocytosis; Therefore, CD47 depletion may enhance phagocytic clearance. Red cells infected with *Plasmodium falciparum* and *Plasmodium vivax* have been shown to display higher amounts of CD47 than uninfected red cells; however, the mechanism behind this increased expression remains unclear. Furthermore, parasites can avoid phagocytosis by modifying complement regulatory proteins, which protect infected host cells from complement-mediated damage. They can, for example, inactivate C3b on the surface of infected erythrocytes, preventing complement-mediated phagocytic clearance of parasites. Moreover, monocytes and macrophages express less complement receptor 1 (CR1) during infection. Surprisingly, infected red blood cells preferentially bind CR1 produced by uninfected red blood cells to form rosettes, presumably isolating them from phagocyte detection.

Also, by removing superoxide and inhibiting ROS from neutrophils, mosquito salivary proteins can influence neutrophil activity. Ex vivo data demonstrate that neutrophils have a decreased ability to create ROS during malaria (**Figure 1**, Plasmodium spp.). In vitro evidence suggests that neutrophil phagocytosis of parasite products reduces their ability to engulf bacteria [1].

It was similarly shown that ex vivo monocytes from children with acute malaria had lower opsonic phagocytosis than their own monocytes 6 weeks later [2].

Finally, parasites in Kupffer cells during rodent malaria have been shown to directly trigger phagocyte death [4].

Humans are infected by parasite sporozoites, which enter hepatocytes and grow rapidly. *Plasmodium spp.* requires nutritional input to the parasitophorous vacuole to reproduce successfully, which implies the existence of host cell manipulation mechanisms. It has been shown that there are membrane connections of the parasitophorous vacuole to the Golgi membranes that were maintained throughout the growth stage in hepatocytes, which are believed to enhance the nutritional supply of hepatocytes. RAB11, a small GTPase, is important for organelle morphological changes during *Plasmodium berghei* infections, and functional alterations of this protein reduced this impact.

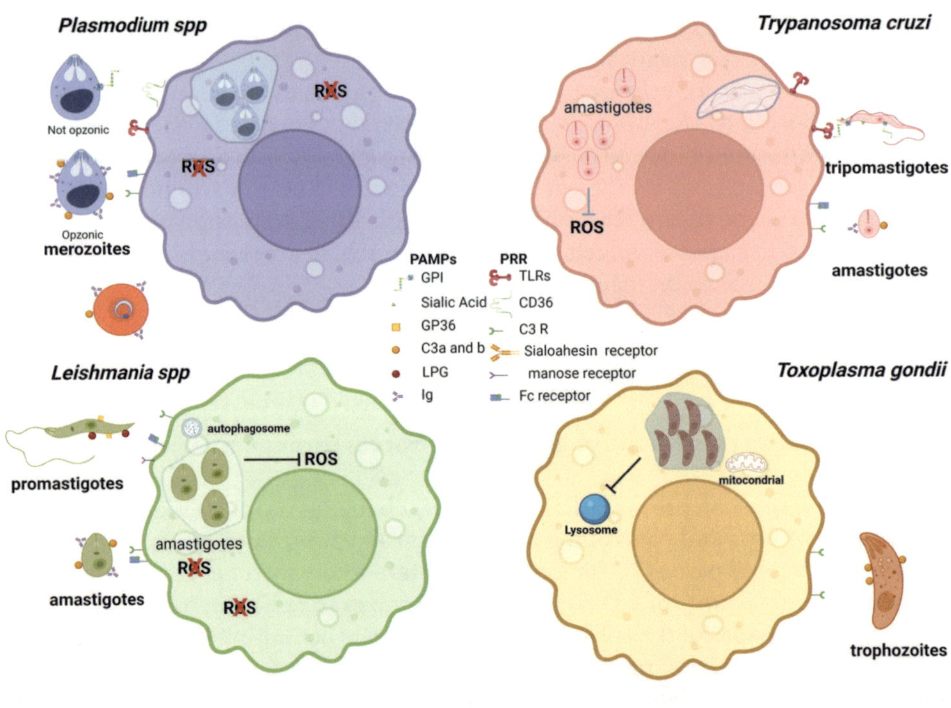

Figure 1.
The image shows the molecules involved in the phagocytosis of pathogenic protists and the evasion mechanisms that evolve to resist in the host cell. Created with BioRender.com.

Mature trophozoites within infected red blood cells can circulate to organs such as the brain, spleen, placenta, and lungs, where they can be sequestered as part of an immune evasion strategy [4].

3.2 Resist the oxidative response, the smart strategy of *T. cruzi*

T. cruzi, in vertebrate hosts, develops a variety of immune evasion strategies. Protection against direct cytotoxic effects of O2•/H_2O_2• on parasite mitochondria within the macrophage phagosome (**Figure 1**, *T. cruzi*); suppression of ONOO production in NO-exposed parasites, and regulation of NO-exposed parasites are among these methods. To resist host-derived oxidants, *T. cruzi* has an arsenal of detoxifying antioxidant defenses, as well as redox metabolism. Trypanothiol (T[SH]2), the main thiol used by the antioxidant system of trypanosomatids, is one of the most important. This system is considered an interesting target route for drug development.

Fe-dependent superoxide dismutases (Fe-SODs) from *T. cruzi* readily remove O2 • and may help to survive intracellularly [32].

TcAPxCcP, a type A hybrid peroxidase that employs ascorbate and cytochrome C as reducing substrates for H_2O_2 detoxification, has also been reported in *T. cruzi* [33]. TcAPxCcP is a membrane-bound peroxidase found in the endoplasmic reticulum and mitochondria throughout the parasite's life cycle, as well as in the plasma membrane during the infective stages of the *T. cruzi* life cycle [34]. Lastly, *T. cruzi* has two GSH-like peroxidases (GPX) that can metabolize fatty acids and phospholipid hydroperoxides despite the absence of selenium in the active site [35]. In the non-infectious epimastigote, GPX-I is found in the cytosol while GPX-II is found in the endoplasmic reticulum. In general, *T. cruzi*'s antioxidant arsenal works as a virulence factor by detoxifying reactive species in the phagosomal compartment.

Furthermore, it has been demonstrated in *T. cruzi* that peroxiredoxins, a family of proteins with antioxidant and redox signaling functions, were upregulated in the infective metacyclic trypomastigote stage and that their expression levels correlated with parasitemia in mice, implying that peroxiredoxin levels mediate *T. cruzi* virulence.

Another pathogen-encoded virulence strategy depends on repair mechanisms that restrict the potentially damaging oxidation of proteins and DNA. Methionine oxidation is mediated by a variety of reactive species such as H_2O_2, peroxynitrite, HOCl, and metal-catalyzed oxidation systems, yielding methionine-(S) and methionine-(R)-sulfoxide (Met-SO) epimers. Enzymatic pathways for methionine oxidation have also been identified. Methionine sulfoxide reductases (Msr) have been identified in a variety of pathogenic organisms, and these enzymes reduce Met-SO by using the reducing equivalents of Trx/TrxR and NADPH [36]. MsrA and MsrB, two distinct enzymes, catalyze the reduction of oxidized methionine diastereomers. MsrA action in proteins is confined to Met(S)-SO residues, whereas MsrB decreases Met(R)-SO. Another essential component for *T. cruzi* pathogenicity is the sanitization of oxidized bases in DNA. Guanine is highly oxidizable, and its most frequent oxidation product is 7,8-dihydro-8-oxo-29-deoxyguanosine (8-oxoG), which has the potential to be mutagenic owing to its structural similarities to thymine [37]. Trypanosomes have effective DNA repair mechanisms as well [38].

3.3 Leishmania subversion of phagocytosis favors the infection

After inoculation, *Leishmania* promastigotes are swiftly phagocytosed, but they can survive and change into immobile amastigote forms that can remain as intracellular parasites. The parasitophorous vacuole is an acidic intracellular compartment where *Leishmania* amastigotes proliferate. Although the amastigote cytoplasm is controlled to near-neutral pH by an active process of proton extrusion, pH plays an important role in the developmental changeover between the promastigote and amastigote phases. Amastigotes are metabolically more active when their environment is acidic. Endosomes, phagosomes, and autophagosomes can all fuse with the parasitophorous vacuole. *Leishmania* amastigotes have evolved to survive in the particular ecological niche of mammalian macrophage phagolysosomes. The parasitophorous vacuole contains a highly hydrolytic and acidic environment, which the parasite does not appear to mitigate. While the parasite's cytoplasm is deliberately kept at a neutral pH, the amastigote's surface membrane adapts to operate efficiently in an acidic mileu, allowing the parasite to collect nutrition while being exposed to extraordinarily high external proton concentrations [39].

It is remarkable how the parasite avoids this harmful surge of ROS generation: it may counteract endogenous ROS production via antioxidant systems or by actively lowering ROS production (**Figure 1**, Leishmania spp) [40].

Although promastigotes and amastigotes enter macrophages by phagocytosis, the oxidative burst that occurs is very different. After infection, both stages show a rise in O2• production of macrophages, although the reaction is significantly stronger in promastigotes than in amastigotes. The discrepancy can be attributed to a decrease in NADPH oxidase activity following amastigote infection. Only once the gp91phox precursor has matured to its full-length molecule, the NADPH oxidase complex can be successfully assembled. This stage of development is dependent on the availability of heme. Infection with *L. pifanoi* amastigotes causes the production of heme oxygenase-1, the rate-limiting enzyme for heme degradation, which inhibits the development of gp91phox and precludes the assembly of NADPH oxidase. *L. donovani* amastigotes also affected another component of the NADPH oxidase complex. Amastigotes caused barely detectable amounts of p47phox phosphorylation, which resulted in p67phox and p47phox phagosomal recruitment defects. Interestingly, protein kinase C (PKC) mediates p47phox phosphorylation, which is suppressed by *Leishmania* promastigotes and amastigotes. This action has been linked to the lipophosphoglycan (LPG) present in promastigotes; in amastigotes, the mechanism responsible for PKC inhibition is uncertain. Moreover, *L. donovani* amastigotes affect the phagosomal lipid raft integrity, which may lead to defective NADPH oxidase assembly [41].

Lastly, infection with *Leishmania* amastigotes can result in reduced O2• generation by inhibiting inositol phosphate buildup and calcium release in infected macrophages. While promastigotes have little effect on overall O2• generation in macrophages, they have been shown to locally impede the assembly of NADPH oxidase at the phagosomal membrane, a defensive system reliant on the presence of LPG repeat units. Moreover, LPG glycoconjugates can influence macrophage iNOS expression. When LPG is administered before IFN-γ, NO generation is decreased compared to control cells. LPG suppresses the production of NO in macrophages in a time and dose-dependent manner. It clearly shows that LPG may regulate iNOS expression in macrophages [42].

Leishmania has an antioxidant defense mechanism as well. Trypanothione/trypanothione reductase has been described in *L. major*, which is crucial for its antioxidant ability against H_2O_2, ONOO, and •NO. $T(SH)_2$ was also discovered to be required for H2O2 elimination in trypanosomatids. $T(SH)_2$ requires the proteins triperedoxin (TXN) and peroxiredoxin (PRX) (which has triperedoxin peroxidase activity) to decrease H_2O_2. The presence of the enzyme ascorbate peroxidase has also been shown to reduce H_2O_2, this is also present in *T. cruzi*. Trypanothione S-transferase and 5,6,7,8-tetrahydrobiopterin superoxide dismutase are among the main antioxidant mechanisms [40].

In summary, the parasite protects itself from the macrophage's oxidative burst by expressing antioxidant enzymes and proteins and inhibiting the synthesis of O2• and •NO in the macrophage. Surprisingly, promastigotes and amastigotes have opposing inhibitory effects. Amastigotes produce a widespread drop in O2• levels in the macrophage, whereas promastigotes lower O2• production just locally in the phagosome. Amastigotes decrease the synthesis of IL-12, O2•, and •NO in addition to their impact on macrophage redox biology. Unlike promastigotes, where LPG was identified as a parasite effector, no chemical associated with amastigotes has been identified as being responsible for the drop in O2• levels. Finally, parasites of *Leishmania* have evolved to live and multiply within ROS-producing macrophages. They do this not just through the use of antioxidant mechanisms, but also by decreasing ROS generation in macrophages [43, 44].

L. donovani infection also activates nuclear translocation and (Nuclear factor erythroid 2-related factor 2) Nrf2 activity, which reduces oxidative stress, but there is no evidence of which molecular partners are required to trigger this signaling yet. What is known in particular is that Nrf2 expression and activation occur upon initial contact with the host cell by increasing the number of gene products related to an antioxidant profile and turning macrophages into an anti-inflammatory spectrum. Knockdown or inhibition of Nrf2 is also known to decrease parasitic infection. But despite the antioxidant effect on cells, continued Nrf2 activation can greatly decrease ROS levels, which is also essential for cellular homeostasis. One of Nrf2's targets is the ferritin gene, which sequesters Fe^{2+}, reducing iron metabolism for parasite growth [41].

An acid phosphatase found in *Leishmania* has been shown to inhibit superoxide anion generation in chemoattractant-stimulated neutrophils. The parasite's LPG was also found to suppress protein kinase C (a regulator of macrophage oxidative metabolism). It has been proposed that *Leishmania* parasites could block lysosomal hydrolases by producing polyanionic compounds capable of forming complexes with positively modified hydrolases or binding to calcium ions.

3.4 *T. gondii* established a unique vacuole to avoid host cell defenses

As previously observed, microorganisms avoid important host defense processes such as phagocytosis, allowing them to establish themselves in the host cell and growth. In mouse macrophages (where this parasite survives), the organelle containing *T. gondii* appears to be arrested, unable to fuse with lysosomes, unless the organism has been coated with antibodies prior to phagocytosis, in which case it is easily destroyed [29]. *T. gondii* also uses tiny Rab-family GTPases for nutrient delivery, demonstrating that intracellular pathogens use host pathways components to promote proliferation. In *T. gondii*-infected cells, for example, mitochondria are organelles that interact with the membrane of the parasitophorous vacuole. The parasites have a mitochondrial association factor 1 (MAF1) locus, which encodes numerous proteins involved in host cell mitochondrial association and immune evasion, with the MAF1b protein serving as the primary mediator. *T. gondii*'s interaction with host cell organelles is most likely due to a requirement for nutritional input, which allows the parasitophorous vacuole to spread. Pernas et al. discovered that *T. gondii* infection had an indirect effect on mitochondrial morphology (**Table 1**) [45].

	Parasite molecules involved in phagocytosis	Pathogen recognition receptors on phagocytic cells	Evasion mechanisms
Plasmodium spp	Merozoites Not opsonic: • GPI • Nucleic acids • Hemozoin Opsonic: • IgG1 and IgG3 that recognize the MSP protein	Not opsonic: • CD36 • TLRs • CR3 Opsonic: • FCg • CR1 y CR3	Can prevent phagocytosis. Removing superoxide and inhibiting ROS.
Trypanosoma cruzi	Tripomastigotes Sialic acid GPI DNA Amastigotes C3a and b Ig G	Sialoadhesin receptor TLR 2 TLR4	*Exit* from the parasitophore vacuole. detoxifying antioxidant defense and redox metabolism. Repair mechanisms that restrict the oxidation of proteins and DNA.
Leismania spp	Tripomastigotes Gp36 LPG Amastigotes C3a and b Ig G	CR1 CR3 TLRs Manose receptor Fc Receptor	Reduced formation of the NADPH oxidase complex. Resistance to hydrolysis and multiply within the phagolysosome, proliferating in the acidic environment. reduced the O2 • generation. antioxidant systems.
Toxoplasma gondii	C3a and b	CR	Inhibition of phagosome-lysosome fusion

Table 1.
Summary of the phagocytosis of pathogenic protists and the evasion mechanisms that evolve to resist in the host cell.

Author details

María Cristina Vanrell* and Patricia Silvia Romano*
Facultad de Ciencias Médicas, Universidad Nacional de Cuyo, Instituto de Histología y Embriología de Mendoza IHEM-CONICET, Argentina

*Address all correspondence to: vanrellcristina@gmail.com and promano@fcm.uncu.edu.ar

References

[1] Aitken EH, Alemu A, Rogerson SJ. Neutrophils and Malaria. Frontiers in Immunology. 2018;**9**. DOI: 10.3389/FIMMU.2018.03005

[2] Dobbs KR, Crabtree JN, Dent AE. Innate immunity to malaria: The role of monocytes. Immunological Reviews. 2020;**293**:8-24. DOI: 10.1111/IMR.12830

[3] World Malaria Report 2021. Geneva: World Health Organization; 2021. Licence: CC BY-NC-SA 3.0 IGO. Available from: https://www.who.int/teams/global-malaria-programme/reports/world-malaria-report-2021

[4] Chua CLL, Ng IMJ, Yap BJM, Teo A. Factors influencing phagocytosis of malaria parasites: The story so far. Malaria Journal. 2021;**20**. DOI: 10.1186/S12936-021-03849-1

[5] Romano PS, Cueto JA, Casassa AF, Vanrell MC, Gottlieb RA, Colombo MI. Molecular and cellular mechanisms involved in the Trypanosoma cruzi/host cell interplay. IUBMB Life. 2012;**64**:387-396. DOI: 10.1002/iub.1019

[6] Melo RCN. Acute heart inflammation: Ultrastructural and functional aspects of macrophages elicited by Trypanosoma cruzi infection. Journal of Cellular and Molecular Medicine. 2009;**13**:279-294. DOI: 10.1111/J.1582-4934.2008.00388.X

[7] David Sibley L. Invasion and intracellular survival by protozoan parasites. Immunological Reviews. 2011;**240**:72-91. DOI: 10.1111/J.1600-065X.2010.00990.X

[8] Rassi A, Rassi A, Marin-Neto JA. Chagas disease. Lancet (London, England). 2010;**375**:1388-1402. DOI: 10.1016/S0140-6736(10)60061-X

[9] Báez A, Presti MSL, Rivarola HW, Mentesana GG, Pons P, Fretes R, et al. Mitochondrial involvement in chronic chagasic cardiomyopathy. Transactions of the Royal Society of Tropical Medicine and Hygiene. 2011;**105**:239-246. DOI: 10.1016/J.TRSTMH.2011.01.007

[10] Sacks D, Noben-Trauth N. The immunology of susceptibility and resistance to Leishmania major in mice. Nature Reviews. Immunology. 2002;**2**:845-858. DOI: 10.1038/NRI933

[11] Yangzom T, Cruz I, Bern C, Argaw D, Den Boer M, Vélez ID, et al. Endemic transmission of visceral leishmaniasis in Bhutan. The American Journal of Tropical Medicine and Hygiene. 2012;**87**:1028-1037. DOI: 10.4269/AJTMH.2012.12-0211

[12] Herwaldt BL. Leishmaniasis. Lancet (London, England). 1999;**354**:1191-1199. DOI: 10.1016/S0140-6736(98)10178-2

[13] Kaye P, Scott P. Leishmaniasis: Complexity at the host-pathogen interface. Nature Reviews. Microbiology. 2011;**9**:604-615. DOI: 10.1038/NRMICRO2608

[14] Ribeiro-Gomes FL, Sacks D. The influence of early neutrophil-Leishmania interactions on the host immune response to infection. Frontiers in Cellular and Infection Microbiology. 2012;**2**:59. DOI: 10.3389/FCIMB.2012.00059

[15] Kautz-Neu K, Noordegraaf M, Dinges S, Bennett CL, John D, Clausen BE, et al. Langerhans cells are negative regulators of the anti-Leishmania response. The Journal of Experimental Medicine. 2011;**208**:885-891. DOI: 10.1084/JEM.20102318

[16] Dvorin JD, Goldberg DE. Plasmodium Egress across the parasite life cycle. Annual Review of Microbiology. 2022;**76**:67-90. DOI: 10.1146/ANNUREV-MICRO-041320-020659

[17] Robert-Gangneux F, Dardé ML. Epidemiology of and diagnostic strategies for toxoplasmosis. Clinical Microbiology Reviews. 2012;**25**:264-296. DOI: 10.1128/CMR.05013-11

[18] Rosales C, Uribe-Querol E. Phagocytosis: A fundamental process in immunity. BioMed Research International. 2017;**2017**. DOI: 10.1155/2017/9042851

[19] O'Flaherty K, Ataíde R, Zaloumis SG, Ashley EA, Powell R, Feng G, et al. Contribution of functional antimalarial immunity to measures of parasite clearance in therapeutic efficacy studies of artemisinin derivatives. The Journal of Infectious Diseases. 2019;**220**:1178-1187. DOI: 10.1093/INFDIS/JIZ247

[20] Turrini F, Giribaldi G, Carta F, Mannu F, Arese P. Mechanisms of band 3 oxidation and clustering in the phagocytosis of Plasmodium falciparum-infected erythrocytes. Redox Report: Communications in Free Radical Research. 2003;**8**:300-303. DOI: 10.1179/135100003225002943

[21] Medina CM, Ferreira ÉR, Bonifácio BS, Mortara RA, Bonfim-Melo A. Trypanosoma cruzi extracellular amastigotes engage Rac1 and Cdc42 to invade RAW macrophages. Microbes and Infection. 2021;**23**. DOI: 10.1016/J.MICINF.2021.104837

[22] Bonfim-Melo A, Ferreira ÉR, Mortara RA. Rac1/WAVE2 and Cdc42/N-WASP participation in actin-dependent host cell invasion by extracellular amastigotes of *Trypanosoma cruzi*. Frontiers in Microbiology. 2018;**9**. DOI: 10.3389/FMICB.2018.00360

[23] Horta MF, Andrade LO, Martins-Duarte ÉS, Castro-Gomes T. Cell invasion by intracellular parasites—The many roads to infection. Journal of Cell Science. 2020;**133**. DOI: 10.1242/JCS.232488

[24] Akiyama HJ, Haight RD. Interaction of Leishmania donovani and hamster peritoneal macrophages. A phase-contrast microscopical study. The American Journal of Tropical Medicine and Hygiene. 1971;**20**:539-545. DOI: 10.4269/AJTMH.1971.20.539

[25] Aikawa M, Hendricks LD, Ito Y, Jagusiak M. Interactions between macrophagelike cells and Leishmania braziliensis in vitro. The American Journal of Pathology. 1982;**108**:50-59

[26] Mauel J. Macrophage-parasite interactions in Leishmania infections. Journal of Leukocyte Biology. 1990;**47**:187-193. DOI: 10.1002/JLB.47.2.187

[27] Argueta-Donohué J, Wilkins-Rodríguez AA, Aguirre-García M, Gutiérrez-Kobeh L. Differential phagocytosis of Leishmania mexicana promastigotes and amastigotes by monocyte-derived dendritic cells. Microbiology and Immunology. 2016;**60**:369-381. DOI: 10.1111/1348-0421.12325

[28] Fortéa OY, Prina E, De La Llave E, Lecoeur H, Lang T, Milon G. Unveiling pathways used by Leishmania amazonensis amastigotes to subvert macrophage function. Immunological Reviews. 2007;**219**:66-74. DOI: 10.1111/J.1600-065X.2007.00559.X

[29] Mauel J. In vitro induction of intracellular killing of parasitic protozoa

by macrophages. Immunobiology. 1982;**161**:392-400. DOI: 10.1016/S0171-2985(82)80097-1

[30] Werk R. How does Toxoplasma gondii enter host cells? Reviews of Infectious Diseases. 1985;7:449-457. DOI: 10.1093/CLINIDS/7.4.449

[31] Sikorski PM, Commodaro AG, Grigg ME. A protective and pathogenic role for complement during acute toxoplasma gondii infection. Frontiers in Cellular and Infection Microbiology. 2021;**11**. DOI: 10.3389/FCIMB.2021.634610

[32] Estrada D, Specker G, Martínez A, Dias PP, Hissa B, Andrade LO, et al. Cardiomyocyte diffusible redox mediators control Trypanosoma cruzi infection: Role of parasite mitochondrial iron superoxide dismutase. The Biochemical Journal. 2018;**475**:1235-1251. DOI: 10.1042/BCJ20170698

[33] Wilkinson SR, Meyer DJ, Taylor MC, Bromley EV, Miles MA, Kelly JM. The *Trypanosoma cruzi* enzyme TcGPXI is a glycosomal peroxidase and can be linked to trypanothione reduction by glutathione or tryparedoxin. The Journal of Biological Chemistry. 2002;**277**:17062-17071. DOI: 10.1074/JBC.M111126200

[34] Hugo M, Martínez A, Trujillo M, Estrada D, Mastrogiovanni M, Linares E, et al. Kinetics, subcellular localization, and contribution to parasite virulence of a Trypanosoma cruzi hybrid type A heme peroxidase (Tc APx-CcP). Proceedings of the National Academy of Sciences of the United States of America. 2017;**114**:E1326-E1335. DOI: 10.1073/PNAS.1618611114

[35] Wilkinson SR, Kelly JM. The role of glutathione peroxidases in trypanosomatids. Biological Chemistry. 2003;**384**:517-525. DOI: 10.1515/BC.2003.060

[36] Piacenza L, Peluffo G, Alvarez MN, Martínez A, Radi R. Trypanosoma cruzi antioxidant enzymes as virulence factors in Chagas disease. Antioxidants & Redox Signaling. 2013;**19**:723-734. DOI: 10.1089/ARS.2012.4618

[37] Aguiar PHN, Furtado C, Repolês BM, Ribeiro GA, Mendes IC, Peloso EF, et al. Oxidative stress and DNA lesions: The role of 8-oxoguanine lesions in *Trypanosoma cruzi* cell viability. PLoS Neglected Tropical Diseases. 2013;**7**. DOI: 10.1371/JOURNAL.PNTD.0002279

[38] Piacenza L, Trujillo M, Radi R. Reactive species and pathogen antioxidant networks during phagocytosis. The Journal of Experimental Medicine. 2019;**216**:501-516. DOI: 10.1084/JEM.20181886

[39] Burchmore RJS, Barrett MP. Life in vacuoles—Nutrient acquisition by Leishmania amastigotes. International Journal for Parasitology. 2001;**31**:1311-1320. DOI: 10.1016/S0020-7519(01)00259-4

[40] Santi AMM, Murta SMF. Antioxidant defense system as a rational target for Chagas disease and Leishmaniasis chemotherapy. Memórias do Instituto Oswaldo Cruz. 2022;**117**. DOI: 10.1590/0074-02760210401

[41] de Vivarini A, Lopes UG. The potential role of Nrf2 signaling in Leishmania infection outcomes. Frontiers in Cellular and Infection Microbiology. 2020;**9**. DOI: 10.3389/FCIMB.2019.00453

[42] Proudfoot L, Nikolaev AV, Feng GJ, Wei XQ, Ferguson MAJ, Brimacombe JS, et al. Regulation of the expression of nitric oxide synthase and leishmanicidal activity by glycoconjugates of Leishmania lipophosphoglycan in murine macrophages. Proceedings of the National Academy of Sciences of the

United States of America. 1996;**93**:10984-10989. DOI: 10.1073/PNAS.93.20.10984

[43] Van Assche T, Deschacht M, Da Luz RAI, Maes L, Cos P. Leishmania-macrophage interactions: Insights into the redox biology. Free Radical Biology & Medicine. 2011;**51**:337-351. DOI: 10.1016/J.FREERADBIOMED.2011.05.011

[44] von Stebut E, Tenzer S. Cutaneous leishmaniasis: Distinct functions of dendritic cells and macrophages in the interaction of the host immune system with Leishmania major. International journal of medical microbiology: IJMM. 2018;**308**:206-214. DOI: 10.1016/J.IJMM.2017.11.002

[45] Blank ML, Xia J, Morcos MM, Sun M, Cantrell PS, Liu Y, et al. Toxoplasma gondii association with host mitochondria requires key mitochondrial protein import machinery. Proceedings of the National Academy of Sciences of the United States of America. 2021;**118**. DOI: 10.1073/PNAS.2013336118

Chapter 11

Phagocytosis: Inflammation-Obesity Relationship

Jeanet Serafín López, Ursino Pacheco García, María Eugenia Castro Mussot and Ernesto Pacheco Ramírez

Abstract

Obesity is a chronic, multifactorial disease with increasing worldwide prevalence. It is characterized by excessive adipose tissue accumulation in the body, which decreases the patient's life expectancy and has been associated with a higher incidence of chronic degenerative diseases, including type 2 diabetes mellitus, systemic arterial hypertension, cancer, and cardiovascular disease. Several investigations have found that the adipose tissue of obese humans and rodents is infiltrated by a high number of macrophages. These cells interact with apoptotic adipocytes, which internalize and accumulate lipids to become foam cells. These processes lead to the release of proinflammatory mediators that promote insulin resistance. In addition, individuals with obesity have higher levels of circulating neutrophils; however, these individuals also have a higher incidence of infection, indicating that the phagocytic function of these cells is affected. This chapter describes several studies that could partly explain the phagocytic mechanisms affected by obesity. Therapeutic alternatives to favor phagocytic capacity are also discussed.

Keywords: obesity, phagocytosis, inflammation, macrophages, insulin, neutrophils

1. Introduction

Obesity results from an energetic balance alteration caused by the abnormal or excessive accumulation of triglycerides in the adipose tissue (AT). It is a chronic and multifactorial ailment and is considered a serious public health illness. Its prevalence is on the rise, and the World Health Organization (WHO) estimates that since 1975, obesity has increased almost thrice worldwide, reaching epidemic proportions. It is considered the epidemic of the twenty-first century [1–3].

The body mass index (BMI) is the most accepted parameter to determine clinically overweight and obesity and is frequently used to identify overweight and obesity in adults using the relationship between weight and stature. It is calculated by dividing the person's weight in kilograms by his/her squared stature in meters (kg/m^2).

The WHO defines overweight and obesity for adults as follows:

- Overweight: BMI equal to or above 25.
- Obesity: BMI equal to or above 30.

Although the BMI is not an ideal indicator because it does not allow the exact determination of an individual's adiposity, it is the most recommended for clinical use by international health organizations due to its easy usage [4].

Different diseases are associated with obesity because there are alterations in the immune response generated by an inflammatory process, which is also related to the following:

- Metabolic disorders such as insulin resistance (IR), type 2 diabetes mellitus (T2DM), cholesterol or triglycerides increase, and metabolic syndrome (MetS).
- Cardiovascular diseases such as hypertension, atherosclerosis, heart failure, and cerebrovascular disease.
- Respiratory diseases such as hypoventilation or sleep apnea/hypopnea syndrome.
- Increased risk for some cancer types and osteoarticular pathologies [1, 5].

2. Inflammation and obesity

The AT can be classified into different compartments: subcutaneous tissue and visceral adipose tissue (VAT). In obesity, VAT is highly associated with the increment of cardiovascular risk and the development of MetS, hypertension, insulin resistance, and T2DM [6].

The VAT is composed of a greater number of adipocytes, but it is a tissue with plentiful immune infiltrate with the presence of eosinophils, neutrophils, macrophages, regulatory T lymphocytes (Treg), CD4+ T lymphocytes, CD8+ T lymphocytes, and type 2 innate lymphoid cells (ILC2). In the VAT in homeostasis, there is a microenvironment rich in IL-4, IL-5, and IL-13, as well as the presence of Treg cells, eosinophils, and ILC2 that promote a Th2 phenotype and M2 macrophage polarization, which express arginase-1 (ARG-1) that inhibits the activity of the inducible enzyme nitric oxide synthase (iNOS) and increase IL-10 production. In obesity, the adipocyte's number and size are increased due to the accumulation of fatty acids inside the cells. This fact demands a higher oxygen concentration, and if it is not attained, it favors the adipocytes' death by apoptosis. That, in turn, causes alterations in the tissue's number and type of immune cells [1, 7–10].

One of the populations that are diminished under the above-described situation is the Treg lymphocytes, which depend on the presence of IL-33 and the nuclear factor PPAR-gamma. In normal conditions, these lymphocytes produce large amounts of IL-10, but when these cells decrease in number, the amount of tumor necrosis factor alpha (TNF alpha), IL-6, and RANTES (CCL5) increases [11]. There is also a mobilization of macrophages into the AT to eliminate dead cells and "remove" their lipid content. These increase the presence of inflammation mediators in the tissue as most of the macrophages change from an M2 phenotype to an M1, which promotes the secretion of proinflammatory cytokines (TNF alpha, IL-6, and IL-12). Other cellular subpopulations (CD8+ T lymphocytes, Th1 CD4+ lymphocytes, B-lymphocytes, and granulocytes) are also activated and secrete cytokines such as TNF alpha, interferon (IFN) gamma, and IL-6, which also contribute to the amplification of the inflammatory response (**Figure 1**) [12–14]. In this way, the increase of these mediators is relevant during the adaptation process

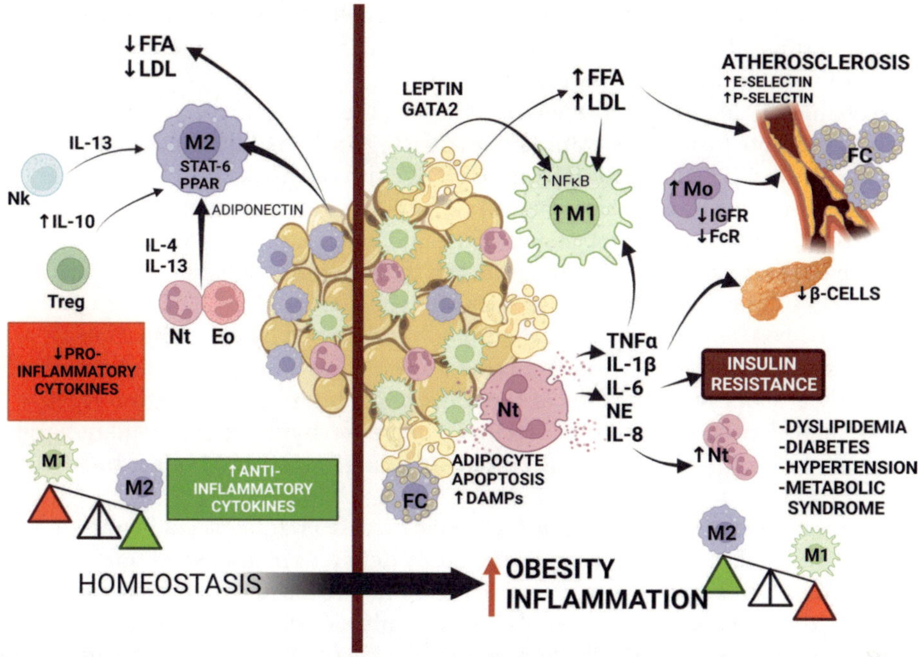

Figure 1.
Adipose tissue in homeostasis and obesity. The adipose tissue (AT) is infiltrated by diverse immune cells that communicate with each other. In homeostatic conditions, the cells present in the tissue include eosinophils (Eo) and neutrophils (Nt), which secrete IL-4 and IL-3; regulatory T lymphocytes (Treg), which produce IL-10; Natural Killers (Nk), which release IL-13; and adipocytes, which release adiponectin. Together, these cytokines generate an anti-inflammatory Th2 microenvironment, and macrophages (Mo) polarize towards an M2 phenotype characterized by the transcription factors STAT-6 and PPAR. In obesity and hyperglycemic states, AT adipocytes undergo hypoxia and cell damage, leading to apoptosis and the release of damage-associated molecular patterns (DAMPs). Moreover, leptin expression increases in obesity, shifting the Mo phenotype towards an inflammatory profile (M1) and increasing transcription factor NFκB. Mo counteract DAMPs through the phagocytosis of apoptotic adipocytes, thereby transforming into foam cells (FC), which are associated with metabolic complications. Upon activation, the cells of this microenvironment secrete more proinflammatory cytokines like TNFα and IL-1β, which, in the long term, decrease insulin production and damage pancreatic β-cells. Higher levels of IL-6 and Nt elastase (NE) produce systemic insulin resistance, and higher IL-8 increases Nt infiltration, further increasing inflammation. Finally, the excess of proinflammatory cytokines, along with the increase in LDL and FFAs, damage the vascular endothelium, increasing the expression of adhesion molecules and the deposition of foam cells that cause atherosclerosis and other pathologies. Created with BioRender.com.

to the gain in fat mass [15]. Nevertheless, when this inflammatory process is not resolved, chronic obesity ensues, which leads to tissue fibrosis and discharge of the extracellular matrix, which prevents the adipocyte enlargement and storing of lipids with the consequent liberation of fatty acids that increase the inflammatory process associated with the loss of insulin sensitivity. These alterations help to the establishment of a state of low-degree chronic inflammation characteristic of individuals with obesity [16].

3. Insulin resistance, metabolic syndrome, and type 2 diabetes

Insulin is a hormone secreted by the pancreatic beta cell in response to diverse stimuli, glucose being the most relevant. Its principal function is to maintain glycemic homeostasis. In this way, after each meal, insulin suppresses the liberation of fatty acids while favoring triglyceride synthesis in the adipose tissue [17].

Insulin resistance (IR) refers to a state in which cells do not respond normally to insulin, and thus, glucose cannot enter the cells with the same easiness, causing its accumulation in the blood (hyperglycemia) [18].

The changes happening in the VAT that lead to the liberation of proinflammatory mediators promote insulin resistance by interfering with insulin signaling through the activation of the c-JUN N-terminal kinase (JNK) and the nuclear factor kappa B (NF-kB) at a local level (AT and macrophages). When these mediators escape into circulation and reach the insulin target tissues (skeletal muscle and the liver), they unchain a systemic IR diminishing the insulin effect in these organs. This process precedes the development of metabolic diseases such as MetS [19–21].

MetS has been defined as a clinical entity characterized by a combination of risk factors. Individuals suffering from this disease show a metabolic disorder that includes visceral obesity and some of the following alterations: IR, triglycerides increase, high-density lipoproteins (HDL-C) decrease, hypertension, and hyperglycemia. This pathology confers a high risk of suffering from T2DM or cardiovascular diseases [8, 22].

Diabetes mellitus is an endocrine-metabolic disease characterized by raised blood glucose levels or hyperglycemia caused by deficient insulin secretion or action. Evidently, the most severe consequence is the damage caused to beta cells caused by lipotoxicity. The excessive accumulation of triglycerides in the pancreatic islets increases the expression of iNOS, raising nitric oxide (NO) levels, which causes alterations in the beta cells function and, finally, apoptosis of these cells, which gradually lose their capacity to compensate for IR with higher insulin secretion. Glucose blood levels increase progressively in prediabetic stages first, leading finally to T2DM [23].

4. Phagocytosis general aspects

The phagocytosis process includes several sequential stages, which are common to macrophages and neutrophils that comprise chemotaxis, adhesion, endocytosis, and the intracellular physical and biochemical changes that prepare the phagocytes to ingest, kill, and digest microorganisms: increment in the cell's general metabolism, phagosome formation, the interaction of the phagosome with endosomes and lysosomes to form the mature phagosome (phagolysosome), phagolysosome acidification, generation of reactive oxygen and nitrogen intermediates, activation of lysosomal hydrolases, and, finally, the elimination of waste materials through exocytosis.

4.1 Chemotaxis

An infection or trauma situation favors a tissue microenvironment, which gives rise to the formation of materials, both exogenous (microorganism derived) and endogenous (coming from damaged tissue), with chemotactic activity. In order for the phagocytic cells to go to the injury site, they must come out of the blood vessels, which involves the participation of adhesion molecules both in phagocytic (integrins and selectins) and endothelial (selectins and adhesins) cells. Some of these molecules are constitutive of the cellular membrane, while others are induced by chemotactic factors or some cytokines. Cells come out of the blood vessels by diapedesis, attracted by factors with chemotactic activity [24, 25].

Chemotaxis requires energy in the form of adenosine triphosphate (ATP) and the presence of calcium and magnesium, which indicates that it is an active metabolical process. As with all cellular functions that imply mobility, chemotaxis depends on the function of contractile structures of the cells that constitute the cytoskeleton.

The interaction of the cells with their external ligand occurs through membrane receptors, which generate biochemical signals that activate several G proteins and protein kinases that result in the polymerization of actin with the consequent cell movement (chemotaxis and phagocytosis) [26].

4.2 Opsonization

Opsonization improves the endocytosis process and requires the interaction of the ingestible particles with serum factors called opsonins. These include antibodies (usually IgG), complement components (C3b, C4b, or iC3b), and other proteins present in the serum, such as colectins and C reactive protein. Opsonins promote phagocytosis through specific receptors against them on the membranes of phagocytic cells [27, 28].

4.3 Endocytosis

Endocytosis is a process by which particles enter the cells due to the presence of receptors on the surface of the phagocytes. These receptors can be pathogen recognition receptors (PRR), which recognize components that are unique to microorganisms or receptors for opsonins.

The cross-linking of receptors for the immunoglobulin Fc region gives rise to signals with the participation of protein kinases, GTPase, ATPase, adaptor proteins, and other associated proteins that lead to actin polymerization, endocytosis, and cellular movement [29].

Among the PRRs, we can consider the Toll-like receptors (TLRs), which have an intracytoplasmic domain and are able to transmit signals. Ten TLRs have been identified, and although there are cellular activation pathways depending on the involved TLR, the mechanism representative of the events is described as follows:

The interaction of TLR with its ligand promotes the recruitment of the signal adaptors MyD88, a protein associated with the intracellular receptor called Toll/IL-1 (TIR) and the adaptor molecule that contains TIR (TRAM) or TIR domain-containing adaptor molecule inducing interferon-beta (TRIF). These events occur in the TIR domain of the TLRs. Depending on the type of adaptor involved, this binds to the interleukin 1 receptor-associated kinases (IRAKs) are a family of related signaling intermediates (IRAK1, IRAK2, IRAK4), TANK-binding kinase (TBK) 1 and an IkappaB kinase (IKK)-related kinase epsilon, which, in turn, binds to the TNF-6 receptor-associated factor (TRAF-6), which becomes activated and stimulates TAK1. This kinase sets in motion the Mitogen-activated protein kinase (MAPK) kinase protein signalization that phosphorylates other kinases such as JNK, which activates and translocates nuclear factors such as PA-1 and NF-κB, with the consequent transcription of the genes coding for proinflammatory cytokines. The importance of the TLRs lies in the fact that if there are defects in signalization, there will be high susceptibility to infections [30].

Within the metabolic changes associated with endocytosis, we can mention that in the phagocytic cells, as a result of the interaction with the ingestible particle, a series of events occur associated with the morphological and biochemical changes that include engulfment of the particle, formation of the digestive vacuole, and lysosomal degranulation with the release of enzymes and other components inside the vacuole.

The morphological events associated with vacuolization and degranulation are similar both in neutrophils and in macrophages, except for the following differences:

macrophages can synthesize more granules in their Golgi complex, they can get rid of the microorganisms' remains by exocytosis, and, finally, they survive the phagocytosis process, while neutrophils generally die [31].

4.4 Phagocytosis events and microbicidal activity

A few seconds after the interaction of the phagocytic cell with chemotactic agents and microorganisms, biochemical alterations are generated, which indicate the presence of metabolic changes related to membrane potential, production and release of cyclic adenosine monophosphate, release of superoxide anion, and later escape of several lysosomal enzymes. Some of these metabolic changes are related to oxygen and nitrogen metabolism, while others are of a nonoxidative nature.

Among the nonoxidative changes accompanying the endocytosis process, we can find an increment in oxygen and glucose consumption and an increase in the activity of the pentose or hexose monophosphates cycle; there is also superoxide anion and hydrogen peroxide production. The set of these changes is what is known as the "respiratory burst" [32].

The destruction of microorganisms occurs through these mechanisms, both oxygen-dependent and independent. The former includes the participation of radicals generated by the nicotinamide adenine dinucleotide phosphate (NADPH) oxidase system, which transforms molecular oxygen into superoxide anion, which, in turn, is transformed into hydrogen peroxide and then into hydroxyl radicals, which, along with the oxygen singlets, constitute the reactive oxygen intermediates (ROIs). The enzymatic system that catalyzes these oxidative changes is named "NADPH oxidase." In neutrophils, the microbicidal activity is increased by the myeloperoxidase that uses hydrogen peroxide as the substrate to produce, along with halide, highly toxic compounds [33].

Nitric oxide (NO) is generated in macrophages from the L-arginine metabolism; generally, its production is regulated by the effects of some cytokines such as gamma interferon. Given its unstable nature and in the same way as the ROI, NO interacts avidly with various chemical groups present in many molecules, causing functional and structural alterations and molecular breakdowns in them. In the target cells, NO inhibits DNA synthesis and respiratory activity [31].

Oxygen-independent mechanisms include lysosomal enzymes that intervene in the digestion of severely damaged microorganisms, and proteins with microbicidal activity. Cathepsin B, cathepsin D, glucuronidase, mannosidase, and phosphatase A2 are acid hydrolases; elastase, cathepsin G, proteinase 3, and collagenase are neutral proteases; and myeloperoxidase, lysozymes, defensins, and lactoferrin are microbicidal factors. Lysosomal hydrolases are activated by the acidification of the phagosomal environment through the activity of an endosomal enzymatic system that functions as a proton pump called "Proton ATPase," which is incorporated into the digestive vacuole's membrane when the phago-endosomal fusion occurs [34, 35].

5. Phagocytosis alterations and their relationship with obesity comorbidities

Lymphocyte subpopulations changes, both for those of the innate and the adaptive immune response, have been reported in obese individuals. These cells accumulate in the obese persons' VAT and could result from a survival increment and proliferation of resident immune cells, as well as greater cellular recruitment toward the VAT or a decrease in the cellular return to peripheral blood [36, 37]. There are also differences in the proportion of these cells among the different fat deposits. It has been observed that there are larger numbers of macrophages, T lymphocytes, and inflammatory molecules in the VAT compared to the subcutaneous tissue of obese individuals. Moreover, it was found that in the VAT from obese individuals with MetS, the number of Tregs is lower [11, 12, 38].

There are several innate immune system cells in the low-intensity chronic inflammation caused by obesity, but since this chapter deals with the phagocytic process and its relation to inflammation obesity, we will focus only on the phagocytic cells.

Alterations of the innate immune system in obesity include, among other aspects, a raised macrophage infiltration in AT, a place where these phagocytes interact with the adipocytes and endothelial cells, forming an inflammatory network. The interaction of these cells promotes the activation of the fat tissue macrophages, which are induced to produce diverse proinflammatory cytokines and chemokines such as TNF alpha and the monocyte chemoattractant protein-1 (MCP-1) [11].

Neutrophils are the first to migrate to the infection sites, and this happens in obesity, where neutrophils are the first cells to respond to inflammation, infiltrate the VAT approximately three days after a high-fat meal, and can stay there for up to 90 days [13, 39, 40].

Neutrophils depend mainly on glucose as the only energy source. In the diabetic patient, there is an excess of advanced glycation end products (AGEs), which are modified proteins that appear at the tissue and plasmatic level as a consequence of the reaction of blood monosaccharides with the protein's amino acids [41]. AGEs are formed in situations of sustained hyperglycemia or high oxidative stress [42]; this is a key part that explains why the neutrophil function is altered in diabetes [43–45].

Several clinical and epidemiological data report a higher incidence and severity of some specific types of infectious diseases, which are more frequent in obese persons than in lean ones. It has also been observed that the risk of developing cutaneous infections is increased, and the capacity to heal wounds is reduced in obese individuals. A decrease in the capacity of polymorphonuclear neutrophils to destroy bacteria was reported, which led to establishing the association of immune system alterations with obesity in children, adolescents, and adults [8, 46].

In obesity, circulating neutrophils are increased (associated with the BMI) as well as in individuals with MetS [47, 48]. These cells present an activated phenotype as indicated by an increase in the plasmatic concentrations of myeloperoxidase and elastase [48–50]. It is not well understood why the activated state of the neutrophils in obese individuals does not result in a more effective antimicrobial function. The following studies might partially explain this conundrum:

Four decades ago, it was described that diabetic patients have defects in their chemotactic response [51, 52]. Nevertheless, other studies showed controversial results, as no differences in the chemotactic response were observed between normal and diabetic patients [45, 53]. On the other hand, experimental studies in alloxan-induced diabetic mice showed that their neutrophils internalized the C-X-C motif chemokine receptor 2, which resulted in a reduced migration [54, 55]. It has also been shown that the administration of insulin to diabetic mice results in the reduction of alfa-1-acid glycoprotein (which is also increased in diabetic persons), restoring cellular migration [54].

Concerning adhesion, hyperglycemic stages increase the adhesion of phagocytic cells, especially for neutrophils, and due to the microenvironment, there is an increment in the protein C kinase (PKC) activator, which favors the expression on the cell membrane of molecules such as P-selectin, E-selectin, and intercellular adhesion molecule-1. The adhesion mechanisms activated in phagocytic and endothelial cells have been associated with the increment in cytotoxic factors (free radicals and TNF alpha) and with transforming growth factor beta-1, fibroblast growth factor, and platelet-derived growth factor. This set of factors is related to the lesions at the vascular level, a bad reparation process, and they increment the appearance of atherosclerosis. Obese and hyperglycemic patients are characterized by presenting vascular and microvascular pathologies [45, 56, 57]. There are not many studies on the alterations of adhesion molecules that affect phagocytosis; it is only known since the 1970s that the presence of hyperglycemic states leads to phagocyte adherence abnormalities. Neutrophils from hyperglycemic patients showed a lower adherence, which is re-established by insulin [58]. Nevertheless, other studies show the opposite; in a diabetic mice and rat model, hyperglycemia (>500 mg/dL) increases the expression of adhesion molecules such as Fc gamma RII/III, ICAM-1, Mac-1, −2 [59, 60].

C3 is a central component of the complement system, and its activation into C3b is critical for bacterial opsonization and phagocytosis. Diabetic patients have elevated levels of C3 and C4 in addition to having a decreased ability to fix complement by IgG [61]. In hyperglycemic conditions, C3 suffers conformational changes that make it unable to initiate the complement pathway or act as an opsonin, despite the fact that it can adhere to bacteria such as *Staphylococcus aureus* [62, 63].

Phagocytic cells display in their cell membranes different types of Fc receptors (FcR), and depending on the activation of these receptors, the phagocyte will exert a different function through second messengers. Insulin can promote changes in the phosphorylation of second messengers, and therefore, it can modify the phagocytic cell response with respect to the glycemia levels based on the presence of the FcR activity, which uses cAMP for signal transduction. In hyperglycemic states, monovalent cations are altered through the FcR functions in the ionic channels so that phagocytosis would be affected by the modifications in the glycolysis pathway [64].

The production of intracellular ROI is often diminished in neutrophils from diabetic persons, which makes them more susceptible to infections. If the glycolysis pathway is modified, phagosome maturation is also altered, mainly with a reduction in the acidification and bactericidal capacity [65]. The molecule C5a has been found incremented in obesity and T2DM [66]. It has been observed that when neutrophils from critical patients are challenged with *S. aureus*, the molecule C5a impacts the phagosome maturation, preventing their acidification [67].

In diabetic rats, a decrease in the activity of the glyceraldehyde-6-phosphate dehydrogenase enzyme is observed, which indicates that the pentose pathway is diminished in the leukocytes from these animals. Leukocytes with reduced activity of this enzyme present damage in phagocytosis, bactericidal activity, and superoxide anion production. In addition, the decreased glucose flux through the pentose phosphate pathway reduces the NADPH and ribose 5-phosphate production, which might be related to a neutrophil malfunction in the diabetic state [65].

Another pathway that affects the bactericidal capacity is the polyol pathway. In hyperglycemic states and obesity, there is stress due to an increase in free radicals, which affects the endoplasmic reticulum of the phagocytic cells; enzymes such as the aldose reductase are activated, which reduces the glucose excess to sorbitol (polyol pathway). This pathway is characterized by an increase in NADPH consumption, leaving less and less substrate for the phagocytic function [68, 69] (**Figure 2**).

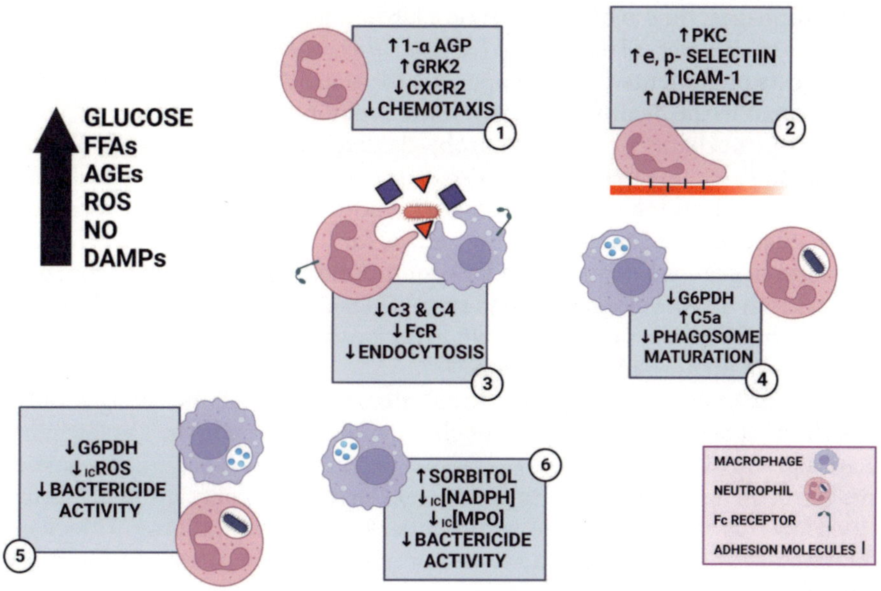

Figure 2.
Phagocytic alterations in obesity. Increased FFAs, ROS, NO, advanced glycation end products (AGEs), DAMPs, and glucose in the microenvironment impact phagocytic cells, especially Nt and Mo. (1) Chemotaxis is decreased due to the high expression of 1 alpha acidic glycoprotein (1-α AGP) and G-2 protein-coupled kinase (GRK-2) and the low expression of the chemotaxis molecule CXCR2. (2) High protein kinase C (PKC) levels increase the expression of adhesion molecules such as e-selectin, p-selectin, and intracellular adhesion molecule 1 (ICAM-1). (3) Endocytosis is affected due to the reduction of opsonins such as C3 and C4 and the decrease in the expression of the immunoglobulin Fc region receptor. (4) Lower function of the enzyme G6PDH and higher C5a prevents the proper maturation of the phagosome. (5) The production of intracellular ROS, which hold bactericidal activity, is also diminished due to decreased G6PDH activity. (6) Excess glucose is reduced to sorbitol, which increases the consumption of NADPH, making it less available for phagocytosis. Created with BioRender.com.

6. Therapeutic strategies

Even though obesity-related metabolic diseases are treated with drugs, some therapeutic alternatives that favor phagocytosis restoration are described here.

In search of improving the phagocytic capacity, which is deficient due to metabolic diseases such as obesity, several solutions have been proposed; among them, the use of probiotics stands out. Probiotics are defined as live microorganisms that have beneficial effects on the host's health when consumed [70]. These beneficial effects result from a wide range of actions that they exert, among which are the regulation of inflammation by increasing IL-10 expression [71] and the modulation of the expression of COX-2, and the activation of TLR4 [72]. In addition, probiotics can modulate insulin sensitivity [73] or decrease the individual's weight or dyslipidemia degree [73, 74], or act directly on the phagocyte, by increasing IFN gamma production, improving phagocytosis and increasing the expression of complement receptors [75].

Probiotics have an immunomodulatory function, and it has been found that their consumption can regulate the macrophage phagocytic activity against several pathogen agents, such as *Aggregatibacter actinomycetemcomitans*, a pathogen bacterium that affects the oral mucosa. When the *Lactobacillus johnsonii* NBRC 13952 probiotic is present, it increments the phagocytic activity and optimizes the bactericidal capacity of the macrophages, thus avoiding infection [76]. In the same way, the consumption of *Lactobacillus rhamnosus* HN001 and *Lactobacillus acidophilus* for four weeks by elderly subjects incremented their phagocytic capacity. With this immune stimulus, an improvement in the health of this population sector is sought [77].

Some of the mechanisms by which probiotics exert their action are still unknown, not to mention that these mechanisms also differ between the strains used for this purpose. Nevertheless, it has been demonstrated that probiotics secrete molecules that can regulate several functions, as is the case for *L. rhamnosus* strain GG (LGG). When macrophages were exposed to LGG-conditioned media, their phagocytic and bactericidal activity was increased up to sixfold. This activity was associated with an increment in free radicals production, with the activation of NADPH oxidase, and a slight increase in nitric oxide generation [78].

Another way that is being explored to counteract the metabolic changes and improve the phagocytic function is through organic compounds such as resolvins. These are a group of molecules derived from omega-3 fatty acids [79] that have a positive effect on decreasing obesity and increasing the phagocytic and bactericidal capacity. How this effect is attained is still under investigation, though a blockade of the Akt pathway and the mitogen activated protein kinase phosphorylation seems to be involved [80].

Macrophages from obese patients exhibit a deficiency in the expression of growth differentiation factor 15 (GDF-15), which is essential for the oxidative metabolism in M2 macrophages and suppresses M1 macrophages, increasing inflammation and

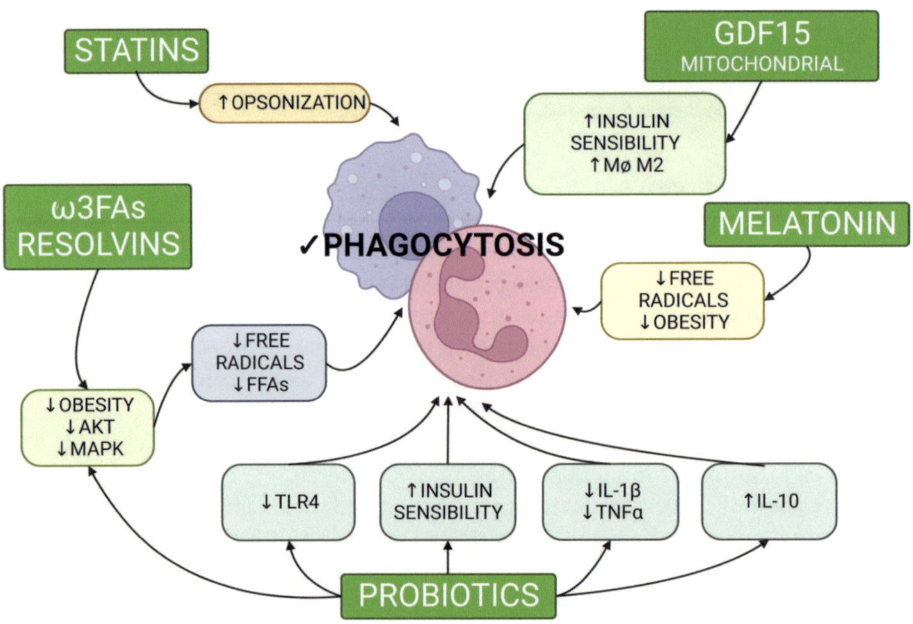

Figure 3.
Alternatives for the recovery of an adequate phagocytosis. Statins increase opsonization improving phagocytosis. The presence of omega-3 fatty acids (ω3FAs) and their derivates, such as the resolvins, reduce obesity, help the M2 differentiation of macrophages, increase phagocytosis, and increase insulin sensitivity. Melatonin increments phagocytosis besides having antioxidant action and modulates obesity. Probiotics generate changes that immunomodulate the microenvironment leading to an improvement in the use of energetic resources, increase the production of anti-inflammatory cytokines (IL-10), diminish the presence of FFAs, and improve all the phagocytic process. Created with BioRender.com

IR. The administration of GDF-15 to obese mice reverts IR, mitochondrial oxidative alterations (improving bactericidal and phagocytosis capacity), and macrophage differentiation, making it a good prospect for obesity treatment [81].

Another condition that can modify the phagocytosis process is the presence of hormones such as melatonin. There is evidence that lactating obese women possess phagocytes with high melatonin concentrations compared to women with a normal BMI. Melatonin promotes the activity of the colostrum phagocytes through G protein-coupled receptors, improving dectin-1 expression, an important type C lectin receptor crucial in proinflammatory responses such as cytokine production, ROI production, and phagocytosis [82]. The melatonin in the colostrum macrophages increases superoxide release in phagocytosis, but it also has cytoprotective effects with an antioxidant function depending on the dose, cellular targets, and exposition time. Considering these functions, the high levels of melatonin present in the colostrum of high-BMI women could be a mechanism of protection against childhood obesity, as obese individuals have reduced melatonin levels. On the other hand, melatonin promotes colostrum phagocytes' activity, which could be important for the protection of the lactating newborn (**Figure 3**) [83, 84].

7. Conclusion

Obesity is a chronic, multifactor illness. Data have been reported that relates obesity to alterations in the immune system in obese children, adolescents, and adults. Neutrophils from obese and diabetic individuals show a deteriorated phagocytic functionality that is manifested by a reduced chemotaxis, phagocytosis, and intracellular reactive oxygen species production.

Some therapeutic alternatives for the recovery of an adequate phagocytosis have been reported, such as probiotics, resolvins, statins, administration of GDF-15, and melatonine, but future research is needed to fully understand the aberrant neutrophil function in obesity and other obesity-related complications.

Acknowledgements

The authors appreciate and acknowledge the observations and support in style correction of Dr. Luis Fabila Castillo.

Conflict of interest

The author has no financial involvement with any organization or entity with a financial interest in or financial conflict with the subject matter discussed in the manuscript.

Author details

Jeanet Serafín López[1*], Ursino Pacheco García[2], María Eugenia Castro Mussot[1] and Ernesto Pacheco Ramírez[1]

1 Department of Immunology, National School of Biological Science, National Polytechnic Institute, ENCB - IPN, Mexico City, Mexico

2 Department of Cardio-Renal Pathophysiology, National Institute of Cardiology "Ignacio Chávez", Mexico City, Mexico

*Address all correspondence to: jeanetserafin09@gmail.com and jserafinl@ipn.mx

References

[1] Rodríguez-López CP et al. Mecanismos inmunológicos involucrados en la obesidad. Investigación Clínica. 2017;**58**(2):175-196

[2] Guilherme A et al. Adipocyte dysfunctions linking obesity to insulin resistance and type 2 diabetes. Nature Reviews Molecular Cell Biology. 2008;**9**(5):367-377. DOI: 10.1038/nrm2391

[3] World Health Organization. 2021. Available from: https://www.who.int/news-room/fact-sheets/detail/obesity-and-overweight

[4] Samson SL, Garber AJ. Metabolic syndrome. Endocrinology and Metabolism Clinics. 2014;**43**:1-23. DOI: 10.1016/j.ecl.2013.09.009

[5] Kanneganti T-D, Dixit VD. Immunological complications of obesity. Nature Immunology. 2012;**13**(8):707-712. DOI: 10.1038/ni.2343

[6] Ibrahim MM. Subcutaneous and visceral adipose tissue: Structural and functional differences. Obesity Reviews. 2010;**11**(1):11-18. DOI: 10.1111/j.1467-789X.2009.00623.x

[7] Bremer AA, Jialal I. Adipose tissue dysfunction in nascent metabolic syndrome. Journal of Obesity. 2013;**2013**:393192. DOI: 10.1155/2013/393192

[8] Andersen CJ, Murphy KE, Fernandez ML. Impact of obesity and metabolic syndrome on immunity. Advances. Nutrition. 2016;**7**:66-75. DOI: 10.3945/an.115.010207

[9] Altintas MM et al. Mast cells, macrophages, and crown-like structures distinguish subcutaneous from visceral fat in mice. Journal of Lipid Research. 2011;**52**(3):480-488. DOI: 10.1194/jlr.M011338

[10] Sartipy P, Loskutoff DJ. Monocyte chemoattractant protein 1 in obesity and insulin resistance. Proceedings of the National Academy of Sciences. 2003;**100**(12):7265-7270. DOI: 10.1073/pnas.1133870100

[11] Wensveen FM, Valentić S, Šestan M, Turk Wensveen T, Polić B. The "Big Bang" in obese fat: Events initiating obesity-induced adipose tissue inflammation. European Journal of Immunology. 2015;**45**(9):2446-2456. DOI: 10.1002/eji.201545502

[12] Johnson AR, Justin Milner J, Makowski L. The inflammation highway: Metabolism accelerates inflammatory traffic in obesity. Immunological Reviews. 2012;**249**:218-238. DOI: 10.1111/j.1600-065X.2012.01151.x

[13] Huh JY, Park YJ, Ham M, Kim JB. Crosstalk between adipocytes and immune cells in adipose tissue inflammation and metabolic dysregulation in obesity. Molecules and Cells. 2014;**37**(5):365. DOI: 10.14348/molcells.2014.0074

[14] Thomas D, Apovian C. Macrophage functions in lean and obese adipose tissue. Metabolism. 2017;**72**:120-143. DOI: 10.1016/j.metabol.2017.04.005

[15] Asterholm IW, Tao C, Morley TS, Wang QA, Delgado-Lopez F, Wang ZV, et al. Adipocyte inflammation is essential for healthy adipose tissue expansion and remodeling. Cell Metabolism. 2014;**20**:103-118. DOI: 10.1016/j.cmet.2014.05.005

[16] Patel P, Abate N. Body fat distribution and insulin resistance. Nutrients. 2013;**5**(6):2019-2027. DOI: 10.3390/nu5062019

[17] Højlund K. Metabolism and insulin signaling in common metabolic disorders and inherited insulin resistance. Danish Medical Journal. 2014;**61**-7:b4890

[18] Lee SH, Park SY, Choi CS. Insulin resistance: From mechanisms to therapeutic strategies. Diabetes & Metabolism Journal. 2022;**46**:15-37. DOI: 10.4093/dmj.2021.0280

[19] Yazıcı D, Sezer H. Insulin resistance, obesity and lipotoxicity. Obesity and Lipotoxicity. 2017;**2017**:277-304. DOI: 10.1007/978-3-319-48382-5_12

[20] Esser N, Legrand-Poels S, Piette J, Scheen AJ, Paquot N. Inflammation as a link between obesity, metabolic syndrome and type 2 diabetes. Diabetes Research and Clinical Practice. 2014;**105**(2):141-150. DOI: 10.1016/j.diabres.2014.04.006

[21] Schmitz-Peiffer C. Protein kinase C and lipid-induced insulin resistance in skeletal muscle. Annals of the New York Academy of Sciences. 2006;**967**:146-157. DOI: 10.1111/j.1749-6632.2002.tb04272.x

[22] Vitale C, Marazzi G, Volterrani M, Aloisio A, Rosano G, Fini M. Metabolic syndrome. Minerva Medica. 2006;**97**(3):219-229

[23] Cieślak M, Wojtczak A, Cieślak M. Role of pro-inflammatory cytokines of pancreatic islets and prospects of elaboration of new methods for the diabetes treatment. Acta Biochimica Polonica. 2015;**62**:15-21. DOI: 10.18388/abp.2014_853

[24] Cockram TOJ, Dundee JM, Popescu AS, Brown GC. The phagocytic code regulating phagocytosis of mammalian cells. Frontiers in Immunology. 2021;**9**(12):629979. DOI: 10.3389/fimmu.2021.629979

[25] Stuart LM, Ezekowitz RAB. Phagocytosis: Elegant complexity. Immunity. 2005;**22**(5):539-550. DOI: 10.1016/j.immuni.2005.05.002

[26] Rojas-Espinosa O, Arce-Paredes P. Fagocitosis: mecanismos y consecuencias. Primera parte. Bioquimia. 2003;**28**(4):19-28

[27] Jaumouillé V, Grinstein S. Receptor mobility, the cytoskeleton, and particle binding during phagocytosis. Current Opinion in Cell Biology. 2011;**23**:22-29. DOI: 10.1016/j.ceb.2010.10.006

[28] Flannagan RS, Jaumouillé V, Grinstein S. The cell biology of phagocytosis. Annual Review of Pathology: Mechanisms of Disease. 2012;7:61-98. DOI: 10.1146/annurev-pathol-011811-132445

[29] Rojas-Espinosa O, Arce-Paredes P. Fagocitosis: mecanismos y consecuencias. Segunda partc. Bioquimia. 2004;**29**:18-31

[30] Brubaker SW, Bonham KS, Zanoni I, Kagan JC. Innate immune pattern recognition: a cell biological perspective. Annual Review of Immunology. 2015;**33**:257-290. DOI: 10.1146/annurev-immunol-032414-112240

[31] Rojas-Espinosa O, Arce-Paredes P. Fagocitosis: mecanismos y consecuencias. Tercera parte. Bioquimia. 2004;**29**(2):55-67

[32] Azevedo EP, Rochael NC, Guimarães-Costa AB, de Souza-Vieira TS, Ganilho J, Saraiva EM, et al. A metabolic shift toward pentose phosphate pathway is necessary for amyloid fibril-and

phorbol 12-myristate 13-acetate-induced neutrophil extracellular trap (NET) formation. Journal of Biological Chemistry. 2015;**290**(36):22174-22183. DOI: 10.1074/jbc.M115.640094

[33] Valenta H, Erard M, Dupré-Crochet S, Nüβe O. The NADPH oxidase and the phagosome. Molecular and Cellular Biology of Phagocytosis. 2020;**153**:177. DOI: 10.1007/978-3-030-40406-2_9

[34] Kissing S, Saftig P, Haas A. Vacuolar ATPase in phago (lyso) some biology. International Journal of Medical Microbiology. 2018;**308**(1):58-67. DOI: 10.1016/j.ijmm.2017.08.007

[35] Wartosch L, Bright NA, Luzio JP. Lysosomes. Current Biology. 2015;**25**(8):R315-R316. DOI: 10.1016/j.cub.2015.02.027

[36] Chatzigeorgiou A, Karalis KP, Bornstein SR, Chavakis T. Lymphocytes in obesity-related adipose tissue inflammation. Diabetologia. 2012;**55**(10):2583-2592. DOI: 10.1007/s00125-012-2607-0

[37] Kammoun HL, Kraakman MJ, Febbraio MA. Adipose tissue inflammation in glucose metabolism. Reviews in Endocrine and Metabolic Disorders. 2014;**15**:31-44. DOI: 10.1007/s11154-013-9274-4

[38] Thyagarajan B, Foster MT. Beiging of white adipose tissue as a therapeutic strategy for weight loss in humans. Hormone Molecular Biology and Clinical Investigation. 2017;**31**:1-17. DOI: 10.1515/hmbci-2017-0016

[39] Xu X, Su S, Wang X, Barnes V, De Miguel C, Ownby D, et al. Obesity is associated with more activated neutrophils in African American male youth. International Journal of Obesity. 2015;**39**:26-32. DOI: 10.1038/ijo.2014.194

[40] Kredel LI, Siegmund B. Adipose-tissue and intestinal inflammation–visceral obesity and creeping fat. Frontiers in Immunology. 2014;**5**:462. DOI: 10.3389/fimmu.2014.00462

[41] Brownlee M. Negative consequences of glycation. Metabolism. 2000;**49**(2):9-13. DOI: 10.1016/S0026-0495(00)80078-5

[42] Yao D, Brownlee M. Hyperglycemia-induced reactive oxygen species increase expression of the receptor for advanced glycation end products (RAGE) and RAGE ligands. Diabetes. 2010;**59**:249-255. DOI: 10.2337/db09-0801

[43] Yan SF, Yan SD, Ramasamy R, Schmidt AM. Tempering the wrath of RAGE: An emerging therapeutic strategy against diabetic complications, neurodegeneration, and inflammation. Annals of Medicine. 2009;**41**(6):408-422. DOI: 10.1080/07853890902806576

[44] Meerwaldt R, Links T, Zeebregts C, Tio R, Hillebrands JL, Smit A. The clinical relevance of assessing advanced glycation endproducts accumulation in diabetes. Cardiovascular Diabetology. 2008;**7**:1-8. DOI: 10.1186/1475-2840-7-29

[45] Dowey R, Iqbal A, Heller SR, Sabroe I, Prince LR. A bittersweet response to infection in diabetes; targeting neutrophils to modify inflammation and improve host immunity. Frontiers in Immunology. 2021;**12**:678771. DOI: 10.3389/fimmu.2021.678771

[46] Chandra RK. Immune response in overnutrition. Cancer Research. 1981;**419**(2):3795-3796

[47] Herishanu Y, Rogowski O, Polliack A, Marilus R. Leukocytosis in obese individuals: Possible link in patients with unexplained persistent

neutrophilia. European Journal of Haematology. 2006;**76**(6):516-520. DOI: 10.1111/j.1600-0609.2006.00658.x

[48] Kim JA, Park HS. White blood cell count and abdominal fat distribution in female obese adolescents. Metabolism. 2008;**57**(10):1375-1379. DOI: 10.1016/j.metabol.2008.05.005

[49] Nijhuis J, Rensen SS, Slaats Y, Van Dielen FM, Buurman WA, Greve JWM. Neutrophil activation in morbid obesity, chronic activation of acute inflammation. Obesity. 2009;**17**(11):2014-2018. DOI: 10.1038/oby.2009.113

[50] Ali M, Jasmin S, Fariduddin M, Alam SM, Arslan MI, Biswas SK. Neutrophil elastase and myeloperoxidase mRNA expression in overweight and obese subjects. Molecular Biology Reports. 2018;**45**(5):1245-1252. DOI: 10.1007/s11033-018-4279-4

[51] Delamaire M, Maugendre D, Moreno M, Le Goff MC, Allannic H, Genetet B. Impaired leucocyte functions in diabetic patients. Diabetic Medicine. 1997;14:29-34. DOI: 10.1002/(SICI)1096-9136(199701)14:1<29::AID-DIA300>3.0.CO;2-V

[52] Gustke CJ, Stein SH, Hart TC, Hoffman WH, Hanes PJ, Russell CM, et al. HLA-DR alleles are associated with IDDM, but not with impaired neutrophil chemotaxis in IDDM. Journal of Dental Research. 1998;**77**(7):1497-1503. DOI: 10.1177/00220345980770070401

[53] Donovan RM, Goldstein E, Kim Y, Lippert W, Kailath E, Aoki TT, et al. A computer-assisted image-analysis system for analyzing polymorphonuclear leukocyte chemotaxis in patients with diabetes mellitus. Journal of Infectious Diseases. 1987;**155**(4):737-741. DOI: 10.1093/infdis/155.4.737

[54] Spiller F, Carlos D, Souto FO, De Freitas A, Soares FS, Vieira SM, et al. α1-acid glycoprotein decreases neutrophil migration and increases susceptibility to sepsis in diabetic mice. Diabetes. 2012;**61**(6):1584-1591. DOI: 10.2337/db11-0825

[55] Seree-Aphinan C, Vichitkunakorn P, Navakanitworakul R, Khwannimit B. Distinguishing sepsis from infection by neutrophil dysfunction: A promising role of CXCR2 surface level. Frontiers in Immunology. 2020;**11**:608696. DOI: 10.3389/fimmu.2020.608696

[56] Mastej K, Adamiec R. Neutrophil surface expression of CD11b and CD62L in diabetic microangiopathy. Acta diabetologica. 2008;**45**:183-190. DOI: 10.1007/s00592-008-0040-0

[57] Barouch FC, Miyamoto K, Allport JR, Fujita K, Bursell SE, Aiello LP, et al. Integrin-mediated neutrophil adhesion and retinal leukostasis in diabetes. Investigative Ophthalmology & Visual Science. 2000;**41**(5):1153-1158

[58] Bagdade JD, Stewart M, Walters E. Impaired granulocyte adherence: A reversible defect in host defense in patients with poorly controlled diabetes. Diabetes. 1978;**27**(6):677-681. DOI: 10.2337/diab.27.6.677

[59] Pereira MAA, Sannomiya P, Leme JG. Inhibition of leukocyte chemotaxis by factor in alloxan-induced diabetic rat plasma. Diabetes. 1987;**36**(11):1307-1314. DOI: 10.2337/diab.36.11.1307

[60] Ptak W, Klimek M, Bryniarski K, Ptak M, Majcher P. Macrophage function in alloxan diabetic mice: Expression of adhesion molecules, generation of monokines and oxygen and NO radicals. Clinical & Experimental Immunology. 1998;**114**:13-18. DOI: 10.1046/j.1365-2249.1998.00687.x

[61] Copenhaver M, Yu CY, Hoffman RP. Complement components, C3 and C4, and the metabolic syndrome. Current Diabetes Reviews. 2019;**15**:44-48. DOI: 10.2174/1573399814666180417122030

[62] Hair PS, Echague CG, Rohn RD, Krishna NK, Nyalwidhe JO, Cunnion KM. Hyperglycemic conditions inhibit C3-mediated immunologic control of Staphylococcus aureus. Journal of Translational Medicine. 2012;**10**:1-16. DOI: 10.1186/1479-5876-10-35

[63] Hostetter MK. Handicaps to host defense: Effects of hyperglycemia on C3 and Candida albicans. Diabetes. 1990;**39**(3):271-275. DOI: 10.2337/diab.39.3.271

[64] Abrass CK. Fc receptor-mediated phagocytosis: Abnormalities associated with diabetes mellitus. Clinical Immunology and Immunopathology. 1991;**58**:1-17. DOI: 10.1080/08820538.2017.1353811

[65] Alba-Loureiro TC, Hirabara SM, Mendonca JR, Curi R, Pithon-Curi TC. Diabetes causes marked changes in function and metabolism of rat neutrophils. Journal of Endocrinology. 2006;**188**(2):295-303. DOI: 10.1677/joe.1.06438

[66] Zhang XY, Liu Y, He T, Yang TT, Wu J, Cianflone K, et al. Anaphylatoxin C5a induces inflammation and reduces insulin sensitivity by activating TLR4/NF-kB/PI3K signaling pathway in 3T3-L1 adipocytes. Biomedicine & Pharmacotherapy. 2018;**103**:955-964. DOI: 10.1016/j.biopha.2018.04.057

[67] Wood AJ, Vassallo AM, Ruchaud-Sparagano MH, Scott J, Zinnato C, Gonzalez-Tejedo C, et al. C5a impairs phagosomal maturation in the neutrophil through phosphoproteomic remodeling. JCI Insight. 2020;**5**(15):e137029. DOI: 10.1172/jci.insight.137029

[68] Lecube A, Pachón G, Petriz J, Hernández C, Simó R. Phagocytic activity is impaired in type 2 diabetes mellitus and increases after metabolic improvement. PLoS One. 2011;**6**(8):e23366. DOI: 10.1371/journal.pone.0023366

[69] Tebbs SE, Gonzalez AM, Wilson RM. The role of aldose reductase inhibition in diabetic neutrophil phagocytosis and killing. Clinical and Experimental Immunology. 1991;**84**(3):482

[70] Tsai YL, Lin TL, Chang CJ, Wu TR, Lai WF, Lu CC, et al. Probiotics, prebiotics and amelioration of diseases. Journal of Biomedical Science. 2019;**26**:1-8. DOI: 10.1186/s12929-018-0493-6

[71] Han SK, Shin YJ, Lee DY, Kim KM, Yang SJ, Kim DS, et al. Lactobacillus rhamnosus HDB1258 modulates gut microbiota-mediated immune response in mice with or without lipopolysaccharide-induced systemic inflammation. BMC Microbiology. 2021;**21**:1-15. DOI: 10.1186/s12866-021-02192-4

[72] Li Y, Yang S, Lun J, Gao J, Gao X, Gong Z, et al. Inhibitory effects of the Lactobacillus rhamnosus GG effector protein HM0539 on inflammatory response through the TLR4/MyD88/NF-κB axis. Frontiers in Immunology. 2020;**11**:551449. DOI: 10.3389/fimmu.2020.551449

[73] Kim SW, Park KY, Kim B, Kim E, Hyun CK. Lactobacillus rhamnosus GG improves insulin sensitivity and reduces adiposity in high-fat diet-fed mice through enhancement of adiponectin production. Biochemical and Biophysical Research Communications. 2013;**431**(2):258-263. DOI: 10.1016/j.bbrc.2012.12.121

[74] Wang R, Sheng M, Shi F, Zhao Y, Zhao L, Wu J, et al. Dysfunctional phagocytosis capacity, granulocyte recruitment and inflammatory factor secretion of Kupffer cells in diabetes mellitus reversed by lidocaine. Diabetes, Metabolic Syndrome and Obesity: Targets and Therapy. 2018;**26**(11):827-834. DOI: 10.2147/DMSO.S186695

[75] Wold AE. Immune effects of probiotics. Näringsforskning. 2016;**45**:76-85. DOI: 10.3402/fnr.v45i0.1787

[76] Jaffar N, Okinaga T, Nishihara T, Maeda T. Enhanced phagocytosis of Aggregatibacter actinomycetemcomitans cells by macrophages activated by a probiotic Lactobacillus strain. Journal of Dairy Science. 2018;**101**(7):5789-5798. DOI: 10.3168/jds.2017-14355

[77] Ibrahim F, Ruvio S, Granlund L, Salminen S, Viitanen M, Ouwehand AC. Probiotics and immunosenescence: Cheese as a carrier. FEMS Immunology & Medical Microbiology. 2010;**59**:53-59. DOI: 10.1111/j.1574-695X.2010.00658.x

[78] Nanjundaiah YS, Wright DA, Baydoun AR, Khaled Z, Ali Z, Dean P, et al. Modulation of macrophage function by Lactobacillus-conditioned medium. Frontiers in Cell and Developmental Biology. 2020;**8**:723. DOI: 10.3389/fcell.2020.00723

[79] Sommer C, Birklein F. Resolvins and inflammatory pain. F1000 Medicine Reports. 2011;**3**:19. DOI: 10.3410/M3-19

[80] Herrera BS, Hasturk H, Kantarci A, Freire MO, Nguyen O, Kansal S, et al. Impact of resolvin E1 on murine neutrophil phagocytosis in type 2 diabetes. Infection and Immunity. 2015;**83**(2):792-801. DOI: 10.1128/IAI.02444-14

[81] Jung SB, Choi MJ, Ryu D, Yi HS, Lee SE, Chang JY, et al. Reduced oxidative capacity in macrophages results in systemic insulin resistance. Nature Communications. 2018;**9**:1-15. DOI: 10.1038/s41467-018-03998-z

[82] Mata-MartínezP, Bergón-GutiérrezM, Del Fresno C. Dectin-1 signaling update: New perspectives for trained immunity. Frontiers in Immunology. 2022;**13**:812148. DOI: 10.3389/fimmu.2022.812148

[83] Morais TC, Honorio-França AC, Fujimori M, de Quental OB, Pessoa RS, França EL, et al. Melatonin action on the activity of phagocytes from the colostrum of obese women. Medicina. 2019;**55**(10):625. DOI: 10.3390/medicina55100625

[84] Bedini A, Fraternale A, Crinelli R, Mari M, Bartolucci S, Chiarantini L, et al. Design, synthesis, and biological activity of hydrogen peroxide responsive arylboronate melatonin hybrids. Chemical Research in Toxicology. 2018;**32**:100-112. DOI: 10.1021/acs.chemrestox.8b00216

Chapter 12

Harnessing Phagocytosis for Cancer Treatment

Alok K. Mishra

Abstract

Phagocytosis is a critical component of the body's immune response, essential for preventing and controlling infections and defending against cancer cells. Macrophages and dendritic cells are the primary immune cells responsible for phagocytosis, recognizing and engulfing abnormal cells, including cancer cells. Although phagocytosis can prevent the spread of cancer cells by destroying them in a healthy immune system, cancer cells may evade this immune mechanism and form tumors. As an emerging therapeutic strategy, boosting phagocytosis is being utilized to target and eliminate cancer cells. This chapter provides an overview of the role of phagocytosis in cancer prevention and progression, highlighting its significance in the body's immune response to cancer. Furthermore, it explores various strategies and approaches to harness the power of phagocytosis in the fight against cancer.

Keywords: phagocytosis, ADCP, immune checkpoints, immunity, tumor microenvironment, rituximab, trastuzumab, dendritic cells

1. Introduction

In the 1880s, Elie Metchnikoff, who studied marine invertebrates, observed special cells that were capable of attacking tiny thorns in starfish larvae. This was his first discovery of phagocytosis. For his pioneering work in cellular immunity, he was awarded the Nobel Prize alongside Paul Ehrlich in 1908 [1].

Phagocytosis is basically referred to as the ingestion of food particles by unicellular organisms, but in multicellular organisms, it is a specialized process carried out by phagocytes, which are a set of specialized cells. The examples of phagocytes in vertebrates include neutrophils, macrophages, monocytes, dendritic cells, osteoclasts, and eosinophils [2].

In the context of cancer, phagocytosis plays a crucial role in the body's defense against malignant cells. Normally, phagocytic cells, such as macrophages are responsible for recognizing and engulfing cancer cells, thereby preventing their spread and growth. However, in some cases, cancer cells can evade the immune system by modifying their surface antigens or secreting cytokines that suppress the recognition ability and activity of phagocytic cells [3, 4].

Macrophages and dendritic cells are the two key components of the innate immune system that play a crucial roles in defending the human body against emerging threats. These cells not only help in eliminating newly transformed cells, but also play a vital role in activating the adaptive immune system when needed. Despite their important role in immune surveillance, there is growing evidence that the polarization of these phagocytes by tumor-derived factors can lead to a pro-tumorigenic response [5, 6].

The recent discoveries of phagocytic immune checkpoints, such as CD47, LILRB1/2, CD24 and PDL-1, has revitalized the field of phagocytosis research [7–10]. These checkpoints can be targeted to enhance phagocytic activity and increase the efficiency of immune surveillance. Additionally, the development of neo-antigen-based cancer vaccines that utilize the phagocytic characteristics of dendritic cells has provided new avenues for cancer treatment [11–14].

In this chapter, I will provide an overview of phagocytic process and its role in tumor biology as well as present the fundamental concepts of this field of research. I will also examine how phagocytes can be harnessed as a tool for cancer therapy and the potential of utilizing these cells in combination with other treatments to achieve improved outcomes.

2. Phagocytosis of cancer cells

Cellular phagocytosis is a complex process that involves the recognition and engulfment of target cells, including cancer cells, by specialized cells known as phagocytes. Phagocytes such as macrophages and dendritic cells are equipped with surface receptors that can recognize pro-phagocytic signals or "eat me" signals on the surface of the target cells. For example, the presentation of calreticulin (CALR) on the surface of cancer cells is one such signal that helps macrophages and dendritic cells to recognize and initiate the phagocytic process.

The process of phagocytosis of cancer cells can be broken down into five main steps: recognition, activation, engulfment, digestion, and elimination. In the recognition step, phagocytes identify and bind to the target cells, leading to the activation of the phagocyte. In the activation step, the phagocyte is stimulated to engulf the target cell, leading to its internalization. The engulfment step is followed by the digestion of the target cell, in which it is broken down and degraded within the phagocyte. Finally, the elimination step involves the removal of the digested material from the phagocyte, which may occur through exocytosis.

In addition to phagocytosis, both macrophages and dendritic cells play an important role in activating the adaptive immune response against cancer cells. These cells can present antigens from cancer cells to T cells, which are responsible for recognizing and eliminating cancer cells in a specific manner. This process is crucial for effective anti-cancer immune responses, and its failure can contribute to cancer progression and the development of immune evasion mechanisms [15–19].

3. Anti-body dependent cellular phagocytosis (ADCP)

The process of phagocytsis is also facilitated by anti-bodies formed against the surface antigen. This form of phagocytosis is called anti-body dependedent cellular phagocytosis or ADCP.

ADCP allows immune cells, such as macrophages and dendritic cells, to recognize and engulf cancer cells. This is achieved through the binding of specific antibodies to the cancer cells, creating a bridge that enables the immune cells to phagocytose the cancer cells. These antibodies can either be naturally produced by the body or artificially engineered to target cancer cells.

Fcγ receptors play a crucial role in cancer cell phagocytosis by antibody-dependent cell phagocytosis (ADCP). These receptors are present on the surface of macrophages and other immune cells and recognize the constant region (Fc region) of antibodies bound to antigens on the surface of cancer cells. This recognition event triggers the phagocytosis of the cancer cell by the immune cells [20, 21].

ADCP plays a crucial role in the body's natural defense mechanism against cancer and is a key component of some immunotherapies used for cancer treatment. For instance, monoclonal antibody therapy utilizes engineered antibodies that target specific cancer cells and trigger ADCP, leading to the destruction of the cancer cells by immune cells (**Table 1**) [20, 21, 43, 44].

3.1 Anti-CD20 (Rituximab)

Rituximab, also known as Anti-CD20, is a monoclonal antibody targeting the CD20 antigen expressed on the surface of malignant B-cells. CD20 is a transmembrane glycoprotein found on the surface of pre-B and mature B-lymphocytes and is used as a therapeutic target for the treatment of B-cell malignancies such as non-Hodgkin's lymphoma (NHL) and chronic lymphocytic leukemia (CLL) [23, 45].

Rituximab works by binding to the CD20 antigen on the surface of cancer cells, leading to antibody-dependent cellular phagocytosis (ADCP) and subsequent destruction of the cancer cells by immune cells. ADCP is a mechanism in which immune cells, such as macrophages and dendritic cells, are able to recognize and engulf cancer cells through the binding of antibodies to the cancer cells [46–48].

Monoclonal Antibody	Target	Cancer type	Trigger of ADCP	Ref.
Rituximab	CD20	Non-Hodgkin lymphoma, chronic lymphocytic leukemia	Fcγ receptors	[22, 23]
Trastuzumab	HER2	HER2-positive Breast Cancer HER2-positive gastric	Fcγ receptors	[24–26]
Cetuximab	EGFR	Colorectal cancer, head neck cancer	Fcγ receptors	[27, 28]
Bevacizumab	VEGF	Colorectal cancer, non- small cell lung cancer, glioblastoma	Not well defined	[29–31]
Alemtuzumab	CD52	Chronic lymphocytic leukemia	Fcγ receptors	[32, 33]
Ofatumumab	CD20	Chronic lymphocytic leukemia	Fcγ receptors	[34, 35]
Atezolizumab	PD-L1	Non-small cell lung cancer, bladder cancer	Fcγ receptors	[36–38]
Durvalumab	PD-L1	Non-small cell lung cancer, bladder cancer	Fcγ receptors	[39, 40]
Avelumab	PD-L1	Non-small cell lung cancer, bladder cancer	Fcγ receptors	[41, 42]

Table 1.
lists some examples of clinically used monoclonal antibodies that utilize ADCP to treat cancers.

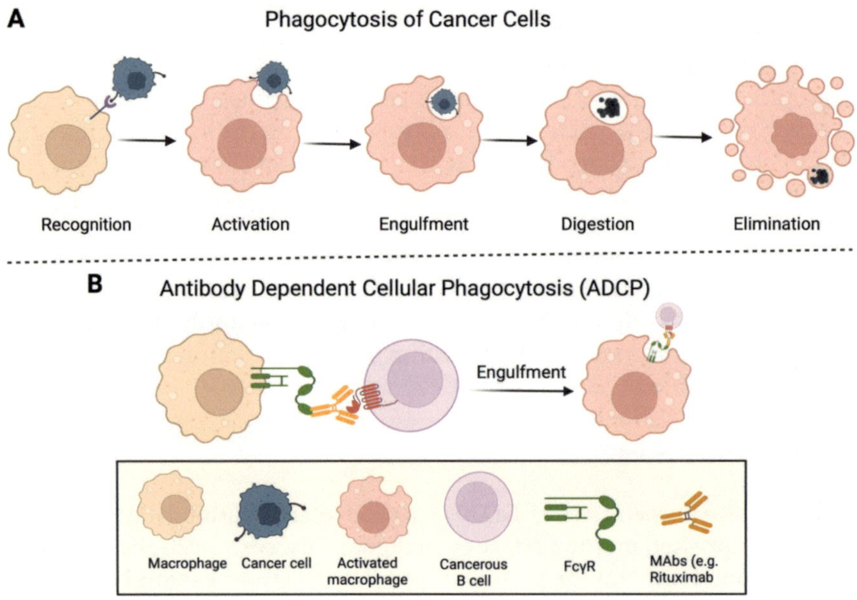

Figure 1.
(A) Steps involves in phagocytosis mediated killing of cancer cells, and (B) antibody-dependent cellular phagocytosis. (ADCP); Monoclonal antibodies (mAbs) (e.g., Rituximab) can bind to both macrophages and tumor cells, leading to the formation of a complex that triggers ADCP. As a result, macrophages engulf the tumor cells that are opsonized by antibodies. The figure was created using BioRender.com.

3.2 Anti-HER2 (Trastuzumab)

Trastuzumab is a monoclonal antibody targeting the human epidermal growth factor receptor 2 (HER2) protein. This protein is overexpressed in some breast cancers and is associated with an aggressive form of the disease. Trastuzumab works by binding to HER2 on the surface of cancer cells, leading to antibody-dependent cellular phagocytosis (ADCP). This process signals immune cells to engulf and destroy the cancer cells [49].

Trastuzumab has been shown to improve response rates and survival outcomes in patients with HER2-positive breast cancer [25, 26]. It is often used in combination with chemotherapy (e.g. paclitaxel, doxorubicin) and/or radiation therapy. Studies have demonstrated its clinical efficacy, such as the "HERA" trial which showed improved disease-free survival in HER2-positive breast cancer patients receiving Trastuzumab and chemotherapy (**Figure 1**) [50].

4. Mechanism of evasion of cellular phagocytosis by cancer cells

Phagocytosis plays a vital role in preventing the spread and growth of cancer cells by eliminating them. However, cancer cells can often evade the immune system, reducing the effectiveness of phagocytosis. They empoly several molecular and cellular mechanisms to evade phagocytosis mediated killing by phagocytes [51–56].

I. **Modifying surface antigens:** Cancer cells can modify their surface antigens to evade recognition by phagocytic cells. This can include changes to proteins, lipids, or carbohydrates on the cell surface.

II. **Suppressing phagocytic activity**: Cancer cells can secrete cytokines and chemokines that suppress the activity of phagocytic cells. This can reduce the efficiency of phagocytosis and allow cancer cells to proliferate.

III. **Inducing immune tolerance**: Cancer cells can induce immune tolerance by producing molecules that activate regulatory T cells, which suppress the immune response. This can reduce the phagocytic activity of immune cells and allow cancer cells to evade destruction.

IV. **Hiding in immune privileged sites**: Some cancer cells can hide in immune privileged sites, such as the central nervous system or the eye, where they are protected from the immune response and phagocytosis.

V. **Expressiong phagocytic checkpoints**: Cancer cells can also stimulate a phagocytosis-resistant phenotype by altering the expression of surface proteins and other molecular markers that can acts as immune checkpoint. These immune checkpoint are popularly known as "Do not eat me signal" these signals can make the cancer cells less recognizable to phagocytic cells and reduce the efficiency of phagocytosis. Following are the known immune checkpoints axes that have been extensively studies and targeted for cancer tratement.

4.1 The immune checkpoints and inhibitors

Immune checkpoints help regulate immune responses and prevent overactive immune responses.

One type of immunotherapy is checkpoint inhibition, which targets immune checkpoint molecules to release the brakes on the immune system and enhance its ability to attack cancer cells. ICIs have shown promising results in preclinical studies and is being actively investigated as a potential treatment for cancer.

Checkpoint inhibition is currently a highly active area of research in the field of cancer treatment, with the aim of developing effective immunotherapies that can help improve patient outcomes and provide new treatment options for cancer patients. Following are some examples of the phagocytic immune checkpoint axes that has been targeted to treat various types of cancers.

4.2 CD47- SIRPα

CD47 is a protein that can be found on the surface of various cells, including cancer cells. Its primary function is to act as a "do not eat me" signal that prevents phagocytosis, the process by which phagocytic cells destroy other cells. This is achieved by CD47 interacting with its receptor, SIRPα, which inhibits the activation of phagocytic pathways, ultimately blocking phagocytosis. The CD47-SIRPα interaction is a crucial component of immune tolerance, helping to differentiate between self and non-self and prevent the destruction of healthy cells. Despite its role in immune tolerance, researchers are investigating the potential for using the CD47-SIRPα interaction as a strategy for cancer therapy. By blocking this interaction, the phagocytic ability of the immune system can be enhanced, which may lead to increased removal of cancer cells. This can be achieved through the use of

Inhibitor	Type	Target	Mechanism of action	Clinical status	Cancer types being studied	Ref.
Hu5F9-G4 (5F9)	Monoclonal antibody	CD47	Blocks CD47-SIRPα interaction, promoting phagocytosis of cancer cells	In clinical trials	Various types	[57]
TTI-621	Fusion protein	CD47	Blocks CD47-SIRPα interaction, promoting phagocytosis of cancer cells	In clinical trials	Hematologic malignancies	[58]
CC-90002	Monoclonal antibody	CD47	Blocks CD47-SIRPα interaction, promoting phagocytosis of cancer cells	In preclinical development	Various types	[59]
AO-176	Monoclonal antibody	CD47	Enhances phagocytosis of cancer cells by macrophages	In preclinical development	Various types	[60]
ALX148	Fusion protein	CD47	Blocks CD47-SIRPα interaction, promoting phagocytosis of cancer cells	In clinical trials	Various types	[61]
JTX 8064	Humanized anti-LILRB2 IgG4 mAb	LILRB2	Blocks LILRB2 interaction with its ligands, promoting phagocytosis of cancer cells	Phase I/II NCT04669899	Various types	[14]
Anti-CD24(SN3)	Monoclonal antibody	CD24	Targets and Induces phagocytosis of CD24+ cancer cells by TAMs	In preclinical development	Breast cancer, Ovarian cancer	[8]

Table 2.
Some examples of immune check point inhibitors that induces cellular phagocytosis.

anti-CD47 monoclonal antibodies or small molecule inhibitors of the CD47-SIRPα interaction, such as Hu5F9-G4 or Sen177. This approach has promising potential as a cancer therapy strategy (**Table 2**) [14, 45, 56, 62–66].

4.3 CD24-SIGLEC10

CD24 and SIGLEC10 are cell surface markers expressed on immune cells. CD24 is primarily expressed on certain B cells and SIGLEC10 is expressed on immune cells called macrophages and myeloid-derived suppressor cells. Both CD24 and SIGLEC10 have been shown to act as immune checkpoint molecules, meaning they help regulate immune responses and prevent overactive immune responses.

Targeting CD24 and SIGLEC10 with immunotherapies has shown promising results in preclinical studies and is being actively investigated as a potential treatment for cancer [8, 9].

4.4 LILRB1/2

LILRB1 and LILRB2 are members of the leukocyte immunoglobulin-like receptor (LILR) family of receptors and are expressed on phagocytic cells such as macrophages, dendritic cells, and monocytes. These receptors serve as phagocytic checkpoints by regulating the phagocytic activity of these immune cells and modulating their ability to engulf and degrade pathogens and cellular debris. LILRB1 and LILRB2 can also regulate the immune response by modulating the activation and function of T cells and natural killer cells. In this way, they play a crucial role in maintaining immune homeostasis and preventing overactive immune responses. Studies have shown that LILRB1 and LILRB2 can also be exploited by cancer cells to evade the immune system and persist in the body. In light of these findings, the targeting of these receptors as phagocytic checkpoints has gained attention as a promising strategy in cancer immunotherapy. Inhibiting the activity of LILRB1 and LILRB2 has been shown to enhance the phagocytic activity of immune cells and improve their ability to target and clear cancer cells. This has led to ongoing research in the field of cancer immunotherapy to further explore the potential of targeting these receptors as phagocytic checkpoints [14, 67, 68].

4.5 PDL-1-PD1

PD-1 (programmed cell death protein 1) and its ligand PD-L1 (programmed cell death ligand 1) are proteins that are involved in regulating the immune response. They are known as immune checkpoint molecules because they prevent the immune system from overreacting and attacking healthy tissues. Traditionally, PD-1/PD-L1 has been viewed as a T cell immune checkpoint, where PD-1 on the surface of T cells interacts with PD-L1 on the surface of other cells, including cancer cells and antigen-presenting cells. This interaction leads to the inhibition of T cell activity, which prevents the immune system from attacking healthy tissues and can allow cancer cells to evade the immune system. However, recent research has also shown that PD-1/PD-L1 is involved in regulating phagocytosis. PD-L1 can be expressed on the surface of tumor cells and other cells, and when it interacts with PD-1 on the surface of phagocytes, it inhibits their ability to perform phagocytosis. This means that by blocking the interaction between PD-1 and PD-L1, it may be possible to enhance the ability of phagocytes to remove foreign particles and to enhance the immune response against cancer cells. As a result, there is growing interest in the development of drugs that target PD-1/PD-L1 for the treatment of cancers [18, 69].

5. Small molecule inducers of Phagocytosis

Small molecule activators of macrophages offer a potential alternative to traditional cancer treatments, such as chemotherapy and radiation therapy, and may also be used in combination with other cancer treatments for a more comprehensive approach to cancer therapy. The goal of using small molecule activators is to enhance the natural ability of macrophages to recognize and eliminate cancer cells, potentially leading to cancer elimination. This type of therapy is still in the early stages of development, but has shown promising results in preclinical studies and early clinical trials.

Some examples of small molecule activators of macrophages include:

1. *CSF-1R inhibitors*: These are drugs that target the colony-stimulating factor 1 receptor (CSF-1R), a protein that regulates the growth and survival of macrophages. By inhibiting CSF-1R, these drugs can deplete the pro-tumerogenic tumor associated macrophages or repolarize them to anti-tumerigeneic thereby, enhancing their ability to phagocytize cancer cells (e.g. Emactuzumab, Pexidartinib) [70, 71].

2. *Toll-like receptor (TLR) agonists*: TLRs are proteins found on the surface of immune cells that help to detect and respond to pathogens. TLR agonists are drugs that mimic the action of pathogens and activate TLRs, leading to increased activation and phagocytic capacity of macrophages (e.g., IMO-2125) [72–74].

5.1 Cell-based therapies

Phagocyte-based cell therapies are a type of cancer treatment that leverage the phagocytic properties of immune cells to eliminate cancer cells. One example of such a therapy is dendritic cell (DC) vaccines, which involve extracting dendritic cells from the patient's blood, enriching them with tumor-associated antigens, and then reintroducing them into the patient. The enriched DCs then travel to the lymph nodes, where they display the antigens to T-cells, eliciting an immune response against the cancer cells [75–77].

Additionally, researchers have developed enginnered macrophages and CAR (chimeric antigen receptor) macrophages as alternative forms of phagocyte-based cell therapy to combat cancer [78, 79].

5.2 Dendritic cells based cancer vaccines

Dendritic cells (DCs) are specialized antigen-presenting cells that originate from bone marrow progenitors. They can take up and process antigens through various mechanisms such as phagocytosis, receptor-mediated endocytosis, or micropinocytosis, depending on the type of antigen and their activation status. DCs can recognize antigens associated with pathogen-associated molecular patterns (PAMPs) or damage-associated molecular patterns (DAMPs). These processed antigens are presented on the surface of DCs by MHC I or MHC II molecules to CD4+ or CD8 + T-cells, respectively (**Figure 2**).

DCs can activate various immune cells including naïve and memory T-cells, natural killer (NK) cells, and natural killer T (NKT) cells, making DC vaccines a promising approach for cancer immunotherapy. Recent clinical trials have shown that tumor-antigen-preloaded DCs can initiate anti-tumor immune responses in patients, indicating the potential of DCs in cancer therapy.

The production of a DC vaccine involves several steps. First, tumor cells are obtained during surgical resection of the patient's tumor. These tumor cells contain specific antigens that are unique to that patient's tumor.

Next, the patient's peripheral blood monocytes are obtained through a process called leukapheresis. These monocytes are then differentiated ex vivo (outside the body) into dendritic cells, which are antigen-presenting cells that can activate the immune system's T-cells. The dendritic cells are then "trained" to recognize the patient's tumor cells. This is done by ex vivo pulsing the dendritic cells with tumor lysate or peptides derived from the patient's own tumor cells.

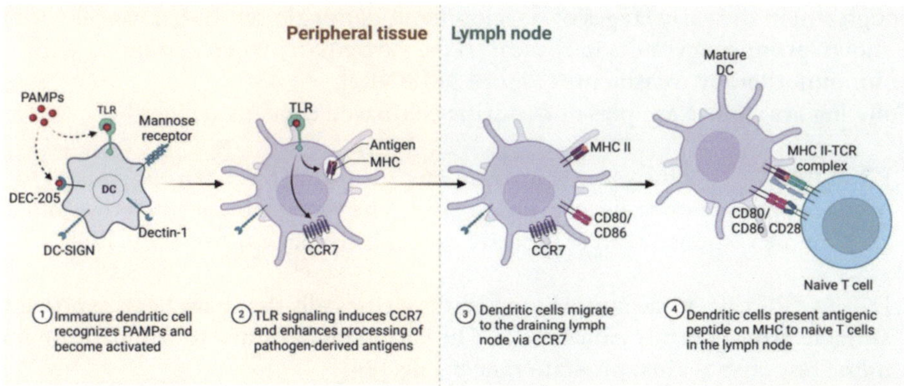

Figure 2.
Illustration of dendritic cell maturation and antigen presentation to T cells. Figure downloaded from Biorender. com(on 02.15.2023).

After the dendritic cells are trained, they are injected back into the patient. The injected DC-vaccine enables the dendritic cells to present the tumor antigens to the patient's CD4 and CD8 T-cells, which are part of the adaptive immune system. The T-cells then become activated a exerts highly specific immune response against the patient's tumor cells. This specific immune response can lead to the killing of the tumor cells, as well as the prevention of further tumor growth (**Figure 3**).

The aim of these vaccines is to activate the patient's immune system against the cancer cells, with the hope of inducing remission or eradication of the cancer.

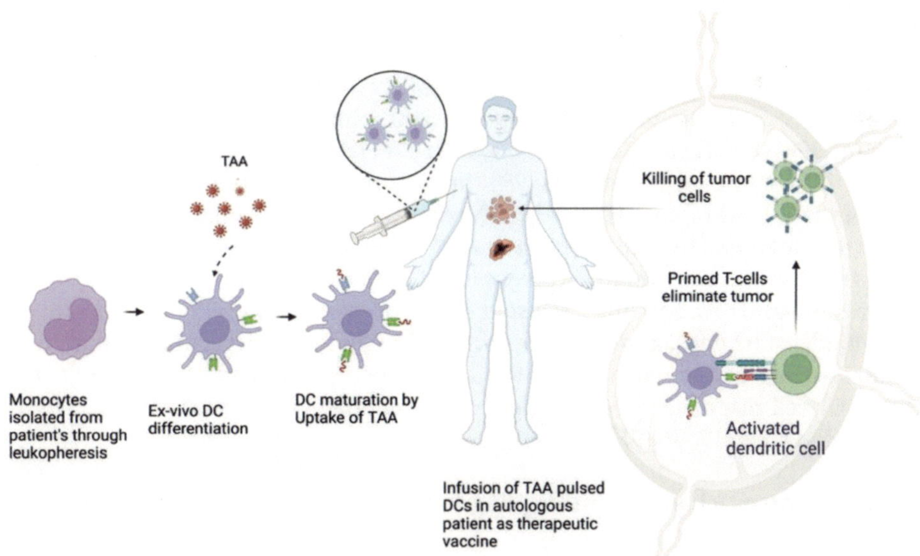

Figure 3.
Illustrates the mechanism of action of a DC vaccine in the body. The vaccine involves the ex vivo maturation and loading of dendritic cells with tumor-associated antigens (TAA). Once the vaccine is administered, the activated T cells that are specific to the TAA circulate throughout the body, searching for cancer cells that express the same antigen. Upon encountering a cancer cell, the T cells attach to it and unleash their cytotoxic activity. The figure was created using BioRender.com.

Although still in the early stages of development, dendritic cell-based cancer vaccines have shown promising results in clinical trials, particularly when combined with other immunotherapy treatments (**Figure 3**) [80–82].

Follwing are some examples of dendritic cell-based cancer vaccines.

1. PROSTVAC-V/F: This vaccine is based on a virus that has been engineered to produce prostate-specific antigens (PSAs). The vaccine is designed to stimulate an immune response against prostate cancer cells that express PSAs [83].

2. DCVAC/PCa: This vaccine is based on dendritic cells that have been exposed to antigens from prostate cancer cells. The vaccine is designed to stimulate an immune response against prostate cancer cells [84].

3. DCVax-L: The experimental vaccine therapy known as DCVax®-L is created using dendritic cells that are loaded with cell extracts or lysates from the cancer cells of the patient. Its purpose is to trigger the patient's immune system to generate a response against the particular cancer cells of the patient. This treatment is intended for brain tumor patients (NCT00045968) [85].

5.3 CAR-macrophages

CAR (Chimeric Antigen Receptor) macrophages are a type of genetically modified macrophages that have been engineered to enhance their phagocytic ability. CAR macrophages are created by introducing a CAR gene into the macrophages, which codes for a chimeric antigen receptor. This CAR allows the macrophages to specifically target and phagocytize specific cells, such as cancer cells, by recognizing specific antigens present on their surface [79]. The goal of this technology is to create a new way to fight cancer and other diseases by harnessing the natural abilities of macrophages to engulf and destroy unwanted cells.

CAR-M therapies have demonstrated the ability to eliminate tumor cells both in vitro and in preclinical in vivo models. In vitro, human CAR-M have been shown to exhibit antigen-specific phagocytosis, as well as secretion of cytokines/chemokines and the ability to kill target antigens [79]. In two immunodeficient NSG xenograft models, a single dose of anti-HER2 CAR-M significantly reduced the burden of tumors and prolonged overall survival against HER2+ SKOV3 tumors. Additionally, CAR-M that were administered intravenously (IV) were found to localize to tumors in several xenograft models and persisted in tumor-free mice (primarily within the liver) for at least 62 days, as detected by whole-body bioluminescent imaging. In vitro analysis further demonstrated that CAR-M were capable of coordinating an antitumor T cell response by recruiting T cells and cross-presenting antigens from phagocytosed cells [19, 86, 87].

5.4 Using nanoparticles to promote phagocytosis

Another way to potentially enhance the phagocytic response is through the use of nanoparticles. Nanoparticles have been extensively studied for their ability to induce macrophage polarization states, as different types of nanoparticles can influence macrophage polarization toward either a pro-inflammatory (M1) or anti-inflammatory (M2) phenotype. When tumor-associated macrophages (TAMs) recognize nanoparticles as foreign, they will engulf them via phagocytosis, releasing the contents of the nanoparticle within the TAMs. Therefore, nanoparticles can be loaded with drugs or contents designed to induce macrophage polarization toward a more phagocytic phenotype, reprogramming them with an affinity for phagocytosis. This makes nanoparticles a potentially attractive vehicle for delivering therapeutic agents that can boost the immune response against cancer [88, 89].

Additionally, recent studies have shown that nanoparticles can be designed to not only enhance the phagocytic response, but also to help stimulate an anti-tumor T cell response by recruiting T cells and cross-presenting antigens from phagocytosed cells. This highlights the potential for nanoparticles to be used in combination with other immunotherapies, such as CAR-T cells or checkpoint inhibitors, to further enhance the immune response against cancer [55, 88, 89].

6. Conclusion

Macrophages and dendritic cells play a crucial role in preventing the growth of cancer cells by recognizing, engulfing, digesting, and eliminating them through phagocytosis. This process is a key aspect of the body's defense against cancer, but cancer cells can develop various mechanisms to evade immune-mediated killing. Understanding these immune evasion mechanisms is important for developing strategies to improve phagocytic activity in cancer patients and enhance the effectiveness of cancer treatments. In recent years, there has been growing interest in using immune checkpoint inhibitors and engineered cell-based immunotherapies to enhance phagocytic activity in cancer patients. In conclusion, phagocytosis is an important cellular process in the body's defense against cancer, and it plays a crucial role in the development of immunotherapies for the treatment of cancer. Overall, this chapter underscores the importance of phagocytosis in cancer prevention and treatment, and highlights the potential for using this process to develop novel and effective cancer therapies.

Acknowledgements

I acknowledge Late Prof. Michael Green, and the Department of Molecular Cell and Cancer Biology, UMass Chan Medical School, for providing all the necessary resources and support.

Conflict of interest

The author declare no conflict of interest.

Author details

Alok K. Mishra
Department of Molecular, Cell and Cancer Biology, UMass Chan Medical School, Worcester, USA

*Address all correspondence to: alok.mishra@umassmed.edu

IntechOpen

References

[1] Tauber AI. Immunity: How Elie Metchnikoff changed the course of modern medicine by Luba Vikhanski. Bulletin of the History of Medicine;**91**(1):140-142. DOI: 10.1353/bhm.2017.0015

[2] Rabinovitch M. Professional and non-professional phagocytes: An introduction. Trends in Cell Biology. 1995;**5**:85-87. DOI: 10.1016/S0962-8924(00)88955-2

[3] Wagner M, Koyasu S. Cancer immunoediting by innate lymphoid cells. Trends in Immunology. 2019;**40**(5):415-430. DOI: 10.1016/j.it.2019.03.004

[4] Dunn GP, Old LJ, Schreiber RD. The immunobiology of cancer immunosurveillance and immunoediting. Immunity. 2004;**21**(2):137-148. DOI: 10.1016/j.immuni.2004.07.017

[5] Sica A, Larghi P, Mancino A, Rubino L, Porta C, Totaro MG, et al. Macrophage polarization in tumour progression. Seminars in Cancer Biology. 2008;**18**(5):349-355. DOI: 10.1016/j.semcancer.2008.03.004

[6] Ma Y, Shurin GV, Peiyuan Z, Shurin MR. Dendritic cells in the cancer microenvironment. Journal of Cancer. 2013;**4**(1):36-44. DOI: 10.7150/jca.5046

[7] Pouliliou S, Nikolaidis C, Drosatos G. Current trends in cancer immunotherapy: a literature-mining analysis. Cancer Immunology, Immunotherapy. 2020;**69**:2425-2439. DOI: 10.1007/s00262-020-02630-8

[8] Barkal AA, Brewer RE, Markovic M, Kowarsky M, Barkal SA, Zaro BW, et al. CD24 signalling through macrophage Siglec-10 is a target for cancer immunotherapy. Nature. 2019;**572**(7769):392-396. DOI: 10.1038/s41586-019-1456-0

[9] Yin SS, Gao FH. Molecular Mechanism of Tumor Cell Immune Escape Mediated by CD24/Siglec-10. Frontiers in Immunology. 2020;**11**:1324. DOI: 10.3389/fimmu.2020.01324

[10] Mantovani A, Allavena P, Marchesi F, Garlanda C. Macrophages as tools and targets in cancer therapy. Nature Reviews. Drug Discovery. 2022;**21**(11):799-820. DOI: 10.1038/s41573-022-00520-5

[11] Steinman RM, Banchereau J. Taking dendritic cells into medicine. Nature. 2007;**449**(7161):419-426. DOI: 10.1038/nature06175

[12] Yu J, Sun H, Cao W, Song Y, Jiang Z. Research progress on dendritic cell vaccines in cancer immunotherapy. Experimental Hematology & Oncology. 2022;**11**(1):3. DOI: 10.1186/s40164-022-00257-2

[13] Marciscano AE, Anandasabapathy N. The role of dendritic cells in cancer and anti-tumor immunity. Seminars in Immunology. 2021;**52**:101481. DOI: 10.1016/j.smim.2021.101481

[14] Mishra AK, Ali A, Dutta S, Banday S, Malonia SK. Emerging trends in immunotherapy for cancer. Diseases. 2022;**10**(3):60. DOI: 10.3390/diseases10030060

[15] Gordon S. Phagocytosis: An immunobiologic process. Immunity. 2016;**44**(3):463-475. DOI: 10.1016/j.immuni.2016.02.026

[16] Rosales C, Uribe-Querol E. Phagocytosis: A Fundamental Process in Immunity. BioMed Research

International. 2017;**2017**:9042851. DOI: 10.1155/2017/9042851

[17] Uribe-Querol E, Rosales C. Phagocytosis: Our Current Understanding of a Universal Biological Process. Frontiers in Immunology. 2020;**11**:1066. DOI: 10.3389/fimmu.2020.01066

[18] Feng M, Jiang W, Kim BYS, Zhang CC, Fu YX, Weissman IL. Phagocytosis checkpoints as new targets for cancer immunotherapy. Nature Reviews. Cancer. 2019;**19**(10):568-586. DOI: 10.1038/s41568-019-0183-z

[19] Mishra AK, Banday S, Bharadwaj R, Ali A, Rashid R, Kulshreshtha A, et al. Macrophages as a Potential Immunotherapeutic Target in Solid Cancers. Vaccines. 2022;**11**(1):55. DOI: 10.3390/vaccines11010055

[20] Nimmerjahn F, Ravetch JV. Fcγ receptors: Old friends and new family members. Immunity. 2006;**24**(1):19-28. DOI: 10.1016/j.immuni.2005.11.010

[21] Musolino A, Gradishar WJ, Rugo HS, Nordstrom JL, Rock EP, Arnaldez F, et al. Role of Fcγ receptors in HER2-targeted breast cancer therapy. Journal for Immunotherapy of Cancer. 2022;**10**(1):e003171. DOI: 10.1136/jitc-2021-003171

[22] Cartron G, Dacheux L, Salles G, Solal-Celigny P, Bardos P, Colombat P, et al. Therapeutic activity of humanized anti-CD20 monoclonal antibody and polymorphism in IgG Fc receptor FcgammaRIIIa gene. Blood. 2002;**99**(3):754-758. DOI: 10.1182/blood.v99.3.754

[23] Tedeschi A, Vismara E, Ricci F, Morra E, Montillo M. The spectrum of use of rituximab in chronic lymphocytic leukemia. Oncotargets and Therapy. 2010;**3**:227-246. DOI: 10.2147/OTT.S8151

[24] Hofmann M, Stoss O, Shi D, Büttner R, van de Vijver M, Kim W, et al. Assessment of a HER2 scoring system for gastric cancer: Results from a validation study. Histopathology. 2008;**52**(7):797-805. DOI: 10.1111/j.1365-2559.2008.03028.x

[25] Vogel CL, Cobleigh MA, Tripathy D, Gutheil JC, Harris LN, Fehrenbacher L, et al. Efficacy and safety of trastuzumab as a single agent in first-line treatment of HER2-overexpressing metastatic breast cancer. Journal of Clinical Oncology. 2002;**20**(3):719-726. DOI: 10.1200/JCO.2002.20.3.719

[26] Romond EH, Perez EA, Bryant J, Suman VJ, Geyer CE Jr, Davidson NE, et al. Trastuzumab plus adjuvant chemotherapy for operable HER2-positive breast cancer. The New England Journal of Medicine. 2005;**353**(16):1673-1684. DOI: 10.1056/NEJMoa052122

[27] Cunningham D, Humblet Y, Siena S, Khayat D, Bleiberg H, Santoro A, et al. Cetuximab monotherapy and cetuximab plus irinotecan in irinotecan-refractory metastatic colorectal cancer. The New England Journal of Medicine. 2004;**351**(4):337-345. DOI: 10.1056/NEJMoa033025

[28] Vermorken JB, Mesia R, Rivera F, Remenar E, Kawecki A, Rottey S, et al. Platinum-based chemotherapy plus cetuximab in head and neck cancer. The New England Journal of Medicine. 2008;**359**(11):1116-1127. DOI: 10.1056/NEJMoa0802656

[29] Funakoshi Y, Hata N, Kuga D, Hatae R, Sangatsuda Y, Fujioka Y, et al. Update on Chemotherapeutic Approaches and Management of Bevacizumab Usage for Glioblastoma. Pharmaceuticals (Basel). 2020;**13**(12):470. DOI: 10.3390/ph13120470

[30] Fujita K, Sano D, Kimura M, Yamashita Y, Kawakami M, Ishiguro Y, et al. Anti-tumor effects of bevacizumab in combination with paclitaxel on head and neck squamous cell carcinoma. Oncology Reports. 2007;**18**(1):47-51

[31] Qu CY, Zheng Y, Zhou M, Zhang Y, Shen F, Cao J, et al. Value of bevacizumab in treatment of colorectal cancer: A meta-analysis. World Journal of Gastroenterology. 2015;**21**(16): 5072-5080. DOI: 10.3748/wjg.v21.i16.5072

[32] Robak T. Alemtuzumab for B-cell chronic lymphocytic leukemia. Expert Review of Anticancer Therapy. 2008;**8**(7):1033-1051. DOI: 10.1586/14737140.8.7.1033

[33] Fraser G, Smith CA, Imrie K, Meyer R. Hematology disease site groupof cancer care Ontario's program in evidence-based care. Alemtuzumab in chronic lymphocytic leukemia. Current Oncology. 2007;**14**(3):96-109. DOI: 10.3747/co.2007.118

[34] Wu Y, Wang Y, Gu Y, Xia J, Kong X, Qian Q, et al. Safety and efficacy of Ofatumumab in chronic lymphocytic leukemia: a systematic review and meta-analysis. Hematology. 2017;**22**(10):578-584. DOI: 10.1080/10245332.2017.1333974

[35] Frustaci AM, Tedeschi A, Picardi P, Cairoli R, Montillo M. Clinical utility and patient considerations in the use of ofatumumab in chronic lymphocytic leukemia. Biologics. 2015;**9**:75-86. DOI: 10.2147/BTT.S60503

[36] Inman BA, Longo TA, Ramalingam S, Harrison MR. Atezolizumab: A PD-L1–blocking antibody for bladder cancer. Clinical Cancer Research. 2017;**23**(8):1886-1890. DOI: 10.1158/1078-0432.CCR-16-1417

[37] Socinski MA, Jotte RM, Cappuzzo F, Orlandi F, Stroyakovskiy D, Nogami N, et al. Reck M; IMpower150 Study Group. Atezolizumab for First-Line Treatment of Metastatic Nonsquamous NSCLC. The New England Journal of Medicine. 2018;**378**(24):2288-2301. DOI: 10.1056/NEJMoa1716948

[38] Vansteenkiste J, Wauters E, Park K, Rittmeyer A, Sandler A, Spira A. Prospects and progress of atezolizumab in non-small cell lung cancer. Expert Opinion on Biological Therapy. 2017;**17**(6):781-789. DOI: 10.1080/14712598.2017.1309389

[39] Murakami S. Durvalumab for the treatment of non-small cell lung cancer. Expert Review of Anticancer Therapy. 2019;**19**(12):1009-1016. DOI: 10.1080/14737140.2019.1699407

[40] Brower V. Anti-PD-L1 inhibitor durvalumab in bladder cancer. The Lancet Oncology. 2016;**17**(7):e275. DOI: 10.1016/S1470-2045(16)30242-X

[41] Rosell R, Karachaliou N. Avelumab in non-small-cell lung cancer. The Lancet Oncology. 2018;**19**(11):1423-1424. DOI: 10.1016/S1470-2045(18)30683-1

[42] Rao A, Patel MR. A review of avelumab in locally advanced and metastatic bladder cancer. Therapeutic Advances in Urology. 2019;**11**:1756287218823485. DOI: 10.1177/1756287218823485

[43] Tay MZ, Wiehe K, Pollara J. Antibody-dependent cellular phagocytosis in antiviral immune responses. Frontiers in Immunology. 2019;**10**:332. DOI: 10.3389/fimmu.2019.00332

[44] Su S, Zhao J, Xing Y, Zhang X, Liu J, Ouyang Q, et al. Immune checkpoint inhibition overcomes ADCP-induced

immunosuppression by macrophages. Cell. 2018;**175**(2):442-457.e23. DOI: 10.1016/j.cell.2018.09.007

[45] Advani R, Flinn I, Popplewell L, Forero A, Bartlett NL, Ghosh N, et al. CD47 Blockade by Hu5F9-G4 and Rituximab in Non-Hodgkin's Lymphoma. The New England Journal of Medicine. 2018;**379**(18):1711-1721. DOI: 10.1056/NEJMoa1807315

[46] Press OW, Leonard JP, Coiffier B, Levy R. John Timmerman; immunotherapy of Non-Hodgkin's Lymphomas. Hematology. American Society of Hematology. Education Program. 2001;**2001**(1):221-240. DOI: 10.1182/asheducation-2001.1.221

[47] Cerny T, Borisch B, Introna M, Johnson P, Rose AL. Mechanism of action of rituximab. Anti-Cancer Drugs. 2002;**13**(Suppl 2):S3-S10. DOI: 10.1097/00001813-200211002-00002

[48] Grillo-López AJ, White CA, Varns C, Shen D, Wei A, McClure A, et al. Overview of the clinical development of rituximab: first monoclonal antibody approved for the treatment of lymphoma. Seminars in Oncology. 1999;**26**(5 Suppl 14):66-73

[49] Vu T, Claret FX. Trastuzumab: updated mechanisms of action and resistance in breast cancer. Frontiers in Oncology. 2012;**2**:62. DOI: 10.3389/fonc.2012.00062

[50] Cameron D, Piccart-Gebhart MJ, Gelber RD, Procter M, Goldhirsch A, de Azambuja E, et al. 11 years' follow-up of trastuzumab after adjuvant chemotherapy in HER2-positive early breast cancer: final analysis of the HERceptin Adjuvant (HERA) trial. Lancet. 2017;**389**(10075):1195-1205. DOI: 10.1016/S0140-6736(16)32616-2. Erratum in: Lancet. 2019 Mar 16;393(10176):1100

[51] Vinay DS, Ryan EP, Pawelec G, Talib WH, Stagg J, Elkord E, et al. Immune evasion in cancer: Mechanistic basis and therapeutic strategies. Seminars in Cancer Biology. 2015;**35**(Suppl):S185-S198. DOI: 10.1016/j.semcancer.2015.03.004

[52] Crispen PL, Kusmartsev S. Mechanisms of immune evasion in bladder cancer. Cancer Immunology, Immunotherapy. 2020;**69**(1):3-14. DOI: 10.1007/s00262-019-02443-4

[53] Wang H, Xu Q, Zhao C, Zhu Z, Zhu X, Zhou J, et al. An immune evasion mechanism with IgG4 playing an essential role in cancer and implication for immunotherapy. Journal for Immunotherapy of Cancer. 2020;**8**(2):e000661. DOI: 10.1136/jitc-2020-000661

[54] Ghasempour S, Freeman SA. The glycocalyx and immune evasion in cancer. The FEBS Journal. 2023;**290**(1):55-65. DOI: 10.1111/febs.16236

[55] Chen S, Lai SWT, Brown CE, Feng M. Harnessing and enhancing macrophage phagocytosis for cancer therapy. Frontiers in Immunology. 2021;**12**:635173. DOI: 10.3389/fimmu.2021.635173

[56] Takimoto CH, Chao MP, Gibbs C, McCamish MA, Liu J, Chen JY, et al. The Macrophage 'Do not eat me' signal, CD47, is a clinically validated cancer immunotherapy target. Annals of Oncology. 2019;**30**(3):486-489. DOI: 10.1093/annonc/mdz006

[57] Sikic BI, Lakhani N, Patnaik A, Shah SA, Chandana SR, Rasco D, et al. First-in-Human, First-in-Class Phase I Trial of the Anti-CD47 antibody Hu5F9-G4 in patients with advanced cancers. Journal of Clinical Oncology.

2019;**37**(12):946-953. DOI: 10.1200/JCO.18.02018

[58] Ansell SM, Maris MB, Lesokhin AM, Chen RW, Flinn IW, Sawas A, et al. Phase I study of the CD47 blocker TTI-621 in patients with relapsed or refractory hematologic malignancies. Clinical Cancer Research. 2021;**27**(8):2190-2199. DOI: 10.1158/1078-0432.CCR-20-3706

[59] Zeidan AM, DeAngelo DJ, Palmer J, Seet CS, Tallman MS, Wei X, et al. Phase 1 study of anti-CD47 monoclonal antibody CC-90002 in patients with relapsed/refractory acute myeloid leukemia and high-risk myelodysplastic syndromes. Annals of Hematology. 2022;**101**(3):557-569. DOI: 10.1007/s00277-021-04734-2

[60] Puro RJ, Bouchlaka MN, Hiebsch RR, Capoccia BJ, Donio MJ, Manning PT, et al. Development of AO-176, a next-generation humanized anti-CD47 antibody with novel anticancer properties and negligible red blood cell binding. Molecular Cancer Therapeutics. 2020;**19**(3):835-846. DOI: 10.1158/1535-7163.MCT-19-1079

[61] Kauder SE, Kuo TC, Harrabi O, Chen A, Sangalang E, Doyle L, et al. ALX148 blocks CD47 and enhances innate and adaptive antitumor immunity with a favorable safety profile. PLoS One. 2018;**13**(8):e0201832. DOI: 10.1371/journal.pone.0201832

[62] Matlung HL, Szilagyi K, Barclay NA, van den Berg TK. The CD47-SIRPα signaling axis as an innate immune checkpoint in cancer. Immunological Reviews. 2017;**276**(1):145-164. DOI: 10.1111/imr.12527

[63] Murata Y, Saito Y, Kotani T, Matozaki T. CD47-signal regulatory protein α signaling system and its application to cancer immunotherapy. Cancer Science. 2018;**109**(8):2349-2357. DOI: 10.1111/cas.13663

[64] Feng R, Zhao H, Xu J, Shen C. CD47: the next checkpoint target for cancer immunotherapy. Critical Reviews in Oncology/Hematology. 2020;**152**:103014. DOI: 10.1016/j.critrevonc.2020.103014

[65] Zhang W, Huang Q, Xiao W, Zhao Y, Pi J, Xu H, et al. Advances in anti-tumor treatments targeting the CD47/SIRPα axis. Frontiers in Immunology. 2020;**11**:18. DOI: 10.3389/fimmu.2020.00018

[66] Logtenberg MEW, Jansen JHM, Raaben M, Toebes M, Franke K, Brandsma AM, et al. Glutaminyl cyclase is an enzymatic modifier of the CD47-SIRPα axis and a target for cancer immunotherapy. Nature Medicine. 2019;**25**(4):612-619. DOI: 10.1038/s41591-019-0356-z

[67] Zhao J, Zhong S, Niu X, Jiang J, Zhang R, Li Q. The MHC class I-LILRB1 signalling axis as a promising target in cancer therapy. Scandinavian Journal of Immunology. 2019;**90**(5):e12804. DOI: 10.1111/sji.12804

[68] Barkal AA, Weiskopf K, Kao KS, Gordon SR, Rosental B, Yiu YY, et al. Engagement of MHC class I by the inhibitory receptor LILRB1 suppresses macrophages and is a target of cancer immunotherapy. Nature Immunology. 2018;**19**(1):76-84. DOI: 10.1038/s41590-017-0004-z

[69] Havel JJ, Chowell D, Chan TA. The evolving landscape of biomarkers for checkpoint inhibitor immunotherapy. Nature Reviews. Cancer. 2019;**19**(3):133-150. DOI: 10.1038/s41568-019-0116-x

[70] Cannarile MA, Weisser M, Jacob W, Jegg AM, Ries CH, Rüttinger D. Colony-stimulating factor 1 receptor (CSF1R)

inhibitors in cancer therapy. Journal for Immunotherapy of Cancer. 2017;**5**(1):53. DOI: 10.1186/s40425-017-0257-y

[71] Cai H, Zhang Y, Wang J, Gu J. Defects in macrophage reprogramming in cancer therapy: The negative impact of PD-L1/PD-1. Frontiers in Immunology. 2021;**12**:690869. DOI: 10.3389/fimmu.2021.690869

[72] Agrawal S, Kandimalla ER. Synthetic agonists of Toll-like receptors 7, 8 and 9. Biochemical Society Transactions. 2007;**35**(Pt 6):1461-1467. DOI: 10.1042/BST0351461

[73] Adams S. Toll-like receptor agonists in cancer therapy. Immunotherapy. 2009;**1**(6):949-964. DOI: 10.2217/imt.09.70

[74] Urban-Wojciuk Z, Khan MM, Oyler BL, Fåhraeus R, Marek-Trzonkowska N, Nita-Lazar A, et al. The role of TLRs in anti-cancer immunity and tumor rejection. Frontiers in Immunology. 2019;**10**:2388. DOI: 10.3389/fimmu.2019.02388

[75] Ahmed MS, Bae YS. Dendritic cell-based therapeutic cancer vaccines: past, present and future. Clin Exp Vaccine Res. 2014;**3**(2):113-116. DOI: 10.7774/cevr.2014.3.2.113

[76] Palucka K, Banchereau J. Dendritic-cell-based therapeutic cancer vaccines. Immunity. 2013;**39**(1):38-48. DOI: 10.1016/j.immuni.2013.07.004

[77] Guo Y, Lei K, Tang L. Neoantigen vaccine delivery for personalized anticancer immunotherapy. Frontiers in Immunology. 2018;**9**:1499. DOI: 10.3389/fimmu.2018.01499

[78] Biglari A, Southgate TD, Fairbairn LJ, Gilham DE. Human monocytes expressing a CEA-specific chimeric CD64 receptor specifically target CEA-expressing tumour cells in vitro and in vivo. Gene Therapy. 2006;**13**(7):602-610. DOI: 10.1038/sj.gt.3302706

[79] Klichinsky M, Ruella M, Shestova O, Lu XM, Best A, Zeeman M, et al. Human chimeric antigen receptor macrophages for cancer immunotherapy. Nature Biotechnology. 2020;**38**(8):947-953. DOI: 10.1038/s41587-020-0462-y

[80] Wculek SK, Cueto FJ, Mujal AM, Melero I, Krummel MF, Sancho D. Dendritic cells in cancer immunology and immunotherapy. Nature Reviews. Immunology. 2020;**20**(1):7-24. DOI: 10.1038/s41577-019-0210-z

[81] Gardner A, Ruffell B. Dendritic cells and cancer immunity. Trends in Immunology. 2016;**37**(12):855-865. DOI: 10.1016/j.it.2016.09.006

[82] Calmeiro J, Carrascal MA, Tavares AR, Ferreira DA, Gomes C, Falcão A, et al. Dendritic cell vaccines for cancer immunotherapy: The role of human conventional type 1 dendritic cells. Pharmaceutics. 2020;**12**(2):158. DOI: 10.3390/pharmaceutics12020158

[83] Shore ND. PROSTVAC® targeted immunotherapy candidate for prostate cancer. Immunotherapy. 2014;**6**(3):235-247. DOI: 10.2217/imt.13.176

[84] Beer TM, Vogelzang N, Bartůňková J, Miller K, Oh W, Oudard S, et al. Autologous dendritic cell immunotherapy (DCVAC/PCa) added to docetaxel chemotherapy in a Phase III trial (viable) in men with advanced (mCRPC) prostate cancer. Journal for Immunotherapy of Cancer. 2015;**3**(Suppl 2):P164. DOI: 10.1186/2051-1426-3-S2-P164

[85] Polyzoidis S, Ashkan K. DCVax®-L--developed by Northwest Biotherapeutics. Human Vaccines & Immunotherapeutics.

2014;**10**(11):3139-3145. DOI: 10.4161/hv.29276. Erratum in: Hum Vaccin Immunother. 2015;11(7):1881

[86] Sloas C, Gill S, Klichinsky M. Engineered CAR-macrophages as adoptive immunotherapies for solid tumors. Frontiers in Immunology. 2021;**12**:783305. DOI: 10.3389/fimmu.2021.783305

[87] Maalej KM, Merhi M, Inchakalody VP, et al. CAR-cell therapy in the era of solid tumor treatment: current challenges and emerging therapeutic advances. Molecular Cancer. 2023;**22**:20. DOI: 10.1186/s12943-023-01723-z

[88] Dukhinova MS, Prilepskii AY, Shtil AA, Vinogradov VV. Metal oxide nanoparticles in therapeutic regulation of macrophage functions. Nanomaterials. 2019;**9**(11):1631. DOI: 10.3390/nano9111631

[89] Reichel D, Tripathi M, Perez JM. Biological effects of nanoparticles on macrophage polarization in the tumor microenvironment. Nano. 2019;**3**(1):66-88. DOI: 10.7150/ntno.30052